Get Fit,
Feel Fantastic!

Get Fit, Feel Fantastic!

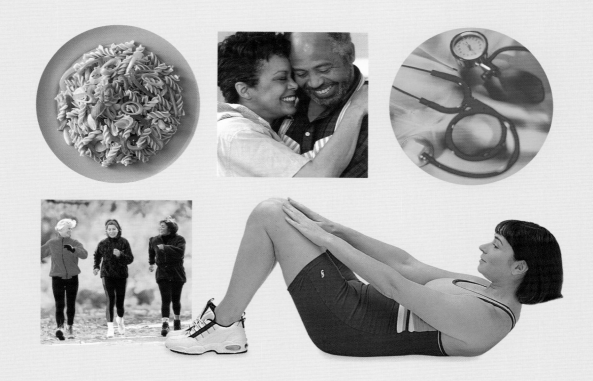

ANNE HOOPER AND DR. MICHAEL PERRING

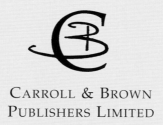

CARROLL & BROWN
PUBLISHERS LIMITED

First published in 2000 in the United Kingdom by:

Carroll & Brown Publishers Limited
20 Lonsdale Road
Queen's Park
London NW6 6RD

Project Editors Jennifer Musset, Nikki Taylor
Art Editor Mercedes Morgan
Designer Finn Lewis

Consultants
Professor Rozalind Gruben AHSI, RSA
Jane Kirby RD

Contributors
Susan Conder BA(Hons), MA(Hons), Dip. Couple Counselling
Clare Hill
Ceri Williams
Ian Wood

Copyright © 2000 Carroll & Brown Limited

A CIP catalogue record for this book is available from the British Library.

ISBN 1-903258-00-6

Reproduced by Colourscan, Singapore
Printed and bound by Imago in Singapore
First edition

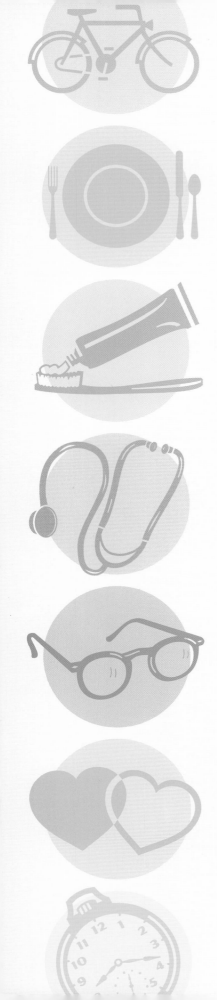

Contents

· ·

Introduction

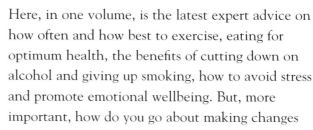

As a new millennium dawns, the great majority of the world's population are living 20 years longer than their parents, according to United Nations' surveys. It's plain to see why – many people now enjoy a better diet, advanced medical care and a healthier lifestyle. Doctors and experts worldwide have made progress in all areas of health to help people stay well for longer. But with advice and treatments coming from all directions, how do you pull it all together? *Get Fit, Feel Fantastic!* arms you with the facts you need to devise your own action plan for greater health and happiness.

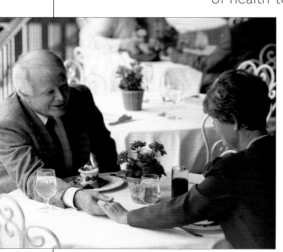

Romance and affection bring vitality into your life, helping you to stay younger for longer.

Here, in one volume, is the latest expert advice on how often and how best to exercise, eating for optimum health, the benefits of cutting down on alcohol and giving up smoking, how to avoid stress and promote emotional wellbeing. But, more important, how do you go about making changes in these areas? The chapters that follow cover all aspects of your life, ranging from exercise and nutrition to emotional health, relationships, sex life and leisure, and tell you everything you need to know to enhance your health and happiness. Most important it doesn't just give you the results of the latest research into all these areas; rather it empowers you to take an active role in determining what you can and want to do to increase the length and quality of your life.

Get Fit, Feel Fantastic! offers expert, practical advice on a wide variety of subjects, including:

▶ How can you meet new people?
▶ What can you do to enhance your sex life?
▶ How does exercise boost your enthusiasm and energy for life?
▶ How can you effectively relieve stress?
▶ What kind of diet keeps you healthy and energised?
▶ How can you boost your mind power and memory?
▶ Will natural remedies control your menopause symptoms?

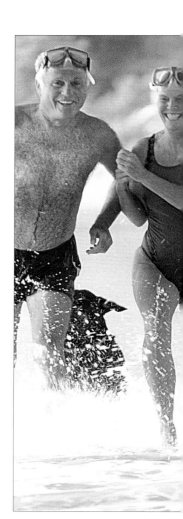

To help you make realistic changes there are action programmes throughout the book that suggest a number of practical steps you can take towards a new, healthy lifestyle: for example, '9 health-giving supplements' and '8 ways to meet new people'. Whether you try out just a couple of suggestions from each programme or all of them, there is a menu of choices so you can pick and choose those that fit in with your budget, schedule and personality. The result? A lifestyle plan that's tailor-made for you.

Limit your exposure to the sun to avoid skin damage and to keep your skin in good condition.

Many of the strategies in this book draw upon complementary therapies – both age-old and new techniques – that use natural substances or the power of your own body to give you a different angle on experiences, induce relaxation, ease pain and help you weather difficult and painful situations.

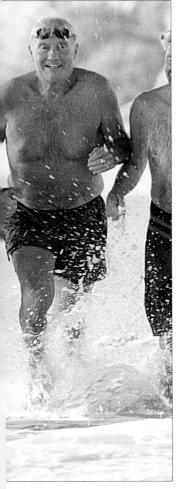

Splashing around with pals combines fun and fitness – both are essential for your wellbeing.

STAYING HEALTHIER FOR LONGER

Medical experts have traditionally defined health as the absence of disease, but we now know that you can do a lot more to improve your health than simply avoiding disease. Broadly speaking, health influences can be categorised as chance (the factors that you can't change, such as your genes) and choice (those that you can, such as your diet).

The 'chance' factors are the environment in which you live (the air and water quality as well as the availability of food and medical care, the pace of society, and so on) and your genetic make-up (your likelihood of developing certain illnesses and the strength and longevity of your organs). There is no doubt that long-lived parents produce long-lived children: if both parents live over the age of 70 then their children are twice as likely as the general population to reach 90 or 100. Genetics, however, can also lead to health problems, including inherited disorders and a propensity to develop certain illnesses or diseases. Unfortunately, you can't change the genes

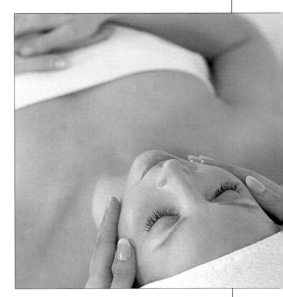

A massage can work wonders for mind and body. Treat yourself – you deserve it.

you were born with (at least not yet!), but being aware of your family's medical history can alert you to illnesses, such as heart disease, to which you may be prone. You can then take appropriate actions to reduce your risk and safeguard your health. For example, you can lower your risk of heart disease by healthy eating, exercise and taking steps to lower high blood pressure.

'Choice' factors are the ones that only you can change, such as your diet, exercise routine and the care you take of your body – that is, your whole lifestyle. This book can help you to make the right decisions for your all-round health, detailing the steps you can take towards a happier, healthier you.

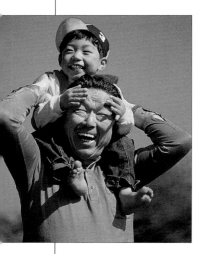

Create a supportive family environment, by promoting involvement with and contact between all family members.

UP-TO-DATE MEDICAL ADVICE

From the latest guidelines on hormone replacement therapy to the 'wonder drugs' that promise to reverse the ill-effects of age, this book sorts out facts from fiction and provides up-to-date information so that you – with your doctor's help where necessary – can develop an effective course of action or treatment.

Increasingly, scientists look to food to provide the secrets to long life; the 'right' food can keep you healthy and ward off (or even cure) disease, while the 'wrong' food promotes ill-health. But it can be hard to find your way through the morass of published material advocating one sort of diet or food over another. *Get Fit, Feel Fantastic!* tells you what foods to eat and in what amounts, how to ensure your quota of essential nutrients, how to keep up your fluid intake and how to become a wise consumer.

Taking control of your health also means being more aware of your body, and this book explains how you can look for early warning signs of physical problems. You know your body best – take time to learn what's normal for you, and be sure to carry out regular self-examinations. Whether it's examining your breasts or testes, or keeping an eye on a mole, be observant and receptive to what your body tells you. By reading this book, you will learn how to check yourself and when to seek professional advice. There are myriad medical tests that can uncover health problems before they become serious, so it's never been easier to keep your body in tip-top physical shape.

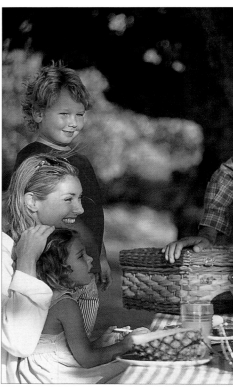

Keep memories alive and share them with others in your family and social circle.

TAKE CHARGE OF YOUR LIFE

Exercise is essential for keeping the body fit and resilient – resistant to disease and the stresses and strains of everyday life. But the wrong kind of exercise or too much is hazardous to your health. Chapter 1 explains how to ascertain the type and amount of exercise that is best for you. You will then learn to assess (and then monitor) your current level of fitness and to set your own goals to become as strong, active and supple as possible. Follow the step-by-step workouts to help build strength, stamina and suppleness.

The importance of a good diet cannot be overemphasised; it affects every aspect of your wellbeing. Chapter 2 looks at the general principles underlying a healthy diet and provides guidelines to help you draw up a realistic eating plan. It also offers simple, common-sense advice on weight management and explains how certain foods can boost your energy levels. Action programmes cover miracle foods that fight disease as well as simple ways to slim down and to energise your life.

How you look is a reflection of how you feel. What does your appearance say about your self-image? Making the most of your looks can go a long way to enhancing your self-confidence. Chapter 3 covers the entire physical form, including face, skin, hair, teeth, body and personal style, and brings together the latest advice on weight loss, diet supplements and exercise to enhance your looks and guard against the damaging effects of time, environment and lifestyle. Recent

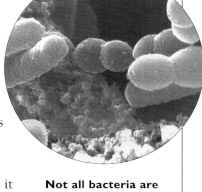

Not all bacteria are harmful; 'friendly' bacteria in yoghurt, for example, can help maintain your body's equilibrium.

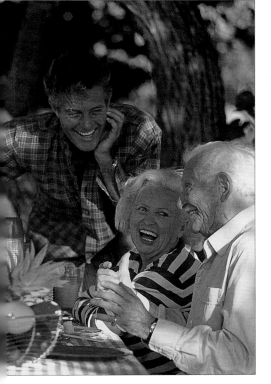

Research shows that you are more likely to exercise if you do something you enjoy. Exercising with a friend is fun and motivational.

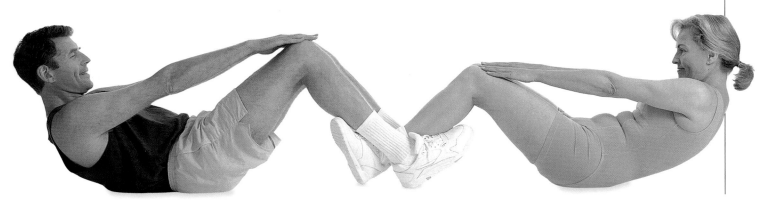

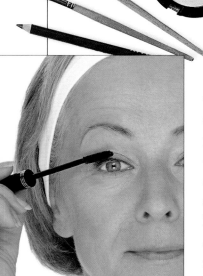

advances in the field of cosmetic surgery – for face and body – are also detailed. Action programmes suggest practical ways to improve your body shape and keep your skin looking younger.

Many diseases and disorders are preventable, and Chapter 4 provides advice on keeping illness at bay. Regular self-examinations and medical check-ups can ensure that problems are caught at an early stage, thereby increasing the chances of successful treatment. Using the guidelines you can detect and monitor any early warning signs. Chapter 4 also shows how, using dietary techniques and other natural health remedies, you can adopt good health habits and stamp out self-destructive ones. It also looks at the options for managing menopause, including hormone replacement therapy and so-called 'natural' approaches. Action programmes suggest ways to reduce the effects of aging and tips to help you give up smoking.

Boost your self-confidence by following the top tips for looking great throughout your life.

The sense of smell is a powerful one; use essential oils and flowers to create different moods in your home.

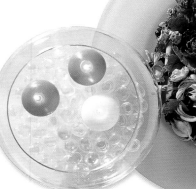

Staying mentally fit and alert is probably the greatest challenge people face, particularly as the predicted life expectancy increases. This book documents not only what is achievable today but also what is on the horizon. Mental deterioration is not an inevitable part of aging, but just as the physical body can become weak through lack of use, the mind needs regular exercise to stay in tip-top condition. Chapter 5 presents the latest research findings on mental agility, memory, and vision and hearing. An action programme suggests ways to enhance your mind power.

How important is a sense of happiness and fulfilment? Emotional health is the core of your wellbeing and directly affects your physical health. The pressures of work, family, relationships and life's unpredictable ups and downs can all take their toll on your health – if you let them. Stress is one of the greatest challenges to health. Negative stress threatens long life, whereas positive stress – sexual and social excitement and physical challenges – can be enjoyable and healthy, and contributes to a long life. Learn how to gauge your current emotional state and how to manage anger, boost your self-esteem and make your life relatively stress-free with the guidance given in Chapter 6.

Although psychoanalysis and psychiatry have enabled many people to overcome emotional problems, not everyone can afford the time and money involved. To make you aware of what's available, Chapter 6 gives the basics of the most popular forms of therapy and how they are best used. Equipped with this information, you'll be in a position to decide which types are suitable for your particular circumstances. Action programmes cover ways to boost your self-confidence and combat stress.

Another important component of a long, healthy life is sex, although researchers aren't certain whether sex keeps you young or you are able to engage in sexual behaviour because you're healthy. But what may be most important is the fact that a continuing sexual life reflects an on-going personal relationship. Did you know that the affection and constant support of a loving partner sometimes makes the difference between life and death for many people? Chapter 6 details tried-and-tested techniques that will help you attain an active and satisfying sex life and solve the problems that inevitably arise in marriage and relationships.

How do you keep your life vital and rewarding as you grow older? Increasing age inevitably leads to changing roles in the family, at work and in society at large. But these should not be seen as lesser roles, as the skills and experience that people

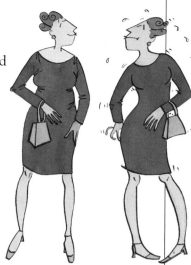

Discover how to accentuate your positive points and play down the negative ones – to create your own personal style.

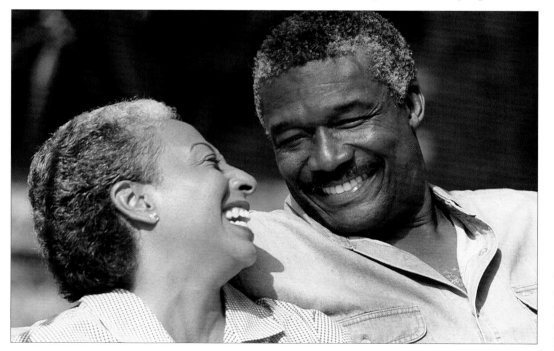

Many experts applaud the benefits of laughter. Ensure you get your daily dose for a happy, healthy life.

accumulate through life can be put to use at any age. Chapter 7 helps you to prepare for these life changes and to take the appropriate action so that your life remains rewarding and fulfilling. Action programmes suggest ways to help you decide what you want to do workwise and socially.

SUCCESSFUL AGING

George Burns said it well: 'You can't help getting older, but you don't have to get old'. That attitude is immensely important in preserving your health and vitality in the prime of your life. To join the club of longer-lived people, you need to develop a positive mind-set: be optimistic, resilient and active. Enjoy your life to the full, and don't let troubles make you depressed, passive or inflexible. It's possible to live not just a long life, nor a long and healthy life, but a long, healthy and happy life.

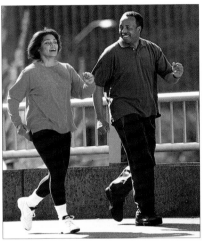

Studies have shown that your attitude accounts for much in life. Making time for enjoyable activities is vital to your wellbeing.

Throughout your life you will experience different inspirations, energies and needs. Gail Sheehy, a writer whose speciality is aging in Western society, has found that in their earlier adult years most people are driven by social ambition, whereas in their middle and later adult life they are inspired more by intellectual quests and interests, and have greater, knowledge, wisdom and direction. It is no coincidence that many great achievements were made by people in their later years; some of the best works by Shakespeare, Beethoven, Goethe, da Vinci and Michelangelo were among their last. Great thinkers, politicians and monarchs often peak after the age of 50, and many scientific advances have been made by researchers in their later years.

Learn a new skill or perfect an existing one. Channelling energy into creative outlets is great for relieving stress.

So, don't sit around at home – get out and about. Being socially involved and mentally active and having a flexible personality are as important as having a fit body. Remember that to be healthy, you need to stimulate your body and your mind. Be happy with yourself and, most important, keep looking forwards.

Chapter 1

Fit for life

Exercise

Physical activity – be it a game of tennis or golf, a gym session or a walk in the countryside – increases your heart rate, improves blood circulation and boosts your health and happiness.

3 REASONS TO EXERCISE REGULARLY

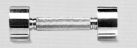

1 It improves lung function, increasing oxygen levels in the body.

2 It strengthens the heart, helping to prevent heart disease and improve blood circulation.

3 It boosts your immune system by speeding up the blood and lymph circulation.

Any exercise in addition to your normal level of activity will benefit your health in a very short time. And the more exercise you do, within reason, the greater the benefits. If you lead a very inactive life, a simple daily 20-minute walk will quickly make you fitter and more energetic, sharpen your mind and senses, and give you that extra zest for life.

You should aim to fit in at least three brisk 20-minute walks each week – in the park, around the block or even on the spot in your own living room – and perhaps add some other sporting activities to improve your strength and suppleness.

IT BOOSTS YOUR ENERGY LEVELS
Daily tasks, such as carrying the shopping or doing housework or home repairs, will seem easier when you exercise regularly, and you will experience fewer aches and pains and minor injuries. You'll also sleep much better and wake feeling really refreshed and ready to take on the day's challenges.

IT MAKES YOU FEEL GREAT
Exercise has many other amazing properties as well. You will feel happier, more relaxed and be less prone to tension headaches, anxiety attacks and stress. Exercise can work as a painkiller and mood enhancer because it causes the body to release chemicals called endorphins. These substances have a similar chemical structure and effect to morphine – only these ones are natural, have no side effects and are excellent for your health and general wellbeing.

Endorphins act on the nervous system in several ways. They reduce pain by blocking pain signals at particular sites in the brain

and spinal cord. However, they also act on special sites in a part of the brain called the hypothalamus, which is responsible for determining mood. It is this action that is thought to give athletes the feeling of euphoria known as jogger's high, experienced particularly after a long run. This feeling can be so pleasurable that athletes may become addicted to training, unwilling to give it up for a single day – even when ill.

In addition to the all-round health benefits of regular exercise, your lovemaking will also improve. You'll feel like having sex more often, it will last longer and you will enjoy it more. These benefits will come to you within weeks of starting regular exercise, and stay with you as long as you continue.

Exercise even helps to alleviate the symptoms of premenstrual syndrome, such as fatigue, abdominal pains, mood swings and water retention, as well as menopausal symptoms, such as hot flushes, sleep disorders, anxiety and depression.

IT STRENGTHENS YOUR BODY
So how does exercise provide all these wonderful health benefits? First, aerobic exercise has a major effect on the heart and lungs. The heart is a large muscle with a specific job to do – to pump blood around the body carrying oxygen, glucose and other nutrients to the major organs and tissues. All muscles get stronger when they are regularly made to do more work, and get weaker when they are underused. The heart is no exception.

Spring-cleaning exercises

The most odious of household chores can provide excellent physical benefits when done properly. For instance:

Scrubbing floors Supporting yourself with one hand on the floor, use the other to make long, sweeping strokes to tone the muscles of the arms and chest.

Sweeping Work your abdominal muscles by pulling in your abdomen as you sweep. Tone the buttocks at the same time by tucking in your tail bone. These movements will help to support your spine.

Wiping tables Use your arm muscles vigorously as you work – it will tone the muscles and keep your wrist, elbow and shoulder joints strong.

Vacuuming Keep your back straight and lunge forwards – bend one leg at the knee while keeping the other leg straight – to strengthen your calf muscles and improve your buttocks and thighs. Don't let your bottom drop below the level of your knee.

Weeding or digging the garden Bend your knees, not your waist. This will tone muscles and help prevent back strain. Squatting will tone your buttocks and thighs.

With exercise, the heart muscle gets thicker and stronger, and is able to pump more blood with less effort. You will notice the effect of this change after just a few weeks of regular aerobic exercise. Your heart won't have to beat as fast when you exert yourself – by running up stairs, for example – and it will quickly revert to its normal rate of beating when you stop and rest.

The improvement that exercise brings can be easily demonstrated by comparing the heart rate of a physically fit person with that of someone who is inactive. The heart of an average adult pumps about nine pints of blood around the body each minute. An inactive person's heart has to beat 80 or 90 times a minute to do this, whereas a fit person's heart beats only 50–60 times per minute. A trained athlete's heart may beat as little as 30 times a minute. It's easy to see whose heart is more efficient!

INCREASED LUNG POWER

The lungs, too, are strengthened by regular exercise. Your lungs are, in effect, twin balloons that have a porous lining to absorb the oxygen you need for energy. The more they can inflate, the more oxygen they can absorb. When you are inactive for long periods, you tend to breathe in a shallow way, inflating your lungs only enough to stay alive. This can leave you feeling tired and listless much of the time and make you vulnerable to chest infections.

Regular physical activity improves the elasticity of the lungs, which allows them to inflate with greater ease.

During exercise, your lung capacity increases five to seven times. Some of this increased capacity stays with you when you are not exercising, so you breathe deeper to produce more power for the muscles and fuel for the brain.

THE HEART PROTECTOR

The vessels that carry blood throughout your body – the arteries and veins – also benefit from exercise. These blood vessels are slightly elastic to help with backflows and with minor pressure surges. With inactivity, they start to lose their elasticity and begin to harden up. They also become more vulnerable to the formation of fatty deposits, known as plaques, especially when blood levels of cholesterol

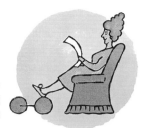

are high. This fatty plaque builds up on the inner walls of the blood vessels, narrowing them and thus slowing the passage of blood through them to the tissues.

This condition, called atherosclerosis, can cause the severe chest pains of angina. It may also lead to the formation of clots that can block blood vessels, resulting in a life-threatening heart attack or stroke. Exercise keeps blood vessels strong and elastic, so that your circulation functions effectively.

A well-known 40-year research project in the US called the Framingham Study investigated the link between exercise and heart disease. It concluded that sedentary people were over five times more likely to die from heart disease than those who fitted even moderate levels of exercise into their weekly routine.

SEDENTARY SPELLS DISASTER

There is another side to the exercise coin, which is the health consequences of leading a sedentary life. For starters, couch potatoes are at far greater risk of developing high blood pressure and high cholesterol, which lead to heart attack and stroke, the biggest killers of middle-aged people.

Lack of exercise weakens the skeleton and increases the risk of developing osteoporosis, a condition that results in fragile bones that fracture easily. Inactive people are more prone to lung ailments, such as bronchitis, and disorders such as diabetes mellitus. In addition, agility and balance can deteriorate as a result of inactivity. A sedentary lifestyle also means that your immune system never works at its peak.

The cornerstone of the body's defence mechanisms is the lymphatic system, which relies on physical activity to push lymph fluid around the body, along with the white blood

ACTIVE MUSCLE

Developing stronger muscles through exercise means you'll burn up more kilojoules (calories), even when sitting still! This is because muscle is metabolically active – it uses fuel even if you're not actually doing anything. If you exercise regularly, your increased musculature will boost your metabolism, meaning your body becomes more efficient at converting fuel to energy and is therefore less likely to store it as fat.

BODY FLUIDS

Replenishing your body's fluid – called rehydration – is vital during any exercise, even if you've only gone for a brisk 30-minute walk. The body constantly dehydrates, losing fluid as vapour in the breath, in sweat and in urine – at least 1 litre (2 pints) per day. This water must be replaced. Even more fluid is lost during any activity that increases the breathing rate and raises body temperature. In hot weather, as much as 1 litre (2 pints) of water may be lost during a 30-minute workout. This may lead to dizziness, exhaustion and even collapse.

To stay hydrated:

▶ Drink a tall glass of water 20 minutes before exercising.

▶ Take small sips from a bottle of water every 10 minutes during your workout.

▶ Drink a glass of water when you finish.

This chart shows the amount of fluid lost in the breath and through sweating, depending on the temperature and activity.

0.5–1 LITRE (1–2 PINTS) PER DAY on a mild day with moderate activity.

0.5–1 LITRE (1–2 PINTS) PER HOUR on a mild day doing moderate activity, such as gardening or housework.

1–1.5 LITRES (2–3 PINTS) PER HOUR on a hot day during moderate exercise, such as brisk walking.

1.5–2 LITRES (3–4 PINTS) PER HOUR on a hot day during vigorous activity, such as jogging or an aerobics session.

cells and antibodies that fight infection. If you are inactive much of the time, your lymphatic system becomes sluggish and ineffective, leaving you more prone to infectious diseases, both minor and major, and a number of other serious conditions.

FREE HEALTH AND FITNESS

The amazing things that exercise offers are free – you don't have to go far to do it, it doesn't take much time and it need not disrupt your day. What's more, moderate exercise properly performed has no harmful side effects.

There is no need to engage in marathons or daily gym sessions 'going for the burn'. Less demanding activities can provide excellent fitness and health benefits. Exercising too strenuously can, in fact, be harmful to health. It can damage the joints, leading to osteoarthritis, and it can suppress the immune system, increasing the risk of disease. So don't overdo it.

There are lots of different ways you can become fit, but the two most effective ways are, first, to aim to be generally more active throughout the day and, second, to incorporate set periods of planned exercise into your week. How you do this is entirely up to you. There are an infinite number of activities, exercises, sports, pastimes and leisure pursuits that will help you get fit. Simple daily tasks such as walking the dog, cleaning the house and gardening, for example, can bring important all-round fitness and health benefits. Other suggestions on how to become more active will be given later on in this section.

Once you decide to shape up, choose activities that you are willing to fit into your weekly schedule and perform long-term. Better still, pick the ones you actually enjoy doing. If you find that one form of activity is too hard, or you just don't like doing it, switch to something else. If it hurts, modify the activity or avoid it altogether. If you continue with a physical pursuit that you don't enjoy or find too demanding, you will quickly become discouraged and you may even end up abandoning the idea of exercise altogether.

BE MORE ACTIVE

One way to work out how much more exercise you need is to calculate your current activity level based on the number of energy units (kilojoules or calories) your body uses up doing different activities. The most inactive thing you could do each day is to watch television. As you sit there, your body burns up around 4.2 kilojoules (1 calorie) per minute (kJ/m or cpm), just keeping you alive.

Research shows that your body may actually use more energy if you stare at a blank wall rather than a television.

If you read a book, your rate goes up slightly (5.5 kJ/m or 1.3 cpm). Yet reading is not an active pursuit, so imagine the difference it makes once you start moving.

A walk around the block raises your activity level to 14.7–21 kJ/m (3.5–5.5 cpm). This means that three 10-minute walks a day will burn up around 420–670 kJ (100–160 calories). You use a similar amount of energy washing the car, dusting, vacuum cleaning, clipping hedges or digging the garden. Swimming uses around 21–63 kJ/m (5–15 cpm), a game of tennis pushes the minimum rate up to 25.2–33.6 kJ/m (6–8 cpm), running increases it to 33.6–63 kJ/m (8–15 cpm) and cycling to 42–50.4 kJ/m (10–12 cpm).

Try to find other ways to increase your daily level of activity. For example, get up a little earlier and walk around the block before you sit down to breakfast. At the shopping centre, walk briskly between shops instead of strolling; at work, use the stairs instead of the lift and visit colleagues rather than using the telephone. Driving is not much more active than watching television, so every time you can replace a car journey with a trip on foot or by bicycle you add to your daily level of activity.

Aim to be a little more active about the home, too. Start by putting away the television remote control and getting out of your chair to change the channel or alter the volume.

Exercise to eat

The habit of 'earning' your meals by exercising can be a useful approach to reducing body fat and increasing exercise and fitness levels. In our evolutionary past, after all, we would have had to expend considerable energy obtaining our food before we could eat it.

There are also physiological bonuses to eating after exercise. When food is taken after physical exertion, nutrients are absorbed more readily and stores of glycogen (the form of glucose that is stored in the liver and muscles until it is needed) are efficiently replaced. But make sure that you cool down properly before eating or you may find yourself also 'earning' indigestion.

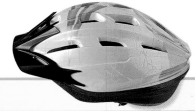

Recreational sports

THE SPORT	THE BENEFITS	THE EQUIPMENT
Tennis or badminton	A casual match demands medium endurance and is a fun way to get fit and lose weight. A serious game can be far more demanding.	You need a racket, balls or shuttlecocks – and a partner. Join your local club, or you can always play casually in a back garden or park.
Aerobics	All-round fitness, depending on the class level.	A class or video and aerobics shoes.
Cycling	Fresh air, free-of-charge transport, improved strength and fitness.	A good bicycle, preferably designed for your purpose.
Squash	Highly demanding, builds strength, flexibility and endurance.	A racket, balls and a squash court.
Dance	An excellent way to reduce stress, have fun and keep fit.	Suitable shoes and clothing, depending on the type of dancing.
Swimming	One of the best sports for developing flexibility and muscle tone.	Comfortable swimwear and goggles (optional).
Cross-country skiing	Builds stamina and strength, especially if continued over long periods.	A cross-country ski path, skis, boots and clothes.
Canoeing, kayaking	Builds strength and endurance, while providing fresh air and great scenery.	A canoe or kayak. Ask your local sports shop about rentals.

While watching television, you could do some simple exercises such as leg rotations, or walk up and down stairs during the commercial breaks. Get a treadmill or exercise bike and use it while watching your favourite show. You could also set aside a little time each morning for a simple warm-up routine and then slowly build this up into regular structured home exercise sessions, perhaps two or three times a week. Before you know it, you'll be making exercise an important part of your lifestyle and enjoying every second.

ASSESSING FITNESS

Before incorporating more physical activity into your life, it may help to assess your current level of fitness so you have a starting baseline. One of the easiest methods of doing this is the walk test.

Find a safe route somewhere, such as a stretch of pavement, a path or a sports track that you know

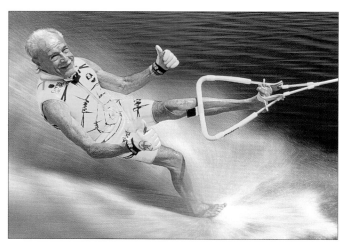

is, say, half a mile or 800 m. You can work this out by measuring it on a map, driving along the route first in your car, using a pedometer (a device for measuring walking distances) or asking the officials at the sports track. Walk the course, there and back, as briskly as you can without stopping – taking care not to get too breathless – and use a watch to time how long you take. It shouldn't take you more than 20 minutes. If it does, don't despair – you now have a starting point.

Once you have begun regular exercise, repeat this test periodically to gauge how you are improving. Consider including it as part of your weekly exercise routine, building up your walking speed and timing it simultaneously. If you are able to complete the test in under 15 minutes, you are fairly fit already, but don't get complacent.

Don't waste any time – get out and get active. There are hundreds of exhilarating pursuits waiting to be mastered.

Fitness rapidly declines if you do not keep up at least a minimum level of activity. Exercising more will improve your fitness and provide many important health benefits at the same time.

Other tests, to measure your stamina, strength and suppleness levels, are covered in later sections of this chapter.

PLAY IT SAFE

To avoid injury and to make exercise more enjoyable, wear clothing that is appropriate for the activity. If you have any queries, ask at your nearest sports shop.

When exercising outdoors on cold days, wear several thin layers so you can discard items of clothing as you warm up. Avoid exercising outdoors in extreme cold or when there is snow or ice on the ground.

Wear appropriate shoes that provide plenty of support for the ankles, with soles that are wide enough to give stability and thick enough to cushion you against impact. Ideally, wear shoes that are designed for your chosen activity. But if you want to do lots of different types of exercise, cross trainers make ideal general-purpose footwear.

BUILDING FITNESS LEVELS

If you're new to exercise, start slow and steady and build up the intensity gradually. The benefits start from the word go, so you don't need to push yourself. A healthy level of exercise will make you breathless – but still able to talk. If exercising with friends, test this by chatting with them at the same time. If exercising on your own, count to ten out loud or sing a song. Exercise should not leave you gasping for breath.

Always seek your doctor's advice before starting regular exercise if you have a medical condition, such as a heart or lung disorder, high blood pressure, diabetes, a spine or joint ailment or an active infection. Your exercise sessions may need to be adjusted according to your personal needs, so seek the advice of a qualified fitness instructor.

No matter what else you plan to do, always start with a gentle warm-up routine and finish with a cool-down session. The amount of time you spend warming up, and the sorts of movements you include, will depend on the activity you are preparing for (see pages 20–21 for a suggested warm-up). In general, a warm-up should last about 10 minutes and include some aerobic activities to raise the heart and breathing rate, and then some stretches to increase the suppleness of the joints and muscle flexibility.

A cooling-down routine involves activities similar to the warm-up, but lasts about half the time, during which you gradually reduce the intensity. It allows your heart and breathing rate to slow down gently and prevents the blood from pooling in the veins, which can cause dizziness. Cooling-down exercises and stretches also help prevent any post-exercise aching, soreness and stiffness, particularly important for those who are new to regular exercise.

While the main reason for these routines is to gently prepare your body for something more active, if you don't have time for a longer exercise session, warming-up exercises are still worth doing for their own sakes. They will get your heart and lungs working harder and limber up the joints and muscles so that you feel livelier and fitter. They also reduce the risk of injury, such as strained joints or muscles.

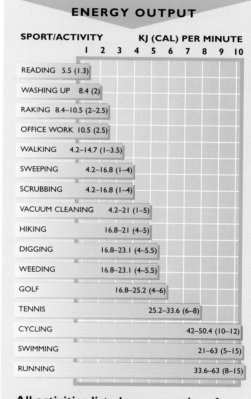

ENERGY OUTPUT

SPORT/ACTIVITY	KJ (CAL) PER MINUTE
READING	5.5 (1.3)
WASHING UP	8.4 (2)
RAKING	8.4–10.5 (2–2.5)
OFFICE WORK	10.5 (2.5)
WALKING	4.2–14.7 (1–3.5)
SWEEPING	4.2–16.8 (1–4)
SCRUBBING	4.2–16.8 (1–4)
VACUUM CLEANING	4.2–21 (1–5)
HIKING	16.8–21 (4–5)
DIGGING	16.8–23.1 (4–5.5)
WEEDING	16.8–23.1 (4–5.5)
GOLF	16.8–25.2 (4–6)
TENNIS	25.2–33.6 (6–8)
CYCLING	42–50.4 (10–12)
SWIMMING	21–63 (5–15)
RUNNING	33.6–63 (8–15)

All activities listed are examples of kilojoule or calorie burners, helping you to keep fit and shed excess weight.

Bounce into the morning with a 10-minute wake-up routine, getting the blood pumping around your body and preparing you for the day ahead. You can also use the routine as a warm-up before physical activity.

DAILY WAKE-UP
and warm-up

These exercises will revitalise your brain, warm your muscles and make your joints more mobile so you are more alert and less prone to aches, pains, strains and sprains.

As you exercise, move smoothly and avoid sudden twists or turns or overstretching any muscle or joint. All forms of exercise need oxygen to fuel them, so it is important to breathe deeply. Find a steady, even rhythm that you can sustain. For a safe and effective warm-up, do some stretches (see pages 36–37) once you have performed some aerobic activity to warm up your body and mobilise your joints. A good guide to being adequately warmed up is that you start to sweat.

Repeat these exercises, but only for 5 minutes, as part of your cooldown. Steadily reduce the amount of effort you put in until you come to a gentle halt. You may want to finish with a few minutes of contemplative deep breathing.

DEEP BREATHING
(to oxygenate the brain and muscles)

Start with deep breathing. Stand with your back lengthened, feet hip-distance apart and arms by your sides. Slowly breathe in (through your nose) as you lift your arms up in a semi-circle until your hands are above your head. Slowly breathe out (through your mouth) as you lower your arms to your sides. Repeat several times.

Breathe slowly and steadily from the bottom of your lungs

Keep your knees slightly bent

ELBOW LIFTS
(to work the arms and upper body)

1 Stand tall with your feet shoulder-width apart and knees slightly bent. Place your fingertips on your shoulders with your elbows close to your body.

Keep your elbows as close to your body as is comfortable

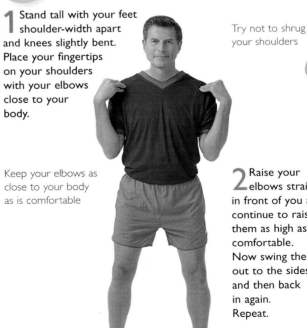

Try not to shrug your shoulders

2 Raise your elbows straight in front of you and continue to raise them as high as is comfortable. Now swing them out to the sides, and then back in again. Repeat.

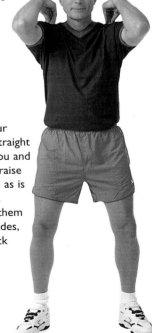

NECK TURN
(to work the upper spine)

Stand comfortably with your back straight and arms relaxed by your sides. Lengthen your neck by lifting the crown of your head towards the ceiling. Turn your head to the left as far as you can comfortably manage. Hold for 2 seconds. Turn back to the front, pause, and repeat on the other side.

TORSO TWIST
(for abdominal muscles)

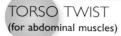

1 Stand with your feet shoulder-width apart and knees slightly bent. Pull in your abdominal muscles, tuck in your tail bone, and fold your arms at shoulder level.

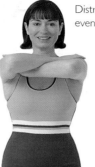

Distribute your weight evenly over both feet

2 Turn your rib cage to the right as far as you can comfortably go, while keeping your hips facing front. Repeat to the left. Alternate until you have completed 8 on each side.

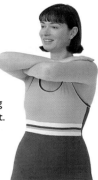

HIP SWING
(to work the hips and sides)

Stand with your feet slightly wider than hip-width apart. Substantially bend the knees towards the toes. With the tail bone tucked underneath you and with both knees remaining equally bent, swing your hips slowly from side to side.

Keep your abdominal muscles pulled in and avoid pushing your bottom out

SIDE BENDS
(to work the upper body)

Stand with your back straight, feet shoulder-width apart, knees slightly bent and hands behind your head. Tucking your tail bone in, bend from the waist to the left and then straighten. Repeat to the right.

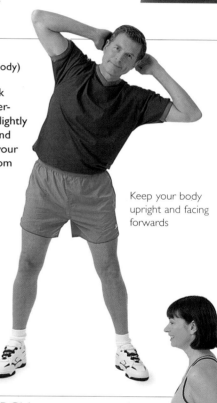

Keep your body upright and facing forwards

Keep your legs just over shoulder-width apart for good balance

SQUATS
(to work legs and lower body)

Place both feet flat on the floor, shoulder-width apart. Bend your knees over your toes while bending slightly forwards at the waist. Return to an upright position. Be sure to look straight ahead throughout. Continue for a minute.

Rest your hands on the top of your thighs as you bend to support the back

WARM-UP MARCH
(to warm muscles and mobilise joints)

Stand tall with your feet slightly apart and arms by your sides. Looking straight ahead, march on the spot, using an easy one-two, one-two rhythm. Lift your knees up and breathe deeply as you march. Continue marching on the spot for 2 or 3 minutes.

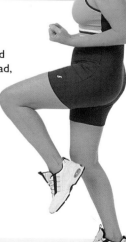

Building stamina

Having the determination to achieve your aims is one of the keys to a happy and successful life. Keep on your toes and be prepared for all that life throws at you by building up your physical stamina.

Studies show that more than 50 per cent of adults in Western countries do little regular stamina-building exercise, and 25 per cent are not physically active in any way. The more sedentary you become in your daily life, the less stamina you have, and this has serious implications for your health. Stamina ensures, for instance, that you can climb a large flight of stairs without puffing or pausing for breath half-way up, or run down the road for a bus if you are late for an appointment. There are other names for this ability, including endurance, cardiovascular fitness and aerobic capacity, but they all mean the same thing – that the heart, lungs and circulation are working efficiently.

While all aspects of fitness are important, improving stamina will have the most immediate and dramatic effects on your health.

A Harvard University study demonstrated that people who expend 6300 kilojoules (1500 calories) a week through stamina-building activities, such as long-distance walking, running or cycling, live the longest.

Sustained, moderate stamina-building exercises burn fat and so help you to shed surplus weight when combined with a weight-reduction diet.

HOW DOES YOUR STAMINA RATE?

The step test is the easiest way of measuring your current stamina before starting regular exercise. This test increases your pulse rate and then measures how well it recovers. First, do the step-ups shown on page 27 for 3 minutes. Stop and wait for 30 seconds before taking your pulse.

Because your heart rate will be falling rapidly, take your pulse for just 15 seconds and then multiply it by four. Compare the figure with the recovery pulse rate chart below to judge your fitness. If you do this test every two to four sessions, you can monitor how your stamina is improving.

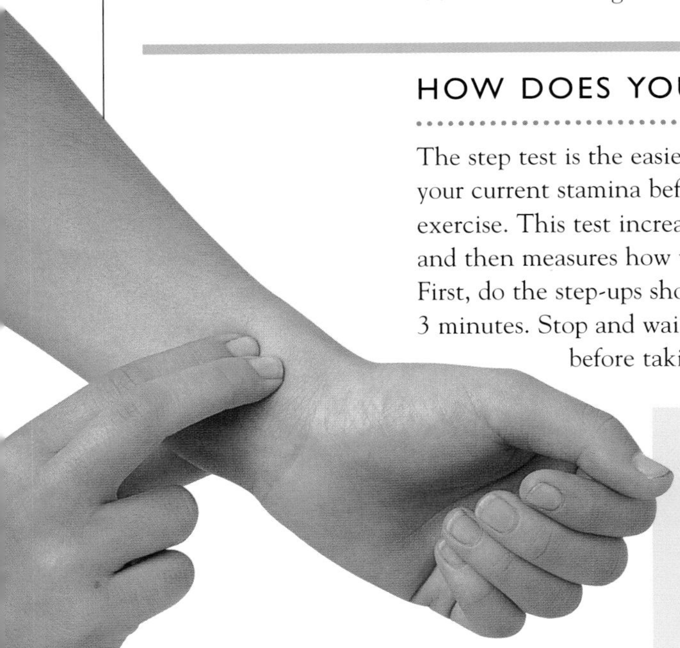

RECOVERY PULSE RATE

WOMEN				
AGE	VERY FIT	FIT	AVERAGE	UNFIT
40–50	<88	88–95	96–115	115+
50+	<91	91–99	100–118	118+
MEN				
AGE	VERY FIT	FIT	AVERAGE	UNFIT
40–50	<80	80–89	90–99	99+
50+	<82	82–92	93–105	105+

Place your first and second fingers just below the base of the thumb. The tip of your second finger should feel a pulse.

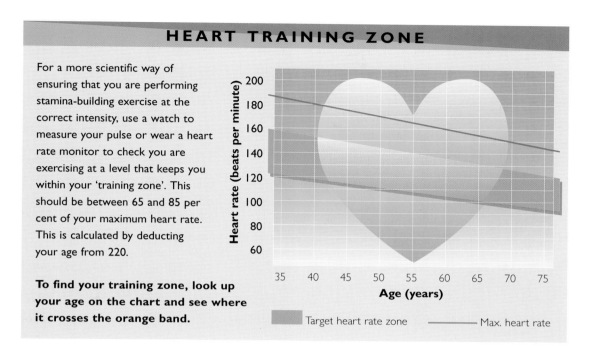

HEART TRAINING ZONE

For a more scientific way of ensuring that you are performing stamina-building exercise at the correct intensity, use a watch to measure your pulse or wear a heart rate monitor to check you are exercising at a level that keeps you within your 'training zone'. This should be between 65 and 85 per cent of your maximum heart rate. This is calculated by deducting your age from 220.

To find your training zone, look up your age on the chart and see where it crosses the orange band.

Target heart rate zone ———— Max. heart rate

PUMP IT UP

Your body makes various physiological adaptations if you perform regular stamina-building exercise. The heart muscle becomes stronger and its pumping capacity increases, which allows more blood to be pumped around the body per heart beat. Because the heart works more efficiently, it beats less often. People who start a programme of regular exercise notice that their pulse becomes slower – even when they are resting – and that after exercise it reverts to its normal rate more quickly.

Regular stamina exercise also expands lung capacity, allowing more oxygen in and removing waste carbon dioxide more rapidly, so that you do not get out of breath as quickly. Blood flow through the lungs and around the body improves, enabling more freshly oxygenated blood to reach the muscles, organs and tissues throughout the body.

To achieve these benefits, the heart, lungs and circulation must work harder, little by little, over a period of weeks and months until they, and you, are fitter than when you started out. Sessions of physical activity that can be sustained for at least 20 minutes (ideally a little longer) and done at a moderate level are the key

TAKE CARE

If you have been inactive for a while, check your condition by measuring your resting pulse rate early in the morning, before getting out of bed. If it is above 100 for a woman or above 90 for a man, see your doctor before starting regular stamina exercises. The doctor may advise against certain activities.

components. Health and fitness experts generally recommend a minimum of 30 minutes of sustained, moderate physical activity at least three times a week.

THE IMPORTANCE OF OXYGEN

Stamina-building activities are sometimes referred to as aerobic exercise. Aerobic literally means 'with oxygen', and refers to all forms of sustained, moderate exercise, including walking, cycling and jogging, not just aerobic step and aerobic dance classes.

We tend to think that all exercise involves oxygen, but, in fact, intensive physical activities such as sprinting and weight lifting are anaerobic, meaning powered 'without oxygen'. This is because it takes several minutes for the heart, lungs and circulation to supply the muscles with oxygen. If the physical activity is very intense, there is no time for oxygen to be produced and the muscles have to perform without it – that is, anaerobically. Instead, they draw upon energy from existing carbohydrate supplies in the muscle through a chemical transformation process. Muscles cannot work this way for very long. If you are able to sustain any specific exercise for a period of 20 minutes, it is evidence that

EXERCISING WITHIN LIMITS

Take note of how easy you find it to talk while exercising. This is sometimes called your perceived rate of exertion (PRE) and shown as a scale.

RATE 1

You can talk and exercise at this rate indefinitely – aim to improve.

RATE 2

You can exercise and still talk in a breathy way – this is the lower rate.

RATE 3

You are more breathless but can still talk at this rate – this is the top rate.

RATE 4

You are uncomfortable talking at this rate of exercise – avoid until you get really fit.

RATE 5

You find it impossible to talk – only trained athletes should attempt this rate.

the muscles are working aerobically. Similarly to aerobic exercise, regular anaerobic exercise increases the body's ability to access and utilise energy.

ENERGY SWITCH-OVER

It is important that exercise is sustained because of the time delay before the body switches from the initial anaerobic energy production systems to the aerobic system. But if you can only manage 10 minutes at a time before tiring, simply do it twice a day. There is no point trying to step up the pace before you are ready. Certainly you need to push your body to get fitter, but attempting anything unrealistic can result in injury or discourage you from continuing.

Start off by walking for 20–30 minutes at the fastest pace with which you feel comfortable. Ideally, walking should make you breathe harder but still enable you to talk out loud. Unless you are monitoring your pulse (see page 22), judging the effort you are putting in may be difficult. You can make a good estimation by gauging the ease with which you can talk. Exercises to build stamina need to be challenging if they are to be effective. Once your current level of activity seems easy, you should start to raise the effort involved. First increase the distance you walk, then the pace, and later include a slight incline in the route. A treadmill can be adjusted to achieve this. Over time (say, 10–20 weeks), you may feel fit enough to jog part of the way.

As you get fitter you will find that you perceive your level of exertion as moderate (rate 2 or 3 – see above left) even though you are now exercising harder. This shows that your

heart, lungs, blood circulation and muscles are adapting to the exercise by becoming stronger and more effective. Perhaps surprisingly, you will find you perspire more freely, too, but this is perfectly natural. It shows that your body's temperature-regulating system is now working more efficiently to dissipate the heat you generate when exercising.

You can make walking and jogging more enjoyable by exercising in attractive or interesting surroundings and by encouraging a friend or partner to come with you. Exercising with a friend has the added advantage of providing mutual support.

EXERCISE CHOICES

Walking and jogging are not the only kinds of stamina-building exercises. Cycling, swimming, dancing and step aerobics are also effective, provided they are sustained for 20 minutes or until mild fatigue sets in. Skipping is another simple form of exercise with major aerobic benefits. You can also combine a range of aerobic exercises, such as step-ups and star jumps (see pages 26–27), into a 20-minute routine to do at home.

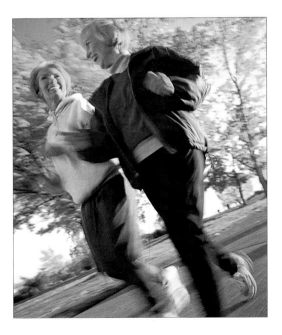

Try to have a companion join you in your workouts. Exercising with friends is fun and keeps you motivated and enthusiastic.

Stamina-building machines

The variety of stamina-building equipment for exercising at home ranges from simple pedal devices to more sophisticated exercise machines. This equipment is also known as cardiovascular machinery because it is particularly beneficial for the heart and blood vessels (cardiovascular system). Machines include stationary bikes, treadmills, climbers and a variety of rowing, step and cross-country skiing machines.

Sources Cardiovascular equipment for home use is available from specialised fitness shops and through mail order catalogues. Before you visit a shop, decide what it is that you want to achieve, and then try out the different types of machine on the market until you find the one that best meets your needs and gives you plenty of room for improvement. Sales staff in specialised stores should be able to offer advice and recommend suitable machines.

Adjustable effort levels The advantage of the more advanced machines is that they can be adjusted to increase the effort involved and so will continue to stretch you as your fitness improves. In the case of stationary bikes, you can increase the amount of friction being applied to the wheel, which makes it more strenuous to pedal. With treadmills and climbers, the front of the device can often be raised so that you are, in effect, walking or jogging up an increasingly steep incline.

Electronic gadgets Top-of-the-range machines usually include computers to monitor both your physical output and your improving fitness levels, thus helping you to fine-tune your

exercise programme. They often include gauges to measure the theoretical distance you have travelled, for example, or the number of kilojoules (calories) burned while exercising. These devices can greatly add to the overall cost and are only a worthwhile investment if you require this level of expertise and know how to use this information in your fitness programme.

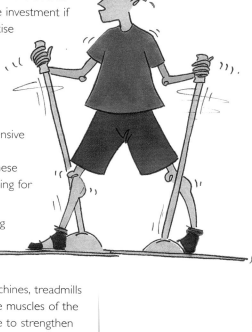

Flywheels vs hydraulics
Machines that incorporate a flywheel are usually more expensive but less strenuous than those involving a hydraulic system. These machines allow you to keep going for longer before tiring.

Muscle toners Stamina-building exercise machines also provide muscle-toning benefits. For example, step machines, treadmills and stationary bicycles tone the muscles of the legs and buttocks. They do little to strengthen the upper body, however, so if using one, ensure that your fitness routine does not neglect other key areas of the body.

Rowing and cross-country skiing machines
These are probably the most effective stamina machines because they exercise the upper body – particularly the arms, chest and abdomen – as well as the legs, and so provide a complete fitness workout.

STAMINA-BUILDING
exercises

Exercises that build endurance are often included in fitness classes and are ideal to do at home. Combine those shown with strength and suppleness exercises (see pages 32–33 and 36–37) for an all-round fitness programme.

You can perform these exercises individually or combine them into a full aerobic workout. Always do a warm-up routine before you start and a cool-down at the end to reduce the risk of injury and aches and pains. After you finish, a breathing exercise may be relaxing.

As your stamina improves, you can increase the time spent on each exercise and repeat the entire workout several times. Aim to increase the total length of the session to at least 20 minutes – preferably 40 minutes – to achieve optimum fitness benefits.

LEG AND ARM CURLS

1 Stand tall with your feet hip-width apart. Keep your elbows at your sides, your hands low in front of you and fists slightly clenched.

Keep your shoulders upright and facing forwards

2 Raise your hands to your shoulders. At the same time, lift your right heel up to your buttocks. Lower your hands as you lower your foot to the floor. Repeat with the other foot. Do this at a steady, even pace. Continue for up to 2–3 minutes.

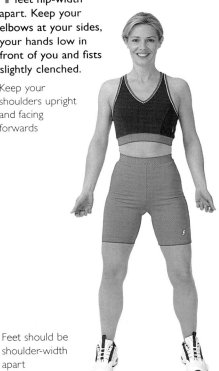

Feet should be shoulder-width apart

Transfer your weight to one foot, then lift the other behind

SWAYS

With feet well apart and knees slightly bent, sway from side to side by transferring your weight from one foot to the other. Swing your arms in front of you at the same time. Do this at a steady, even pace. Continue for 2–3 minutes.

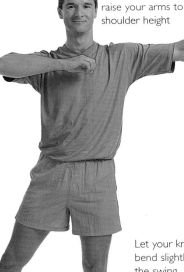

Make sure that you raise your arms to shoulder height

Let your knees bend slightly with the swing

HALF STARS AND STAR JUMPS

1 HALF STARS: Stand with your back straight, knees slightly bent, abdomen pulled in and arms by your sides. Bend your knees, raising both arms to shoulder height at the same time.

2 Lower your arms and bring the feet together with a small jump. Find a rhythm and repeat at least 20 times. Make sure you don't lift your arms above shoulder height.

1 STAR JUMPS: Stand tall with your feet slightly apart and arms by your sides. Bend your knees and then spring upwards, raising both arms above your head at the same time. Land with your feet well apart and knees in line with your toes.

2 Now, spring upwards and land with your feet together and your arms at your sides. Repeat for up to 30 seconds.

Trampolining for health

Bouncing on a mini-trampoline for a few minutes gives the heart and lungs a good workout and strengthens muscles and bones. You can try bouncing on alternate legs, or clapping your hands beneath each raised knee as you jump. Take care not to lose your balance, and make sure that you have a soft landing in case you fall.

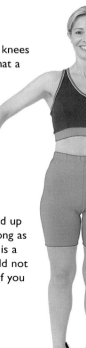

STEP-UPS

Step on and off a sturdy box 10–20 cm (4–8 inches) high (or a step) for up to 3 minutes. First, step up with the left foot, then the right, and then step down with the right foot, followed by the left. Fully straighten the knees each time you step up, but don't lock them. Keep an even, regular pace — up, up, down, down. Continue for up to 3 minutes.

SPRINGING

Stand with your feet together and knees slightly bent. Spring high enough that a piece of paper could be passed under both feet. As you land, be sure to bend the knees and bring the heels down to the floor. Keep the pace moderate. Start off with short sessions of 20–30 springs and pause for a minute between sessions. Once you get the swing of springing, build up to 60–80 springs a minute for as long as you can comfortably manage. This is a high-impact exercise and you should not attempt it without medical advice if you suffer from osteoporosis.

Building muscular strength and endurance

Keep your body ready for action and prepared for strenuous or weighty tasks by regularly exerting your muscles. Strength and endurance training tones and conditions your muscles, as well as improving your fitness.

Strength is the ability to lift, lower, push or carry an object of such mass, weight or resistance that the effort involved can only be sustained for a short time. For example, you need muscular strength to lift a heavy suitcase into the boot of a car, to unscrew the tight lid of a jar or to push a piano. Endurance, on the other hand, is the ability to sustain a level of activity for extended periods, such as carrying heavy shopping home or digging the garden. Improving muscular strength and endurance will provide important benefits to both your health and your quality of life.

On average, men and women are at their strongest at the age of 30. After that, muscle mass and strength tend to go into a steady decline – unless people do something about it and make strength exercises an important part of their lives.

Regular resistance exercises can reduce and even reverse the steady decline in strength with age, no matter how old or unfit you are when you start.

According to scientists at Johns Hopkins University in the United States, older adults who have been doing strength exercises for more than 15 years are as strong or stronger than inactive 20-year-olds. Studies conducted at a nursing home showed that even 80- and 90-year-olds could double their leg muscle strength and improve daily activity levels by 35 per cent after just 10 weeks of strength exercises. Just as aerobic exercises boost the heart and lungs, so strength exercises build up the muscles. Unless muscle is regularly used, its tone diminishes and it becomes weaker. Unfit muscles tire easily, are

MUSCLE-BUILDING MYTHS

TRUE
Many body builders develop muscular bulk without necessarily having the matching strength. They achieve this by using very specific muscle exercises and stretches and keeping to a strict high-protein diet. Unless you're intending to join the body-building circuit, it is better to aim for increased strength.

TRUE
You may need to alter your diet if you want to improve your muscular strength. This is because it is the carbohydrates in your diet, such as bread, pasta, rice, cereals and fruit and vegetables, that fuel muscle development. If you are eating a balanced diet, you do not need extra protein, and you most certainly will not need extra fats or sugars in your diet.

FALSE
A popular misapprehension is that if you stop regular weight training, the muscle you have developed turns to fat. This is an illusion, due to the fact that a return to a sedentary lifestyle invariably means the muscles shrink in size, and more fat is deposited around the body, including around the muscles. The process is quickly reversed by returning to a more active lifestyle.

FALSE
Some people believe strength exercises always make muscles bulkier and less flexible. This, too, is a myth. Good strength-building exercise enhances flexibility by putting muscles through their full range of movement.

prone to injury and limit the amount of activity your body can take. A small amount of thought and effort can save your muscles.

STRENGTH TRAINING

Building strength involves working your muscles against some degree of resistance, such as lifting a weight. But it isn't sufficient to lift a weight only once: You need to work the muscles to their maximum capacity, and this means performing each movement several times – repetitions. This is known as challenging the muscles. By raising the weight or the number of repetitions, you increase the challenge.

Weight lifting isn't the only form of resistance training, however. In fact, every time you sit down or stand up, you work by carrying your body weight against gravity. Other examples include tensile resistance, such as the pull you feel walking through deep mud.

Water offers considerable resistance and swimming is an ideal form of strength exercise – as well as improving stamina.

Although muscles grow larger in response to strength training, it doesn't mean you will gain a body builder's physique, which takes many hours of specialised training and dedicated effort. You will, however, be helping yourself to a fitter, stronger body with firmer muscles and less body fat.

ENDURANCE TRAINING

Muscular endurance refers to a muscle's ability to work repeatedly for an extended period of time. Endurance is needed for tasks that do not pose much of a resistance challenge but require repetitive movements – for example, the repeated brush strokes required when painting a ceiling, the arm movements involved in polishing a car and the leg power used when climbing long flights of stairs all require muscular endurance. The ability to maintain good posture throughout the day, whether sitting, standing or on the move, is also dependent upon muscle endurance.

HOW STRONG ARE YOU?

The abdominal curl (or crunch) test is a good way to help you determine your current level of muscular ability. To do an abdominal curl, lie on your back with your shoulders resting on the floor, arms by your sides. Lift your head and shoulders off the floor so that your hands slide forwards towards your knees and then carefully lower your head and shoulders again. Breathe out as you curl up and breathe in as you come down. Do as many as you can in 1 minute and compare the result with the chart shown below.

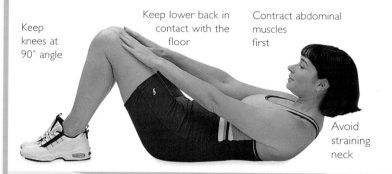

Keep knees at 90° angle | Keep lower back in contact with the floor | Contract abdominal muscles first | Avoid straining neck

ABDOMINAL MUSCLE STRENGTH RATING

WOMEN				
AGE	VERY FIT	FIT	AVERAGE	UNFIT
40–50	35+	31–35	24–30	<23
51–60	30+	26–30	20–25	<19
60+	25+	21–25	15–20	<14
MEN				
AGE	VERY FIT	FIT	AVERAGE	UNFIT
40–50	39+	35–39	29–34	<28
51–60	34+	30–34	24–29	<23
60+	29+	25–29	19–24	<18

In order to build endurance, you need to do exercises that require the muscles not only to overcome moderate resistance but also to continue doing so for an extended period of time. In other words, while strength training involves heavier weights but fewer repetitions, endurance training involves lighter weights but more repetitions, preferably continued for over 20 minutes. Before you start regular strength and endurance exercises, it might help to gauge your current level by doing the abdominal curl test (shown above) so that you can measure your improvements. Your abdominal muscles help you to maintain your posture during various physical activities and thus are good indicators of overall muscular fitness.

STAY BALANCED

Many stamina-building exercises, such as jogging and using treadmills, improve the strength and endurance only of the muscles involved. If you concentrate on these types of exercise, you run the risk of developing an imbalanced physique, with powerful leg and buttock muscles but weak shoulders, chest and arms. To prevent this, make sure your exercise routine includes resistance exercises for the upper body. Alternatively, use stamina-building equipment such as rowing and skiing machines that exercise the upper and lower body at the same time.

Many muscles work in pairs. To create movement in one direction, lifting a glass for example, one muscle in the arm will contract while the other relaxes. To provide movement in the opposite direction, putting the glass down, the muscle actions reverse. Unless both muscles of the pair are exercised evenly, imbalances can occur that reduce the efficiency of the joints and increase the risk of injury. This is a major cause of posture problems, leading to symptoms such as persistent neck and back pain.

You should vary the types of exercise you do so that all the muscles of the body are improved – or conditioned – evenly without concentrating on any particular muscle group.

Certain muscles have important roles as fixating, or stabilising, muscles. This means that their main task is to maintain the body's position or posture while other muscles are doing

Popular resistance aids

Building your strength doesn't have to mean lifting huge weights as these alternatives show:

Dumbbells These can be used singly or in pairs and may be obtained as fixed sizes, available in a range of weights, or adjustable types to which extra weights can be added. They are simple to use, safe and effective. They can be used to provide extra resistance when doing standard exercises, or in exercises designed specifically for dumbbells.

Barbell This is a bar to which weights are attached at either end. Barbells are very effective because they strengthen the support muscles, which help maintain posture and stability, as well as the main muscle groups. However, their use requires training from an experienced fitness instructor for safety.

Elastic training band You can use this in many different ways. For example, sitting on a chair, loop it around one foot and hold the two ends by your hip. Straightening that leg

against the resistance of the band strengthens the muscles in the front of your thigh. For the upper body, take it in your hands, either in front of your chest or behind your back, and stretch it to strengthen arms and shoulders.

Ankle and wrist weights These increase the amount of resistance involved when doing standard strength exercises such as those shown on pages 32–33.

Gym machines Resistance machines are easy to use and simple to adjust when you want to increase the effort involved. Most machines target individual muscles or muscle groups, so take care not to overwork these areas of the body or you could end up with imbalanced muscles. There are multi-purpose gyms available, too, which include a range of different machines that can be worked through systematically. These useful devices are designed to improve all-round muscle strength and endurance.

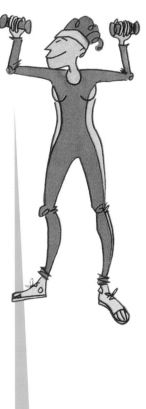

active physical work, such as lifting, pulling or pushing. Varying the exercises and activities you do will ensure that these muscles get a proper workout, too. Strong abdominal muscles, for example, are particularly important when lifting heavy loads (see page 29); they give extra protection to the back and help to prevent a hernia (where the intestine protrudes through a weak area of muscle).

Never do strength exercises when you are tired. You greatly increase the risk of injury if, because of physical or mental fatigue, you are not in total control during an exercise or you are not concentrating on doing the exercise correctly. Poor exercise technique is likely to put excessive strain on muscles, joints and connective tissue that are not prepared or strong enough to cope with it.

BEAT THE PAIN BARRIER

Aim to alternate resistance exercises with aerobic or stamina-building routines. This gives your muscles a chance to recover from the build-up of lactic acid, which is a common side effect of high-intensity activities such as weight lifting or sprinting. In these anaerobic activities, oxygen cannot be delivered to the muscles in time to assist with the breakdown of glycogen (the form in which glucose energy is stored in the muscles). Without the presence of oxygen, glycogen breakdown produces lactic acid. It is the build-up of lactic acid in the muscles that causes the burning sensation associated with intense activity.

The pain eventually builds up to the point where you must rest. As soon as you stop, muscles start to use oxygen to break down the lactic acid. The more lactic acid that has built up, the more oxygen is needed to break it down. This is called the 'oxygen debt' and is why you pant for breath after sprinting. By alternating aerobic exercise with resistance activities you enable muscles to disperse the lactic acid. You will then not have to stop doing strength exercises prematurely because of fatigue or muscle pain.

You can also train to improve your recovery rate by timing each stop to allow yourself

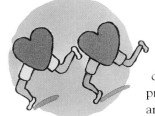

RUNNING WILD

By running just 8 km (5 miles) a week, you can reduce your risk of heart disease – the number one killer in the Western world – by 20 per cent. Running can also help you lose weight, strengthen muscle and bones and slow the aging process. Even your skin and hair will benefit, and you'll feel great, too.

just enough time to breathe evenly and deeply before repeating the exercise. With practice, this will enable you to recover faster and further improve your stamina.

RESISTANCE ACTIVITIES

You do not have to join a gym or go to the pool regularly to develop and maintain good muscle tone. Effective training can be done in the comfort of your own home using your body weight as resistance, with exercises such as push-ups and abdominal curls. Other methods include the use of elastic exercise bands and hand, wrist or ankle weights.

Apart from deliberate, specific exercises, the best way to ensure your muscles remain strong and with good endurance capacity is to use them on a regular basis. Performing tasks yourself rather than relying on labour-saving gadgets, or other people, is your best guarantee of muscle tone.

Try new activities, such as ice skating or ballroom dancing, to exercise more muscles. Every time you use a muscle in a different way, you help your whole body remain healthy and strong.

Ideally, activities to improve strength and endurance should increase the muscles' normal workload moderately. First, increase the number of repetitions you do, and then up the weight; raise both steadily rather than attempt big increases too soon.

TAKE CARE

When doing resistance exercises, don't hold your breath or keep still for more than a few seconds, as this raises your blood pressure. Steadily breathe out when exerting maximum effort and breathe in as you relax the effort. If you have high blood pressure, see a doctor before starting resistance exercises.

Muscle-toning exercises won't turn you into an Arnold Schwarzenegger lookalike. Instead, they will ensure that your muscles stay in good shape and can work more efficiently so that you can do everyday tasks for longer.

MUSCLE-TONING exercises

To avoid developing imbalanced muscles, you need to do a range of muscle-toning exercises. These can be included with aerobic and other exercises as part of a general fitness routine. If new to exercise, do a few of each and slowly build up the number. Always do a warm-up routine before you start and a cool-down at the end to reduce the risk of injury and post-exercise aches and pains. To refresh your muscles, march on the spot between exercises to help prevent a build-up of lactic acid (see page 31).

As you do these exercises, maintain comfortable breathing and do the movements slowly and in a controlled manner. Remember to always breathe out on the exertion. Continue each exercise only to the point of mild fatigue and stop any exercise that causes pain. Seek advice from a qualified fitness instructor if you experience problems with these exercises.

WALL PUSH-UP
(to tone arms and upper body)

1 Stand up straight in front of a wall – almost an arm's length away – with your feet flat on the floor.

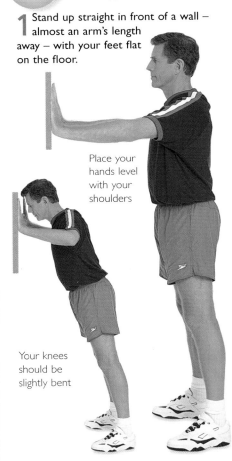

Place your hands level with your shoulders

Your knees should be slightly bent

2 Bend your elbows to lower your body towards the wall. Straighten your elbows to return to the start position. Keep your back straight and your abdominal muscles held in at all times.

BOX PUSH-UP
(to tone arms and upper body)

1 Kneel down with your knees and feet hip-width apart and your arms supporting your upper body.. Keep your hands shoulder-width apart and directly below your shoulders – fingers pointing forwards. Don't lock your elbows straight.

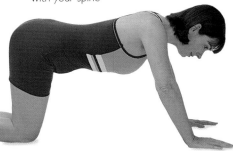

Keep your abdomen pulled in and your head in line with your spine

2 Breathing in, lower your upper body until your nose almost touches the floor. Pause briefly, and then breathe out as you raise your upper body again. Keep your head, neck and spine in line at all times and pull your abdominal muscles in. You can also practise this exercise against a wall.

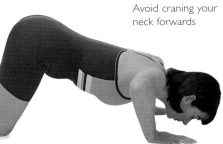

Avoid craning your neck forwards

HEEL RAISES
(to tone calves)

1 Stand facing a wall – about a foot-length away – with back straight and feet together.

2 With your hands resting lightly against the wall for support, lift up on your toes and hold briefly before lowering your heels to the floor.

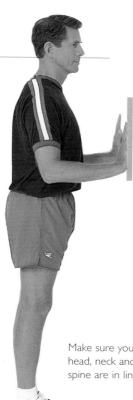

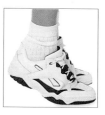

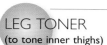

Make sure your head, neck and spine are in line

LOWER BACK RAISES
(to tone lower back)

Lie face down with your legs straight, toes resting on the floor and feet together. Hold your arms by your sides and pull in your abdominal muscles. Breathe in. Breathe out as you slowly raise your upper body off the floor. Breathe in as you hold briefly and then breathe out as you slowly lower to the floor. Keep your chin pointing down at all times. Stop if you feel any strain.

Your feet should be in contact with the floor

Keep your neck in line with your spine

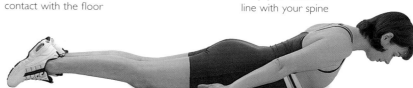

EASY SQUATS
(to tone thighs and buttocks)

Straighten your back and pull in your abdominal muscles

1 Stand with your back straight, hands on hips, feet flat on the floor hip-width apart and facing forwards.

2 Bend at the knees letting your bottom push backwards. Avoid tipping forwards. Pause briefly and then return to the upright position. Don't squat too low – never allow your bottom to go below knee level and always push your knees out over your toes, but not beyond them.

LEG TONER
(to tone inner thighs)

1 You need to wear shoes for this exercise. Standing upright, take a wide step to the left, bending the knee towards the toes as you do so.

2 Draw the left leg back to the centre as you straighten both legs, dragging the foot along the floor. Repeat 10 times, then do the same with the other leg.

Imagine you're wiping chewing-gum off the sole of your shoe

Keep your head, neck and spine in line at all times

Building suppleness

The ability to achieve a full range of movements – to turn, stretch, twist and bend – without stiffness, aching or suffering a spine or joint injury is defined as suppleness, or flexibility.

Suppleness is an important part of everyday life. Being supple means you can reach up to take an item down from a shelf, for example, or bend down to tie your shoe laces, without feeling that your movements are restricted in any way. You tend to take suppleness for granted when you are young, but as you get older, you need to spend a little time enhancing and then maintaining it.

You can start a routine of simple stretches at any age to restore or increase flexibility to muscles and joints. In fact, studies show you are never too old to reverse the reduced level of suppleness that comes with age – no matter how long it has been building up.

Suppleness is achieved by regular stretching of the muscles, either by carrying out specific exercises or by participating in activities that take the joints through their full ranges of movement. Muscles are wrapped in connective tissues, which, rather like chewing gum, are resistant to being stretched when cold.

For this reason, it is very important to attempt stretching exercises only when your muscles are warm. When stretching, a slight degree of tension should be felt in the muscle. Attempting to stretch too far causes physical discomfort or even pain and can result in injury. In order to maintain your flexibility, stretches need to be held for at least 10 seconds. This gives the connective tissue and muscle enough time to lengthen.

Stretches should always be executed slowly. Once you are familiar with the positions, you can develop your flexibility by relaxing in them for progressively longer periods. You will find that as the muscles relax they can be stretched further. If you are not used to doing this sort of activity regularly, you can soon find your joints stiffening up and your range of movement becoming much more limited.

SAFE STRETCHING

Avoid forceful stretches. You should feel only a comfortable tightness, not pain, when a muscle is stretched to its limit. Never go beyond this point. Avoid stretches that put excessive strain on other parts of the body. For example, deep knee bends, in which the bottom drops below the level of the knees, and touching the toes while keeping the legs straight, can be harmful because they put too much strain on the back and joints. Always place your hands on your thighs when stretching the muscles at the back of the leg (hamstrings) as this helps support the lower back, whether standing or sitting.

When stretching, apply only slow, steady pressure and resist the temptation to speed up the stretch by bouncing. This puts more stress on the tendons than the muscles. Muscles are armed with a reflex device to protect them from being over-extended. This

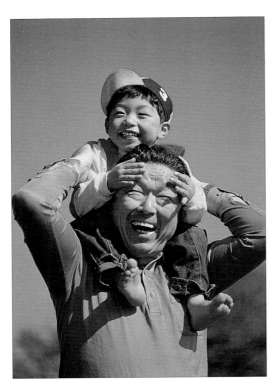

Maintaining your suppleness means you can enjoy life to the full without worrying about muscle aches or injuries.

means that every time you move into a stretch, the initial reaction of the muscle is to contract in order to protect itself. Held for a few seconds, this initial contraction will disperse and the muscle can then relax into a stretch. Bouncing, which is also known as ballistic stretching, repeatedly triggers the reflex action and results in a series of contractions rather than the desired lengthening of the muscle.

It is important that stretches are attempted by moving the joints only in the directions for which they are designed. The knees, for example, are hinge joints and can be damaged if attempts are made to rotate or move them laterally. Ligaments, the bands of fibrous tissue that hold the joints in place, can be damaged if the joint is moved in a direction it is not designed to go.

BENEFITS OF STRETCHING

Stretching is ideal for those times when other kinds of exercise, such as strength- or stamina-building activities, might be inappropriate. You can do stretches at home, while travelling, or in an office while you are reading through a letter, for example. Poor posture and lack of mobility is a common cause of muscle pain among office workers.

By doing simple stretching exercises during the day you can improve posture and joint mobility, reduce muscular tension and avoid muscle pain.

If you suffer intermittent neck- or backache, perhaps because of poor posture or tension, controlled stretching might alleviate the problem (see pages 36–37).

Regular controlled stretches aid relaxation and general wellbeing by loosening muscles that have become tense through physical effort or anxiety, stress or another emotional cause. It may also be important to do carefully controlled stretches when recovering from an injury. This is because muscle damage always leads to the formation of fibrous scar tissue, which does not stretch.

HOW SUPPLE ARE YOU?

Before starting regular stretching exercises, it helps to know how supple you are now. One way to do this is the sit and reach test, which involves attempting to touch your toes from a seated position. To do this test, sit with your feet together and your legs out straight in front of you. Point your toes towards the ceiling. Bending from the waist and keeping your legs on the floor, stretch your arms forwards to reach your toes. An average or below-average result indicates that you should concentrate on improving your suppleness. A good result indicates that, while suppleness is not a major problem for you, you should still include flexibility exercises in your fitness programme to maintain your current level.

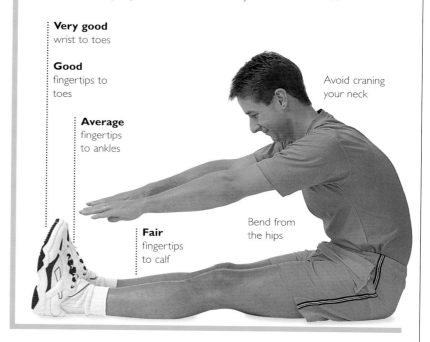

Very good
wrist to toes

Good
fingertips to toes

Average
fingertips to ankles

Fair
fingertips to calf

Avoid craning your neck

Bend from the hips

The presence of scar tissue results in loss of flexibility and increases the risk of future injury. To avoid this, once the muscle starts to heal, it is advisable to ask a qualified fitness instructor or physiotherapist about appropriate exercises you can do.

By stretching before starting a physical activity, including housework, you reduce the risk of joint strains or sudden muscle tears. Besides increasing your range of movement, the flexibility that comes with regular stretching exercises allows you to apply force comfortably over greater distances. This is particularly useful when playing sports such as golf or tennis.

This daily 10-minute stretching routine will ensure that your muscles become more elastic and supple and your joints more mobile. The increased suppleness will improve your posture and help prevent stiffness and injury.

STRETCHING exercises

Always do a thorough warm-up first (see pages 20–21). Move into each stretch position slowly and gently until you reach a point of mild tension. Breathe out as you start the stretch but breathe normally as you hold it.

Your suppleness changes from one day to the next, depending on factors such as mood, motivation, physical and emotional tension, warm-up routine, temperature and muscle fatigue and soreness. So even

if you have done a particular stretching movement before, never force it if it seems difficult. Stop at once if you feel any pain.

You may want to alternate some of the strength-building exercises shown on pages 32–33 with these stretches in order to give your muscles time to recover and ease tension that might otherwise build up in the muscle. The following stretches should be held for approximately 10–15 seconds.

FRONT OF THIGHS
(for the upper legs)

1 Holding onto a wall or chair, lift your right knee up in front of you. 'Soften' the knee that is supporting your weight.

2 Take hold of your right ankle with your right hand and allow your knee to lower until the thigh is vertical and your knees are side by side, and hold the stretch. This may not be possible to begin with but will come as you regularly practise. Repeat on the left.

Pull in your abdominal muscles and tilt your pelvis forwards as you ease your foot up

BACK STRETCH
(for the lower spine)

1 Get on your hands and knees on the floor, hands under shoulders, fingers pointing forwards and knees hip-width apart.

Align your head with your spine and look at the floor

Tilt your pelvis forwards as you curve your back

2 Pull your abdomen up towards your spine and curve your back. Hold for up to 10 seconds and then relax your back.

Keep your hands under your shoulders

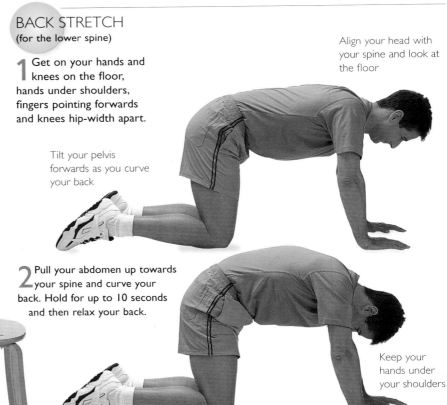

BACK OF THIGHS
(for the upper legs)

1 Sitting on the edge of a chair, place one foot flat on the floor. Extend the other leg in front of you, with your heel on the floor.

2 Placing your hands on your thigh, lean forwards from the hips and feel the stretch in the back of the thigh on the straight leg. Repeat on the other side.

Keep your spine straight and your shoulders square

NECK STRETCH
(for the neck and shoulders)

Sit comfortably on an upright chair. Reach your left hand behind you and grasp the back of the chair seat, behind your left buttock. Slowly tilt your head towards the right shoulder and feel the stretch down the left side of your neck. Repeat on the other side.

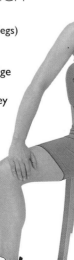

Adopt a balanced and solid sitting position

FRONT OF CHEST
(for the chest and shoulders)

Sitting upright on a chair, place your hands on your lower back. Squeeze your elbows towards each other behind you while lifting your chest up and forwards. Feel the stretch in the chest and front of the shoulders.

ARM STRETCH
(for the upper arms and shoulders)

Sitting upright on a chair, imagine you have an itch between your shoulder blades and attempt to reach it with your right hand by lifting your arm above your head and bending the elbow. Use your left hand apply gentle pressure to the upper part of your right arm. Repeat on the other side.

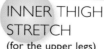

CALF STRETCH
(for the lower legs)

Stand with your feet under your hips. Take a step back with the left leg, placing the foot flat on the floor. Bend your right knee over the toe. Place your hands on the right thigh for support. Make sure your left foot faces forwards and the leg remains straight. Repeat on the other side.

The stretch should be felt in the right calf

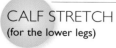

INNER THIGH STRETCH
(for the upper legs)

Sitting upright towards the edge of a chair, position your thighs as far apart as they will comfortably go. Hold on to the inside of the thighs and ease the knees apart from each other further. Feel the stretch in the groin and inside thighs.

Keep your feet flat on the floor

7 ways to **stay fit**

Fitness can be fun if you include plenty of interest and variety in your exercise plan. There are lots of activities to choose from, so be selective. You are more likely to stick with a workout that you enjoy.

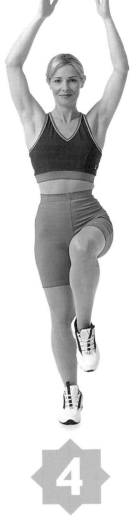

VISIT A FITNESS INSTRUCTOR

1

If you have clear fitness goals, or you need some help staying motivated, a fitness instructor or trainer may be the answer. Qualified instructors can assess your current level of fitness and tailor a suitable programme to your needs and aspirations. They can motivate you to stay on target, or adjust the fitness programme if it is less effective than you had hoped.

JOIN A GYM OR FITNESS CENTRE

2

If you like a lot of variety in your fitness programme, a gym or fitness centre might be the ideal venue for you. There will be a choice of exercise machines, weights and other fitness aids for you to try out, with instructors on hand to explain how to use them. You will also be able to choose from a wide range of exercise classes, including aerobic, dance and step classes, body toning and power workouts. Larger gyms and fitness centres may provide other facilities, such as sauna, jacuzzi, steam room and massage, to leave you feeling relaxed and revitalised.

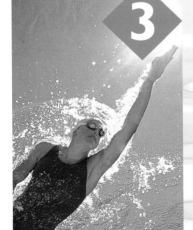

3

EXERCISE IN WATER

Water is a perfect medium for all-round fitness – it offers a resistance, so that water-based exercise builds muscle strength and endurance while aiding stamina and suppleness. Water's buoyancy also reduces impact on the joints. For this reason, exercises performed in water are particularly suitable for overweight people and those with joint or back problems. Water aerobics is a form of exercise that includes the stamina-building properties of conventional aerobic dance classes along with the support and buoyancy of the water. For those who prefer a competitive element to their exercise, there are pool-based sports such as water polo.

4

Pop in an exercise video

There are many different styles of exercise video available, some better than others. Make sure the one you choose is up-to-date, as older videos (especially pre-1990 ones) include exercises now thought dangerous. Select one that matches your current fitness level and one that complements your fitness goals.

START A WALKING CLUB

5

Try involving family, friends and neighbours in a walking club. Encourage members to take turns organising walks along different local routes of interest. Each person could do some research into, say, the local wildlife or historic landmarks and turn the walk into a guided tour. As well as being good exercise, this will make it a social occasion and inspire interesting conversation, too. If you wish, include hilly or rough terrain in the route to make the walk more demanding.

ACTIVITIES COMPARED

All physical activities – from household chores to sports – can improve your stamina, suppleness or strength. Use the chart to guide you to the ideal sport or combination of activities to help you meet your fitness goals.

KEY: 3=EXCELLENT, 2=GOOD, 1=AVERAGE

ACTIVITY	STAMINA	SUPPLENESS	STRENGTH
AT HOME:			
HOUSEWORK	2	2	2
CLIMBING STAIRS	2	1	2
GARDENING	2	1	3
SKIPPING	3	2	1
STEP AEROBICS	3	2	2
OUTDOORS:			
CYCLING	3	1	2
WALKING	2	1	1
JOGGING	3	1	1
AT THE FITNESS CENTRE:			
AEROBICS	3	3	2
CIRCUIT TRAINING	3	3	3
WEIGHT TRAINING	1	2	3
SWIMMING	3	3	3
ROWING MACHINE	3	1	2
EASTERN PURSUITS:			
JUDO	2	2	2
T'AI CHI	2	3	1
YOGA	1	3	1
SPORTS:			
TENNIS	3	3	3
GOLF	1	2	1
FOOTBALL	2	2	2
SQUASH	3	3	2

6

Take up an outdoor sport

Look to the great outdoors for fun ways to get fit. Choose from cross-country skiing, sailing, rock climbing, windsurfing, horse riding, rowing and canoeing among others – whatever your area offers. You can learn the basics of an outdoor sport at any age, but if you took part in a particular activity in your youth, you'll be surprised how quickly you can pick it up again. Depending on your skill level, seek basic instruction or a refresher course. Outdoor sports can also motivate you to stay in shape. For example, canoeing makes demands on the upper body, so an exercise routine could focus on this area.

DANCE THE NIGHT AWAY

Shimmy your way onto the dance floor and build all-round fitness in a social setting by taking up dancing. Dance forms range from ballroom dancing – both Latin American and modern – to jazz and tap, some easier to learn than others. Line dancing and disco dancing are ideal if you don't have a dance partner, because you do the steps in a group rather than as a couple.

7

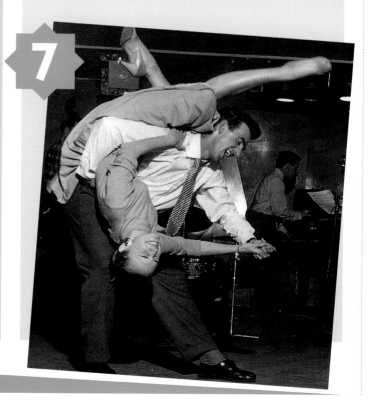

PLANNING YOUR
own home gym

When planning your gym, take into account the space you have available, the amount of money you want to spend and your exercise objectives. If possible, set aside an area as your own personal fitness zone where the equipment is always ready for use. A spare bedroom, study or garage is ideal.

Remove tools and appliances that might cause injury if you fall against them. Ensure the floor is strong enough to take the weight of the equipment and springy enough for you to perform energetic exercises – such as skipping and jogging on the spot – without jarring your knees.

Your personal fitness zone should also be a pleasant environment, to strengthen your resolve to continue with a regular exercise regimen. Make sure the room is heated in winter, draught-free but well ventilated and well lit. It does not have to be very warm, but it should not be cold or you will increase the risk of injuring joints and muscles. A radio, CD-player or TV could keep you entertained and provide the right tempo as you exercise.

Make sure that you have enough time after your programme to recuperate properly before resuming your everyday activities – it is often the best part of a good workout.

EXERCISE CIRCUIT

If you have plenty of space, you might lay out your exercise equipment for circuit training. This involves arranging a series of stations, each for a different exercise, sometimes involving equipment such as a multi-gym, rowing machine, weights or skipping rope. Place a mat in the centre of the circuit so you can include floor-based exercises or stamina-building activities like jogging in place. The idea is to move around the circuit, working at each station in turn. Choose your own pace, but keep it fast to benefit from aerobic exercise. Circuit training promotes all aspects of fitness – stamina, strength and suppleness – and ensures that all parts of the body get a really thorough workout. By altering the number or sequence of the exercises, you can concentrate more on your stamina or strength in preparation for a particular activity.

Exercise equipment

Arrange the equipment so there is plenty of space for general exercises. Use a sturdy chair, table or cupboard for support as needed.

An exercise mat is useful, especially if the fitness area has a hard stone or cement floor. It will make floor exercises more comfortable and ensure that high-impact activities put less strain on the joints. A mini-trampoline, which builds stamina and provides low-impact muscle-boosting exercise, is helpful if space is limited, as it can be folded flat for storage.

Improvise wherever possible. You can buy a brand-name exercise step,

or use a low bench or the bottom stair, for example. A set of dumbbells of different weights is good for muscular endurance and strength, but you can use cans of soup or vegetables, or water-filled plastic bottles. Avoid exercising with barbells at home unless trained in their use by a qualified fitness instructor.

A canvas bag weighted with a bag of flour is ideal for leg-toning exercises. Sit on a sturdy table or worktop with the handles of the bag over your ankle and slowly lift your leg up and down to work the leg muscles.

ROWING MACHINES

Affordable, collapsible and great for whole-body fitness, you can set up a rowing machine in your living room and row to your favourite music.

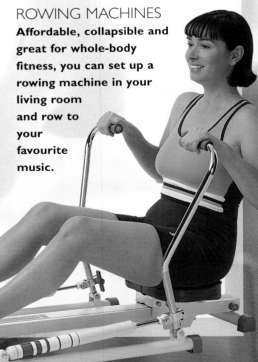

Chapter 2

Healthy diet

Eating for good health

Keeping your body topped up with the right kind of fuels and nutrients boosts your energy levels, maintains body functions and all-round health, and keeps you looking and feeling great.

One of the keys to enjoying a fit and active life is a balanced diet. A good diet keeps you feeling physically energetic and mentally alert, and enhances your general wellbeing. A poor diet, on the other hand, is associated with an increased risk of illness, including heart disease, stroke, diabetes, digestive disorders and certain types of cancer. Two-thirds of natural deaths in the West are believed to be linked to diet, according to leading experts on nutrition and health.

Some people feel dissuaded from following a healthy diet because they associate it with bland, tasteless or dull foods. On the contrary, a good diet encompasses a huge range of delicious foods – a change in diet may even introduce you to a world of exciting new flavours you never knew existed. It can even include your favourite high-fat or high-sugar foods – provided they represent only a small proportion of the diet.

Harvard University studies have found that repeatedly gaining and losing even a moderate amount of weight can raise the risk of heart attack by up to 75 per cent.

All forms of food are made up of a number of nutrients – fat, carbohydrate, protein, water, fibre, vitamins and minerals – each of which plays an important role in a healthy diet. Together they are essential for keeping you fit and well. Your primary aim is to maintain a diet that contains all these essential nutrients in the right proportions. This will not only ensure you have sufficient energy to fuel your daily activities but will help protect you against disease and ill health.

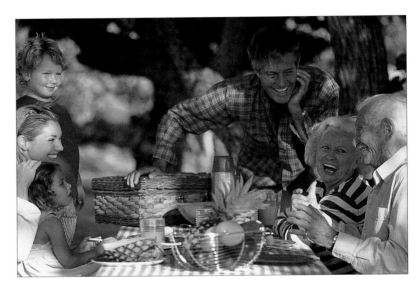

A varied diet that contains all the vital nutrients will help to keep you fit and well throughout life.

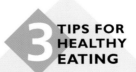

3 TIPS FOR HEALTHY EATING

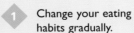

1. Change your eating habits gradually.

2. Limit processed foods because most contribute large amounts of sodium and other additives.

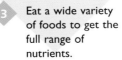

3. Eat a wide variety of foods to get the full range of nutrients.

The good news is that you only need to follow a few simple rules for this to happen. To help you, medical authorities have drawn up guidelines for healthy eating based on a large body of research into the incidence of diet-linked diseases throughout the world. The clear message is that the best way of getting all the nutrients you need is to eat a wide variety of foods in moderation.

DAMAGE LIMITATION

The typical Western diet is high in fat, refined sugar and salt – particularly from meat, dairy products, fried and convenience foods, biscuits and cakes – and low in dietary fibre, which is found in foods such as fruit and vegetables. Fatty foods are usually eaten at the expense of nutrient-rich foods and eating a lot of them can result in obesity and cardiovascular problems, such as coronary heart disease and stroke. Enjoy fatty foods as a rare treat, not as part of your regular diet.

Current health guidelines recommend that added sugar (as opposed to sugar naturally present in fruit and vegetables) should not exceed 10 per cent of your total kilojoule (calorie) intake. It is important, however, not to go to the other extreme and eat only fruit and vegetables – a diet that does not include all the food groups will be deficient in a number of essential nutrients.

The body's most efficient energy source is glucose, best obtained from nutrient-rich carbohydrates, such as bread, pasta, rice and potatoes, and fruit and vegetables. Refined, or added, sugar is a less desirable source of glucose because it represents empty kilojoules, meaning that it provides no nutritional benefits other than an immediate but short-lived energy boost (see page 54).

In many populations around the world, including Japan, Africa and Polynesia, the increase in sugar consumption throughout the 20th century has coincided with a greater incidence of cancer.

FATS AND OILS

Fats and oils (the liquid forms of fat) play an important part in the diet. Besides adding flavour, aroma and texture to food, they assist in the growth, repair and maintenance of cells and nerves, and provide nutrients. Research suggests, however, that the typical Western diet contains too much fat – about 38–40 per cent of a person's total daily kilojoule intake. Leading experts in cardiovascular disease strongly recommend limiting fat consumption to a healthier 30–35 per cent.

As important as not overindulging is being selective about the kinds of fats and oils you consume. There are three main types of fat: saturated, polyunsaturated and monounsaturated. The term 'saturated' means that a fat's molecules have a full complement of hydrogen atoms. If there is one site on the molecule where a hydrogen atom is missing, the fat is known as monounsaturated. If there are more than one of these sites, the fat is referred to as polyunsaturated.

Saturated fats tend to raise the level of cholesterol in the blood – linked to heart disease and stroke – and so should represent only a small proportion of the total fat you eat. You should also avoid trans-fatty acids, found in

Planning a healthy diet

Here's an easy way to obtain the right quantities of the right foods for a healthy diet. Think of what you eat and drink in terms of servings, and follow the guidelines below to plan your daily diet. A typical serving would be a piece of fruit, half a cup of vegetables, pasta or rice, a slice of bread, 55–85 grams (2–3 oz) of lean meat or 55 grams (2 oz) of cheese.

Grain products 5–12 servings Choose whole-grain and enriched products. They are filling and contain vitamins and minerals.

Fruit and vegetables 5–10 servings These are rich in vitamins and minerals and also contain a high percentage of fibre and water to fill you up and prevent constipation. Eat – or drink in juice form – as much fruit and vegetables each day as you like, but no fewer than 5 servings.

Meat and alternatives 2–3 servings Choose lean meats, poultry and fish as well as dried peas, beans and lentils. These are protein-rich foods, which are vital for muscle and nerve function.

Dairy products 2–3 servings Choose low-fat milk products. They contain calcium, which is needed for healthy bones, nerves and teeth.

Other foods to be eaten sparingly These include foods that are mostly oils, such as butter, margarine, cooking oils and lard; foods that are mostly sugar, such as jam, honey, syrup and sweets; and high-fat and/or high-salt snacks such as crisps.

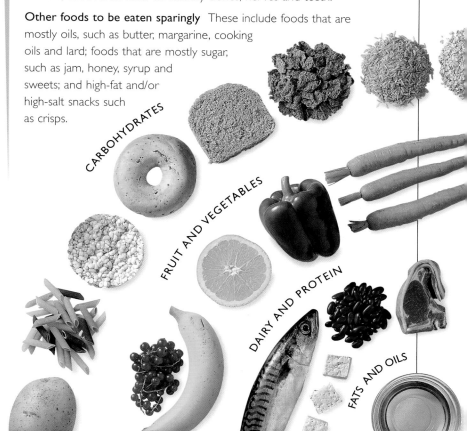

CARBOHYDRATES

FRUIT AND VEGETABLES

DAIRY AND PROTEIN

FATS AND OILS

those margarines and processed foods made from vegetable oils in a process called hydrogenation. These products are as harmful as saturated fats.

Monounsaturated and polyunsaturated fats tend to lower harmful cholesterol levels and so should make up most of the fat you eat. Oily types of salt-water fish (such as herring, tuna, mackerel, salmon and sardines) contain omega-3 fatty acids, a type of polyunsaturated fat that keeps all bodily functions healthy, boosts the immune system, and helps to prevent or alleviate high blood pressure, clogged arteries, heart disease, stroke, arthritis and some cancers.

A study conducted over 11 years by researchers at Harvard Medical School in the U.S. showed that people who eat fish – including shellfish – less than once a month are 52 per cent more likely to die of a heart attack than those who eat seafood at least once a week.

Dietary cholesterol can be found in various foods including eggs and shellfish. Current medical advice is that this form of cholesterol does not pose a significant health risk if eaten in moderation. The level of harmful cholesterol in the blood can be most effectively reduced by cutting down on saturated fats and trans-fats. To help you maintain the right balance, choose poultry and fish over red meat, eat low-fat dairy products, trim off fat from meat, and use vegetable oils in cooking.

SALT

Made up from sodium and chlorine, salt (sodium chloride) is vital for health in small amounts but is often over-consumed in the West. For health, you need to consume only around 500 mg per day in total but the average Western diet contains around 8–12 times as much! Much of this salt is added during food processing or manufacturing, for example in canned, frozen and convenience foods, and fast food. The rest is added during cooking or at the table when flavouring food.

UNSATURATED:

walnuts
almonds
safflower oil
corn oil
sunflower oil
olive oil
soya bean oil
peanut oil
avocados
herring
swordfish
mackerel
tuna

OILS AND FATS

SATURATED:

poultry
beef
pork
egg yolk
palm oil
lamb
cream
butter
cheese
ice-cream
whole-fat milk
cocoa butter
coconut oil

As a basic guide, you can identify saturated fats, which are mostly found in meats and dairy foods, by the fact that they solidify at room temperature. Whereas unsaturated fats from vegetable and fish sources stay liquid at room temperature. For optimum health, increase the proportion of unsaturated fats in your diet and reduce the level of saturates.

A high-salt diet is linked to high blood pressure in people who are predisposed to the disease, increasing the risk of heart disease and stroke. In the West, the drop in rates of stomach cancer over the last 50 years has matched the decline in the eating of smoked, pickled and salted foods. In Japan, where these foods are still widely eaten, stomach cancer rates remain high.

CARBOHYDRATE

The body's most common source of energy is carbohydrates. The two main types of carbohydrates found in food are simple and complex. The simple carbohydrates, also known as sugars, are natural and are found in milk, fruit and vegetables, honey and table sugar. The complex, or starchy, carbohydrates are found in bread, pasta, peas, beans, nuts and root vegetables (carrots, parsnips and turnips), potatoes and rice.

People often eat simple carbohydrates, and refined sugars in particular, for a quick energy boost, but this can backfire (see page 54). Complex carbohydrates provide plenty of easily accessible energy, but without the energy drop common after eating sugars.

PROTEIN

Protein is one of the most important materials in the body, and is vital for growth and health. About 20 per cent of our bodies is made up of proteins, which are found in the muscles and bones, hair and nails, brain, hormones and enzymes. Proteins are made up from a basic set of 20 molecules called amino acids. Twelve of these can be made by the body, while the remaining eight must be obtained directly from food and so are known as essential amino acids. We need a constant supply of protein to replace lost tissue, such as skin and hair, and to renew damaged and worn-out cells. More is needed during illness.

The World Health Organization recommends a daily intake of 45 grams of protein for women and 55 grams for men. These amounts are easily achievable – particularly if you eat a balanced and varied diet – as protein is found in all forms of meat and fish,

The unhealthy Western diet

A comparison of the typical Western diet with Mediterranean, East Asian and African cuisine illustrates the link between food and disease. In the latter regions, rates of heart disease and breast, prostate and colon cancer are low. Mediterranean, East Asian and African people's diets are higher in foods that have strengthening and protective qualities, such as fruit, vegetables, soya, rice, pasta and unsaturated fats, and lower in foods with saturated fats and refined sugar. When people from these cultures move to the West and adopt the Western diet, their rates of heart disease and cancer increase dramatically due to the diet change.

The average Western diet is high in saturated fats and refined sugar. Many common dishes are very low in nutritional value.

The average Japanese diet includes more healthy mono- and polyunsaturated fats, such as soya and vegetable oils. It is also very low in sugar.

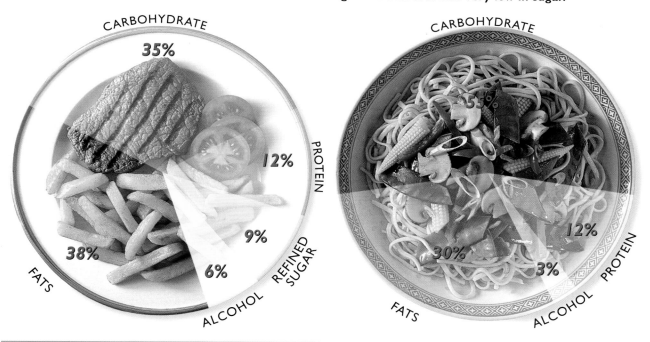

milk, cheese, eggs, soya products, peas, beans, nuts, lentils and whole-grains. In fact, the typical Western diet provides more than enough for good health. However, some protein foods, such as meat, nuts and dairy products, are high in fat, and so if eaten in excess can lead to weight and cardiovascular problems. When there is insufficient carbohydrate or fat to meet the body's energy demands, protein can be used as a last resort. The process of breaking down protein into amino acids and then into glucose and fatty acids stresses the liver and kidneys. Ideally, you should eat no more than two or three servings of protein a day.

WATER

Water is vital for flushing out waste products from the body, keeping the skin, kidneys and bladder healthy and in good working order. Lack of water causes many physical problems and can interfere with mental functioning, leading to fatigue and poor concentration.

Your body works best on about eight glasses of water daily. However, a surprising amount of the fluid you need comes from solid food in your diet. For example, fruit and vegetables, particularly salad, can be as much as 95 per cent water and may contribute up to 18 per cent of an adult's daily water intake. Even seemingly dry foods such as bread and

4 WAYS TO BOOST FIBRE

1. Choose whole-grain bread or pasta.

2. Add beans, lentils, peas or barley to soups and stews.

3. Add raw sliced vegetables to salads.

4. Add fresh or dried fruit to whole-grain breakfast cereals.

cereals contain water, about one-third by weight, while meat, fish, eggs and dried peas and beans may supply around 2 per cent of your daily fluid intake.

For good health, make sure you drink liquids – water, juices and soft drinks – frequently throughout the day. Try to restrict your consumption of caffeine-containing drinks as they have a dehydrating effect. Also, because many drinks contain unwanted sugar or milk fat, it is a good idea to ensure that at least half your fluid intake is in the form of plain water, either straight from the tap or bottled.

IMPORTANCE OF FIBRE

Fibre occurs naturally in all foods of plant origin, such as fruit and vegetables, although it is often removed during the processing of grains. Because it is indigestible, fibre can fulfil several important functions in the diet. For example, it helps to fill you up without providing extra kilojoules (calories).

There are two types of fibre: insoluble and soluble. Insoluble fibre is found in wheat, rice and bran. It absorbs many times its own weight in water and so provides both bulk and lubrication to speed the passage of waste matter through the body. One of the prime causes of constipation is a lack of fibre in the diet. By accelerating waste removal from the body, fibre ensures that carcinogens – cancer-causing substances – do not stay in contact with the lining of the bowel long enough to have a damaging effect.

Colon cancer is one of the major killers in the West – yet there is strong evidence that a high-fibre diet can help to prevent it.

Soluble fibre is found in foods such as oats, peas and citrus fruits, and works in a different way from insoluble fibre. It forms a gel on the inside of the intestinal tract that binds with cholesterol, helping to remove it from the body. This reduces blood cholesterol levels and the risk of heart disease. Most plant foods contain both soluble and insoluble fibre.

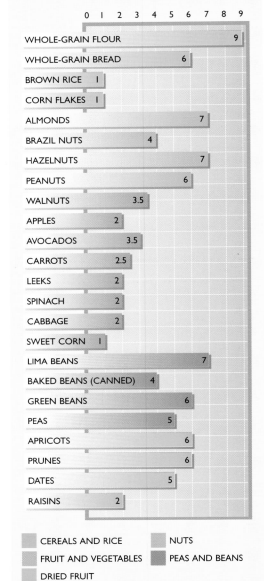

FIBRE CONTENT OF COMMON FOODS

Food	Fibre (g per 100g)
WHOLE-GRAIN FLOUR	9
WHOLE-GRAIN BREAD	6
BROWN RICE	1
CORN FLAKES	1
ALMONDS	7
BRAZIL NUTS	4
HAZELNUTS	7
PEANUTS	6
WALNUTS	3.5
APPLES	2
AVOCADOS	3.5
CARROTS	2.5
LEEKS	2
SPINACH	2
CABBAGE	2
SWEET CORN	1
LIMA BEANS	7
BAKED BEANS (CANNED)	4
GREEN BEANS	6
PEAS	5
APRICOTS	6
PRUNES	6
DATES	5
RAISINS	2

CEREALS AND RICE NUTS
FRUIT AND VEGETABLES PEAS AND BEANS
DRIED FRUIT

The chart above shows how many grams of fibre there are in 100 grams of each food. Increasing your consumption of high-fibre foods helps you prevent constipation and greatly reduces the risk of disease. Rural Africans eat nearly five times as much fibre as most Westerners, which may explain their very much lower rates of colon cancer.

The typical Western diet is low in fibre – less than 12 grams per day, whereas 20–35 grams are recommended for healthy eating – and is associated with colon cancer, high blood cholesterol and obesity. If you are accustomed to a low-fibre diet, be sure to increase your intake gradually to avoid problems such as diarrhoea, bloating, flatulence and abdominal cramps.

VITAMINS

Certain organic chemicals are required in minute amounts by the body. Known as vitamins, they play a part in countless processes in the body. So far, 13 different vitamins have been discovered. The body can make vitamin D through the skin when it is in contact with sunlight, but the others must be obtained from food. In very general terms, vitamins maintain good health in two ways. First, they play an integral part in a range of bodily functions, so that a shortage of vitamins in the diet leads to deficiency diseases. Second, some of these micronutrients actually protect the body against diseases, such as heart disorders and cancer. Most life-threatening vitamin deficiency diseases – such as scurvy, beri-beri and rickets – are rare in Western society. These are caused, respectively, by a lack of vitamins C, B_1 and D. However, many nutritionists believe that the Western diet is too low in vitamins to guarantee optimum health (see end of book).

One group of vitamins that is believed to hold the key to good health is the antioxidants; these include vitamins A, C and E. Antioxidants are chemicals that help protect

Vitamins – miracle micronutrients

VITAMIN	SOURCES	NEEDED FOR
A	Dairy products (choose low-fat versions), deep orange and yellow fruit and vegetables, dark-green vegetables, liver, fish oils	Maintaining proper vision, healthy skin and other tissues – especially the mucus lining of the air passages – and protecting against free radicals.
B1 (thiamin)	Seafood (fish, shellfish), pork	Healthy nerves and muscles, carbohydrate metabolism and maintenance of good memory function.
B2 (riboflavin)	Dairy products (choose low-fat versions), dark-green, leafy vegetables, beef, lamb, pork	Growth, the release of energy from food, and the maintenance of skin and other tissues.
B3 (niacin)	Seafood (fish, shellfish), poultry, nuts, seeds, potatoes	Energy production in the cells; may aid toxin disposal; may help avoid depression.
B5 (pantothenic acid)	Meat, eggs, soya, nuts, peas, beans, whole-grain cereals	Manufacture of some hormones and fatty acids; may alleviate rheumatoid arthritis.
B6 (pyridoxine)	Fish, red meat, poultry, whole-grain cereals, soya products	Growth, healthy blood, protection against disease and coping with stress.
B12 (cyanocobalamin)	Animal products	Healthy blood and nerves.
C (ascorbic acid)	Cantaloupe (rock melon), citrus fruit, cruciferous vegetables (broccoli, Brussels sprouts, cabbage), peppers, potatoes	Healthy tissues, efficient wound healing, protection against free radicals, heart disease, stroke and cancer.
D (calciferols)	Egg yolk, oily fish, fortified milk, sunlight	Strong bones and healthy nerves and muscles.
E (alphatocopherol)	Eggs, nuts, seeds, vegetable oils, dark-green, leafy vegetables	Protection against free radicals, heart disease, stroke, cataracts and cancer.
Folic acid	Dark-green, leafy vegetables, fortified grains	Maintaining a healthy immune system and tissues.
H (biotin)	Liver, eggs, beans, nuts, mushrooms, bananas, peas	The release of energy from food, and the removal of waste by-products.
K (phylloquinone, menadione)	Dark-green, leafy vegetables, cruciferous vegetables, whole-grains, meat, dairy products	Healthy bones and the blood's clotting action.

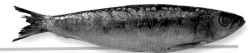

Minerals – the foundation of health

MINERAL	SOURCES	NEEDED FOR
Calcium	Dairy products (choose low-fat versions), green, leafy vegetables, beans, canned sardines with bones	Strong bones and teeth, healthy nerves and muscles.
Copper	Seafood (fish, shellfish), liver, peas, nuts, dried beans	Healthy blood and bones.
Iodine	Seafood (fish, shellfish), seaweed, fortified table salt	Healthy thyroid – the gland that controls metabolism.
Iron	Meat, fish, poultry, dark-green, leafy vegetables, cereals, nuts, beans	Healthy blood and immune system.
Magnesium	Soya, green vegetables, nuts, whole-grain cereals	Healthy tissues and muscle functioning.
Potassium	Whole-grain cereals, bananas, oranges, asparagus, plums, beans, meat and fish	Fluid balance in the body; helps avoid water retention and high blood pressure.
Selenium	Seafood (fish, shellfish), meat, whole-grain cereals, Brazil nuts, dairy foods	Protection against free radicals; may help prevent cancer and preserve male fertility.
Zinc	Seafood (fish, shellfish), meat, eggs, seeds, nuts, whole-grain bread and cereals	Healthy immune system and tissues, wound healing; may promote male fertility.

the body from free radicals – unstable molecules that occur naturally in the body and are also produced by smoking, pollution and sunlight. Free radicals damage the arteries, increasing the risk of atherosclerosis and heart disease; they also disrupt the repair and manufacture of body cells, which can lead to cancer and premature aging.

Vegetables and fruit with the highest vitamin content are those that are freshly picked from your garden or local farm. The longer they spend in transport and storage before you eat them, the more vitamins they lose. Canned and frozen fruit and vegetables retain most of their vitamins, since the produce is harvested at its peak and processed soon after. (While some vitamins are lost during canning and freezing, none are lost in transport and storage.) If fresh produce looks pale and limp it may have been kept too long, in which case choose frozen instead.

BOOST YOUR VITAMIN INTAKE

Many nutrients are also lost from fruit and vegetables in the process of cooking; because of their fragility, they are either destroyed by the heat or they leach out and disperse into the cooking water.

Follow these guidelines to maximise the vitamin content of your food:

▶ **Selection** Choose the most brightly coloured fruit and vegetables, because they have the highest vitamin content. Choose vitamin-enriched breads, breakfast cereals and grains.

▶ **Storage** Keep fruit and vegetables in a cool, dark place (ideally in the crisper or salad bin of the refrigerator) until you eat them. A vegetable such as broccoli loses vitamin C at the rate of 5 per cent per day when kept at room temperature. Light accelerates vitamin depletion, particularly of vitamins A, D and B_2.

▶ **Cleaning** Instead of soaking, which removes vitamins, scrub vegetables under running water or swish in a bowl.

▶ **Preparation** Avoid cutting fruit and vegetables too small – the bigger the pieces, the more nutrients are retained.

▶ ***Cooking time*** Eat vegetables raw or cook them for the shortest time possible in as little water as possible (until just tender-crisp). To retain the nutrients that pass into the cooking water, add it to soups and stews. Always cook potatoes in their skins.

▶ ***Cooking methods*** Fewer vitamins are lost during the cooking process if you steam, microwave or stir-fry vegetables rather than boil them.

MINERALS

Minerals are non-organic substances derived from soils and rocks which are absorbed by plants. We obtain minerals when we eat plants, or consume animals and fish that have eaten plants.

There are two main groups of minerals, macro elements and trace elements. Macro elements, such as calcium, chloride, iron, magnesium, phosphorus, potassium and sodium, are needed in relatively large amounts in the diet. Trace elements, which include chromium, copper, iodine, manganese, molybdenum, selenium and zinc, are needed only in minute quantities. In the right amounts, all minerals are vital to good health, so excesses and deficiencies can contribute to ill health.

Potassium works with sodium to regulate fluid balance in the body. A potassium–sodium ratio of 5:1 is thought best for good health. But while sodium is usually abundant in the average Western diet, many people consume less potassium than they need – a potassium–sodium ratio as low as 1:2 in some cases – which increases the risk of fluid retention and high blood pressure.

Serious mineral deficiencies are rare, but certain elements – calcium, iron, magnesium, selenium and zinc – are often lacking in the Western diet (see end of book).

Calcium is one of the most abundant minerals in the body and makes the bones strong and rigid. Around 99 per cent of calcium in the body is in the skeleton. Osteoporosis, the bone-thinning disorder that is most common in later life, is made worse by a lack of calcium in the diet. (See page 124 for ways to prevent osteoporosis.)

Phytochemicals – the natural health aids

GROUP	PHYTOCHEMICAL	SOURCES	ACTION
Flavonoids	Anthocyanosides	Blackcurrants, dark cherries	Help prevent cancer and are antioxidants.
	Quercetin	Onions, apples, tea, red wine	Helps prevent heart disease and stroke.
	Ellagic acid	Cherries, strawberries, grapes	Helps prevent cell damage/stomach ulcer.
	Capsaicin	Chilli peppers	Helps guard against cancer.
	Coumaric acid	Tomatoes, carrots, green peppers	Helps guard against cancer.
	Resveratrol	Grapes	Reduces harmful cholesterol, protects heart/arteries, boosts immune system.
	Limonene	Citrus fruits	Helps guard against cancer.
Phytoestrogens	Isoflavonoids	Soya products (soya flour, tofu), linseed	Help prevent breast and prostate cancers.
	Lignins	Whole-grain cereals, pulses, fennel	Help prevent breast and prostate cancers.
Carotenes	Alpha, beta, lutein and lycopene	Red, orange and yellow vegetables and fruit, green, leafy vegetables	Help prevent cancer and are antioxidants.
Glucosinolates	Isothiocyanates, indoles	Cabbage, broccoli, Brussels sprouts	Help prevent some cancers.
Allium compounds	Organosulphides	Garlic, onion, leeks, chives	Lower blood pressure and levels of harmful cholesterol, may prevent cancer.

Calcium is contained in many vegetables but is more easily absorbed from dairy products, such as milk, cheese and yoghurt, and fish than from plant sources.

Iron is one of the most widespread minerals in nature, yet many people do not eat enough of it. Iron's most important role is in the blood, where it forms an essential part of the proteins haemoglobin and myoglobin, which transport oxygen from the lungs to the tissues. A shortage of iron results in a type of anaemia, which can cause fatigue, headaches and brittle nails.

Some foods are high in iron but contain chemicals that restrict the body's ability to absorb it. These include whole-grains, which contain phytates, and spinach, which contains oxalates. Iron absorption is also hindered by tannin, found in tea, coffee, and some carbonated drinks and herbal teas.

As well as being an antioxidant, zinc forms part of more than 70 enzymes that regulate cell metabolism in the body, so it is no wonder that a shortage of this mineral can have far-reaching effects. These include loss of appetite, growth retardation, skin changes and abnormalities of the immune system.

Selenium is an antioxidant mineral found in many foods, but in widely varying amounts (the selenium content of plant foods depends largely on the soil type). Many people in the West are believed to eat around half the recommended daily intake (see end of book).

Arizona Cancer Center researchers showed that selenium supplements cut cancer deaths by over 50 per cent, especially those from lung, colon and prostate cancers.

Selenium is an antioxidant that helps to prevent the fats in the cells from turning 'rancid', and so protects cells from premature damage and aging, and cancer.

NATURE'S MEDICINES

One of the most important discoveries made by food scientists this century has been a group of phytochemicals (plant chemicals) with medicinal properties (see chart on page 49). They include flavonoids, bioflavonoids or polyphenols – about 4000 of them have been discovered so far, and there are believed to be many more.

They have various properties – antioxidant, anti-inflammatory, anticancer, antiviral and antibacterial. The flavonoid quercetin, for example, found in onions, apples, tea and red wine, is thought to help prevent heart disease and stroke.

FRIENDLY BACTERIA

Not all bacteria are harmful. Humans and some bacteria have evolved a symbiotic relationship – living together in a way that benefits both of them. Hundreds of different types of bacteria live within the body in equilibrium, some producing important vitamins, others counteracting harmful bacteria. Fungal infections and some bowel disorders can develop if this equilibrium is disturbed – for example, following a course of antibiotics that destroy both good and bad bacteria. Foods that are high in 'friendly bacteria', such as yoghurt with live cultures, can help to restore bacterial balance in the body and improve digestion and bowel function.

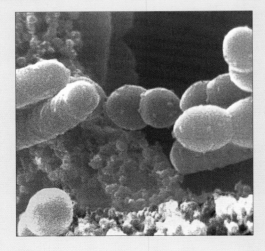

Put your eating habits to the test

Do you pay enough attention to your diet? Answer the following questions to find out whether you are giving your body what it needs or perhaps putting your health at risk. Answer the questions honestly, and then count up how many As, Bs or Cs you have at the end. Read the corresponding advice below to see how your eating habits rate and what you can do to improve them.

How many servings of fruit and vegetables do you usually eat each day?

A Fewer than two
B Two, three or four
C Five or more

How often do you eat fried foods instead of grilled, boiled or oven-cooked?

A Usually or always
B Often or sometimes
C Rarely or never

On average, how many alcoholic drinks do you have every day?

A Four or more
B Two or three
C One or fewer

On average, how many cups of coffee or tea do you drink every day?

A Eight or more
B Between four and seven
C Less than four

How often do you eat whole-wheat bread or pasta instead of the refined white variety?

A Rarely or never
B Often or sometimes
C Usually or always

How often do you eat oily fish, such as tuna, salmon, sardines, herring, mackerel or trout?

A Rarely
B Once every month or two
C At least once a week

How many sugary foods and drinks do you have every day, including sugar in coffee or tea?

A Over eight
B Between three and seven
C Fewer than two

Do you eat more than four eggs per week?

A Usually or always
B Often or sometimes
C Rarely or never

How many times a day do you eat dairy or animal fats, such as in butter, milk, cheese or red meat?

A More than eight
B Three to seven
C Two or less

How often do you eat processed fast foods instead of cooking with more wholesome ingredients?

A Usually or always
B Often or sometimes
C Rarely or never

How many times a day do you eat high-fibre foods, such as whole-grain bread or pasta, fruit or vegetables?

A Two or less
B Three, four or five
C Six or more

How often do you choose low-fat over full-fat alternatives, such as skimmed milk for full-fat milk?

A Rarely or never
B Often or sometimes
C Wherever possible

MOSTLY As

You need to pay more attention to your diet – consuming too much saturated fat, sugar and processed foods with few or no nutrients increases your risk of illness and can lead to weight problems and a loss of health and energy. If you want to live a longer and healthier life, read this chapter and change your eating habits.

MOSTLY Bs

Although you are watching your diet and are probably aware of the health risks involved in eating certain types of food, you need to make a greater effort to eat well most of the time. Look at the questions to which you answered A or B and make a note of the things you need to change.

MOSTLY Cs

Well done! You clearly think about what you eat and are aware of how it affects your body functioning and health. If you answered A or B to any of the questions, however, you should take steps to improve these aspects of your diet.

10 miracle foods **that fight disease**

You can eat your way to better health with a range of foods that provide natural defences against disease. Make a point to serve meals that include the following ingredients.

BANANAS

Ready-packed in their own skins, bananas can be eaten anywhere. They're high in potassium, which counteracts the effects of sodium (salt), thus reducing the risk of high blood pressure. Potassium is particularly important for older people. Bananas also contain starch for energy and vitamins B₃, B₆ and C. For a delicious drink, mix 250 ml (9 fl oz) low-fat milk, 120 ml (4 fl oz) low-fat yoghurt, 1 tbsp honey, ¼ tsp cinnamon and one banana in a blender until smooth.

1

CABBAGE FAMILY

Broccoli, cauliflower, Chinese greens, cabbage and Brussels sprouts are all low in kilojoules (calories) and high in insoluble fibre, helping to prevent colon cancer. They are full of vitamins K and C (a cup of broccoli has twice the minimum recommended daily level of vitamin C), selenium and chromium, and most contain antioxidants such as beta-carotene. They also contain calcium, for strong bones, and potassium, to regulate blood pressure. Their extra-special ingredient is a group of chemicals called isothiocyanates, which counteract cancer-causing agents. The leafy, green members of the family are also rich sources of iron; to aid iron's absorption, partner with foods rich in vitamin C, such as red peppers.

2

Citrus fruits

Oranges, lemons, limes, mandarins, grapefruit and tangerines are high in antioxidant vitamins and flavonoids, such as hesperidin, which strengthen the antioxidant effect, and limonene, which boosts the immune system. Citrus fruits are also a good source of potassium, which helps regulate blood pressure, and pectin, a soluble fibre that helps reduce LDL cholesterol.

3

ONION FAMILY

Garlic, onions, shallots, leeks, spring onions and chives are all members of the onion family and contain allium compounds and flavonoids to help fight cancer. These vegetables also are effective at lowering harmful forms of cholesterol and boosting beneficial ones, reducing the clotting action of the blood and lowering blood pressure. Together these effects reduce the risk of heart disease and stroke. Eating onions regularly may prevent gastric disorders and combat bronchial infections. Garlic is believed to be good for preventing the blood clots that cause heart attacks. Its active ingredients are easily destroyed by cooking, though, so add towards the end of cooking time, or add raw garlic to salads and dips.

4

Chilli peppers

Chilli peppers contain capsaicin, a phytochemical that stimulates the blood circulation and reduces the risk of blood clots. They contain antioxidants, too, which help prevent cell damage. Like all spicy foods, they increase the metabolic rate by up to 25 per cent for several hours, and so can aid weight loss.

5

OILY FISH

Herring, kippers, mackerel, salmon, sardines and tuna — the so-called 'oily fish' — contain large amounts of omega-3 fatty acids, which reduce the risk of high blood pressure and the levels of cholesterol and fats in the blood, thereby decreasing the risk of heart attack and stroke.

6

7

LIVE YOGHURT

Yoghurt is high in calcium to strengthen bones and reduce the risk of osteoporosis. Live yoghurt contains 'friendly bacteria', such as *Lactobacillus acidophilus*, which have a wide range of beneficial effects. They help restore the bacterial balance of the gut. Many women who suffer from recurrent candidiasis (thrush), a yeast infection affecting the vagina, find that yoghurt with live cultures can be beneficial when eaten or applied directly into the vagina. It is thought that both the bacteria and the alkalinity of the yoghurt help keep the yeast organisms in check.

Berries, cherries and grapes

Berries are good sources of antioxidants. Cherries, strawberries and grapes contain ellagic acid, which helps combat cancer. Dark berries, such as blackcurrants, are high in anthocyanosides, which help to fight urinary infections and food poisoning. Cranberries and blueberries are effective at preventing and relieving cystitis. All these fruits are high in potassium, which helps regulate blood pressure, and the soluble fibre pectin, to lower blood cholesterol levels.

8

OLIVE OIL

As a monounsaturated form of fat, olive oil helps to reduce levels of harmful LDL cholesterol in the blood and lowers blood pressure. Serve uncooked, such as in a salad dressing, or use in place of saturated fats, for example to fry foods, but take care not to increase your overall intake of fats and oils. Olive oil is high in the antioxidant vitamin E – which helps fight cancer and reduces the risk of heart disease – but low in acid (less than 1 per cent) for a better flavour. Choose extra virgin olive oil, which is made from the first pressing of olives, often from a single estate.

9

TOMATOES

Rich in potassium, tomatoes help normalise blood pressure and contain the antioxidant vitamins C and E, and beta-carotene, which all protect against heart disease and cancer. Tomatoes also contain lycopene (a type of carotene), which helps to flush out cancer-causing agents. Surprisingly, cooking tomatoes seems to increase their beneficial effects. Studies have shown that eating at least 10 portions of cooked tomato products (including purée, ketchup, tomato soup and tomato-based sauces) each week reduces the risk of prostate cancer. Fat helps the body absorb lycopenes, so serving it with a food such as cheese – in, say, a pizza topping – increases its effectiveness. But take care to keep your diet low in fat.

10

Boosting energy levels

The right balance of foodstuffs and nutrients will keep you powered up all day, while the wrong choice of foods can actually drain you of get-up-and-go, leaving you feeling listless and lethargic.

The energy you need to keep going can only come from the food and drink you consume. While most people in Western countries consume more than enough kilojoules (calories) in a typical day to run a marathon, plant the garden and put up shelves in every room of the house, many complain of feeling drained of energy. This may be compounded if they are trying to lose weight at the same time and not taking in the amount of fuel their bodies are used to.

Some people, on the other hand, want to put on weight and so need to increase their kilojoule (calorie) intake, but without developing complications such as heart disease.

The connection between food intake and energy output is not always an obvious one, but there are some measures that everyone can take to feel generally fitter and livelier. Incorporating more physical activity into your daily life, as described in Chapter 1, can go a long way towards helping you feel more energetic. But you must also ensure that your diet contains the right kinds of energy-boosting foods, at the right times, to provide the high-octane fuel your body needs.

GLUCOSE POWER

The body's primary energy source is glucose. All forms of carbohydrate, both simple and complex, are broken down into glucose through the digestion processes. Some of this glucose is released into the bloodstream for immediate needs – the brain, in particular, needs a constant supply. Some of the glucose is transported into the tissues to fuel the basic cellular processes, and some is converted into a storage form called

THE BLOOD-SUGAR ROLLER COASTER

Feeling tired? It's tempting to pick up a chocolate bar, a fizzy drink or a cup of sugared coffee for a quick energy boost, but this is often the worst thing you could do. The body quickly converts these simple sugars into glucose and then releases extra insulin – the hormone that allows glucose to be carried into the cells. But the sugar is quickly used up, leaving you feeling drained of energy, while the extra insulin in the blood continues to deplete available glucose stores. This results in a craving for more sugar – leading to a blood-sugar roller coaster effect. To prevent this, choose starchy carbohydrate snacks instead, such as whole-grain bread or bananas, which release their energy more slowly but at a steadier rate. If you must eat high-sugar foods, it is best to do so just after a full meal so that your blood-sugar levels remain relatively constant.

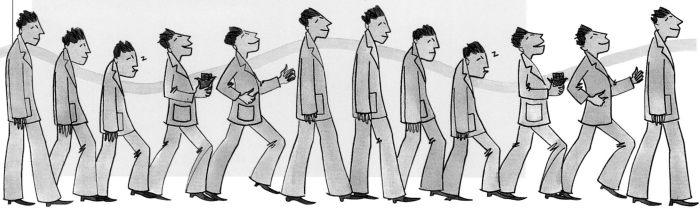

glycogen. This is stored in the liver and the muscles, where it can be called upon to provide energy when necessary.

Although glucose is the body's main fuel, it is not necessarily a good idea to eat or drink pure glucose for energy. As a simple sugar, it causes a rapid rise in blood-sugar levels but is quickly used up again, thus contributing to the blood-sugar roller coaster.

ENERGY FOODS

Complex carbohydrates hold the key to increasing your energy levels because they provide energy that the body can use easily and quickly without undesirable after-effects. The energy boost you get from simple carbohydrates like refined sugar acts like an electrical power surge; it can provide too much energy too quickly, making you feel hyperactive and jittery. It also dissipates just as quickly, leaving you feeling more tired and drained than you did before.

Although the complex forms take longer to convert into energy that the body can use, they also last longer, providing a sustainable source of energy that can keep you active for extended periods of time. Because the sugars in complex carbohydrates are absorbed slowly into the bloodstream, they can help to stabilise blood-sugar levels. This in turn will help you to avoid the sudden energy dips that can strike at certain times of the day.

To ensure that your body has a constant source of readily available energy to fuel all its needs, you should aim to have high-carbohydrate meals throughout the day. This doesn't mean eating a lot of carbohydrates at any one sitting, simply that you should eat smaller meals throughout the day and that carbohydrates should form the major part of every meal. As the basis for a high-energy regimen, eat breakfast, lunch, dinner and a pre-bedtime snack.

POWER SNACKING

In the past, snacking between meals was discouraged because it was thought important not to spoil your appetite for the main meals. Nutritionists and doctors now take a

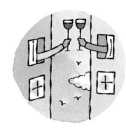

DRINK TO YOUR HEALTH
Researchers have finally concluded that alcohol (in moderation) relieves stress, relaxes you and benefits your all-round health. A glass of red wine, in particular, with a meal aids the digestion of fats, lowers blood pressure and reduces the risk of heart disease. So eat, drink (in moderation) and be merry.

different view, however. Current wisdom is that careful snacking can be beneficial. It ensures that energy is supplied at a constant rate and your blood-sugar levels remain stable, which also helps to prevent overeating at mealtimes, so aiding weight control. Avoid snacks that are high in fat, refined sugar or salt, such as doughnuts, pastries, sweets and crisps. Instead, make each snack a mini-meal based on bread, cereals, fruit and vegetables, and low-fat dairy products. As well as providing a steady supply of energy, healthy snacks increase your intake of fibre, vitamins, minerals and other nutrients.

VITAMIN AND MINERAL DEFICIENCIES

Daily recommended intakes are detailed at the end of the book. Deficiencies may cause low energy levels, as follows:

Thiamin (vitamin B_1), found in wholegrains, pork, beef, peas, beans, lentils, soya products and brown rice, plays a crucial role in carbohydrate metabolism. Even a mild deficiency can result in fatigue, weight loss, depression and sleep disorders.

Riboflavin (vitamin B_2) is needed to release energy from foods. It is found in animal products, fish and dairy foods as well as in enriched and fortified grains. It works in conjunction with niacin and vitamin B_6.

Niacin (vitamin B_3), which is found in meat – particularly beef – fish, whole-grains and milk, plays an important part in the formation of certain enzymes involved in glucose and carbohydrate metabolism, and so is crucial for energy production. Niacin deficiency reached epidemic proportions in the southern US in the late 19th century because corn, the staple food in the region, contains a type of niacin that the body cannot absorb unless the corn is roasted, which is how the Native Americans cooked it; but this was not known at the time. Today, niacin is provided by many foods.

Pantothenic acid (vitamin B_5), found in eggs, meat, fish and whole-grains, plays a major role in the functioning of the adrenal hormones, which regulate metabolism.

continued on page 58

10 ways to **boost energy**

Tap into your extra energy reserves with the following pick-me-ups. You will probably find that some work better than others, or you may want to experiment with techniques of your own.

1

BREATHE DEEPLY

Oxygen is a great source of energy but one we do not exploit to its fullest. The Eastern art of yoga uses a unique system of breathing through alternate nostrils that is designed to energise and strengthen the body and aid the removal of waste products. Start the day with this exercise to give the brain and muscles an immediate boost. You can perform these exercises at other times, too, when you feel tired, lethargic or generally below par. Make sure you are sitting comfortably with your back straight and head level. It may help to sit cross-legged, but this is not essential. Keep your mouth closed and breathe through your nose – drawing the air from deep down in your abdomen. To check that you are breathing correctly, practise while resting one hand on your abdomen; feel it expand first as you breathe in. Rest your other hand on your lower ribcage and feel it expand after your abdomen does.

1 Close your right nostril and breathe in slowly through the left until your chest is expanded to its full capacity.

2 Close both nostrils and hold your breath while you count slowly to 16.

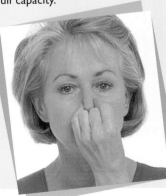

3 Release the right nostril, keeping the left closed, and breathe out slowly until your lungs are empty. Breathe in slowly through the right nostril. Now repeat step 2 and then breathe out slowly through your left nostril. Repeat up to 10 times.

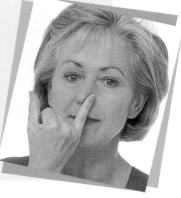

TRY ACUPRESSURE

2

An Eastern therapy, acupressure, aims to cure disorders by restoring the flow of energy through the body. It is similar to acupuncture but uses finger pressure instead of needles at strategic points – known as acupoints – on the body. Proponents of acupressure believe that fatigue is caused by an obstruction in the energy channels. To help clear these pathways, try these exercises: rub your ear lobes between your thumb and forefinger; pull the toe adjacent to the big toe on each foot and then rub it vigorously.

Drink water

Dehydration is a common energy drainer. Drink a glass of water in the morning and at any other time that you need a pick-me-up. Even if you don't feel particularly thirsty, aim to drink 8 glasses every day.

3

SUPPLEMENT YOUR DIET

4 If you think your diet may be deficient in key nutrients, consider taking vitamin and mineral supplements. Choose those that supply 100 per cent of the recommended daily amounts of the important vitamins and minerals (see end of book).

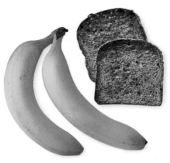

Eat a starchy snack
....

5 A carbohydrate snack such as toast, a bagel or a banana will provide an easy and sustainable source of energy.

TOWEL RUB

For an invigorating rubdown to start each day, try this towel rub. Soak a clean cotton hand towel in hot water and wring it out. Using short, vigorous movements, scrub your skin, starting with your toes and working up to your head. As soon as the towel cools, put it back into hot water.

6

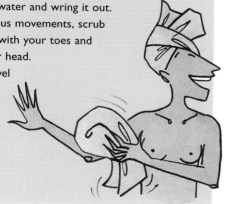

TAKE A SHOWER

7 Spend a minute or two under the shower, first of all really invigorating your face and head under warm water. Then start to alternate the water between warm and cool. This stimulates your circulation and encourages your blood to penetrate deeper into the tissues, carrying energy-giving oxygen and glucose with it. Don't let the water run too hot or cold and avoid wetting your head during this technique as the sudden temperature changes can make you feel dizzy. It also may be inadvisable for anyone with high blood pressure or a heart disorder.

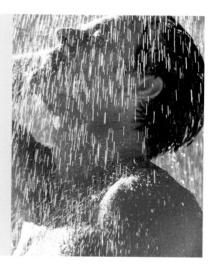

Get physical
....

8 Go for a brisk walk instead of slumping in front of the television. Or get the blood flowing and oxygen carrying to the tissues by jogging on the spot, stamping your feet and shaking your arms. Stretching exercises (see pages 36–37) will also help revitalise you.

Stand tall
....

9 Proponents of the Alexander technique believe good posture helps to enhance the flow of energy in the body. To help improve your energy levels, imagine yourself being lifted up – as though you had a string attached to the top of your head, raise your head up, stand tall and pull your shoulders back. Keep your back straight and your abdomen in and walk forwards in this posture. Avoid holding your shoulders too far back or slouching, as both postures can block the free flow of energy.

TAKE A SIESTA

A 20-minute early- or mid-afternoon rest, or even a snooze (if you are at home), will revitalise both mind and body, especially after lunch. Energy output tends to decline at this time and concentration falls, partly because some of your blood leaves the brain to aid the digestive system. Without a rest, decision-making suffers and mistakes are more likely. The afternoon siesta has been a tradition in Latin countries for many centuries.

10

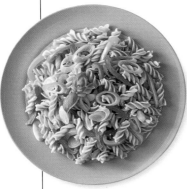

Whole-wheat pasta with sweet peppers

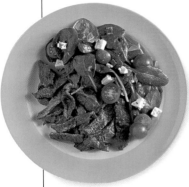

Steak with spinach

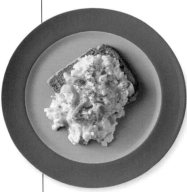

Ham with eggs

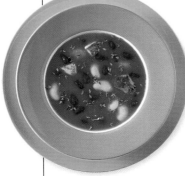

Pork with beans

Minor deficiencies may cause fatigue and supplementing has been found to help cases of chronic fatigue syndrome.

Vitamin B$_6$ (pyridoxine) is needed mainly to break down and release energy from protein, and for many other metabolic processes. Requirements increase with protein intake. Slight deficiencies disrupt both riboflavin and energy metabolism and may cause fatigue and psychiatric problems. Good sources include chicken, pork, soya, nuts and whole-wheat.

Vitamin B$_{12}$ (cyanocobalamin) is found in liver, meat, fish, dairy products and eggs, and is essential for the production of energy. A lack of B$_{12}$ results in a condition called pernicious anaemia, with symptoms of exhaustion and shortness of breath. Those who do not eat animal products, such as strict vegetarians or vegans, run the greatest risk of deficiency.

Vitamin C (ascorbic acid), found in fresh fruit, fruit juices and vegetables, is involved in the production of carnitine, which transports fats into muscle cells for energy. (Athletes often use a carnitine supplement to improve their performance.) As a result, a mild deficiency can lead to fatigue. Modern convenience foods tend to be low in vitamin C, and smoking, stress, illness, injury and surgery increase our need for this vitamin.

Iron deficiency is one of the most common causes of fatigue, as iron is needed for haemoglobin and red blood cell production and functioning. Haemophiliacs and menstruating women, in particular, need a high-iron diet. Rich sources include red meat such as liver, kidney and heart. Eggs, pulses and cocoa also contain iron.

Magnesium maintains the electrical balance in the tissues, and deficiencies can cause

Iron in food becomes more readily available for digestion if eaten in combination with other iron-rich or vitamin C-rich foods. Some good examples are pictured left.

3 WAYS TO BOOST YOUR IRON INTAKE

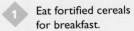

1 Eat fortified cereals for breakfast.

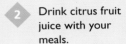

2 Drink citrus fruit juice with your meals.

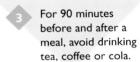

3 For 90 minutes before and after a meal, avoid drinking tea, coffee or cola.

problems with muscle function. Much research shows that a slight deficiency can cause fatigue, and supplements quickly boost energy in many sufferers. Magnesium is a component of chlorophyll, found in all green plants, so green, leafy vegetables are good sources, along with almonds, cashews, whole-grain bread, meat and tofu.

Potassium, found in bananas, apples, potatoes, oranges, asparagus and plums, plays a major role in muscle function, and deficiencies can lead to muscle fatigue. A shortage is most common in people who don't eat enough fresh fruit and vegetables, in alcoholics and in those taking medication for asthma. Deficiencies can also be due to hormonal imbalances.

ENERGY-BOOSTING EATING PLAN

Having the occasional pick-me-up is all well and good, but if you're regularly feeling tired, you may need to change your diet.

Consider the following tips to boost energy levels and keep you going between meals:

▶ *Alcohol* Reduce alcohol consumption; don't drink alcohol on an empty stomach – it can lead to low blood-sugar levels.

▶ *Snacks* Eat a carbohydrate snack, such as a banana, low-salt pretzels or a bagel (avoid high-fat toppings such as full-fat cheese).

▶ *Caffeine* Limit the caffeine from coffee, tea and colas. Caffeine can increase insulin production, which lowers blood-sugar levels.

▶ *Sugary foods* Cut down on sugar in coffee and tea, cakes, biscuits and sweets.

▶ *Regular meals* Eat three meals a day that are high in complex carbohydrates.

▶ *Nutrient-packed foods* Eat highly nutritious foods, such as complex carbohydrates, and avoid processed foods, which have low levels of vitamins and minerals.

Eating to lose weight

By taking a sensible approach, you can shed weight and yet eat full, satisfying and healthy meals without binging, feeling guilty or becoming preoccupied with counting kilojoules (calories).

There are many good reasons for shedding excess weight. Being overweight increases the risk of developing serious disorders such as heart and kidney disease, diabetes, high blood pressure and some cancers, and leads to poor self-esteem. But weight loss should never become a preoccupation. An obsessional attitude to dieting, counting kilojoules (or calories), and rapid weight loss is, at best, counter-productive and, at worst, harmful. Crash diets and yo-yo dieting can lead to nutritional deficiencies, chronic tiredness, increased risk of infections and psychological problems. Eating disorders such as anorexia and bulimia are thought to arise partly as a result of an obsessional desire to be thin.

If excess weight is a problem, your aims should be twofold: first, to reduce your weight in small increments of 0.5–1 kg (1–2 lb) each week and, second, to develop healthy eating habits. Weight-loss goals should always be sensible and long-term.

A programme of weight reduction should run over months rather than weeks and be made up of small, achievable goals that you set (and meet) along the way.

Weight fluctuations are common and demonstrate that the body is a complex and constantly varying system. Your weight is

LOSING WEIGHT SAFELY

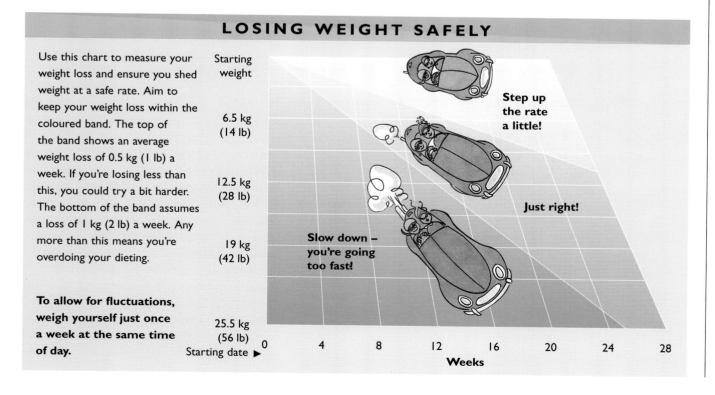

Use this chart to measure your weight loss and ensure you shed weight at a safe rate. Aim to keep your weight loss within the coloured band. The top of the band shows an average weight loss of 0.5 kg (1 lb) a week. If you're losing less than this, you could try a bit harder. The bottom of the band assumes a loss of 1 kg (2 lb) a week. Any more than this means you're overdoing your dieting.

To allow for fluctuations, weigh yourself just once a week at the same time of day.

Starting weight

6.5 kg (14 lb)

12.5 kg (28 lb)

19 kg (42 lb)

25.5 kg (56 lb)

Starting date ▶ 0   4   8   12   16   20   24   28

Weeks

Step up the rate a little!

Just right!

Slow down – you're going too fast!

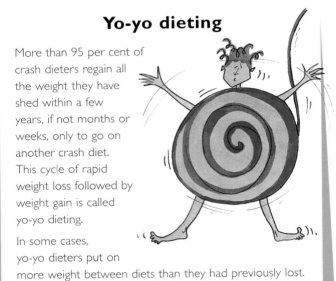

affected by such factors as hormone changes, altered activity levels and physical health. If, for example, you have had a meal or drink, or if your bladder or bowels are full, or (for women) if you are premenstrual, your weight can vary by as much as 1.4 kg (3 lb) over the course of a day.

There are numerous weight-loss methods to choose from and rarely a week goes by without a new 'wonder diet plan' being unveiled to a public desperate for results. Many of these methods are based on sound dietary principles, so if you think one may work for you, give it a try. But be wary of diets that offer a 'quick-fix'. Even if you manage to shed weight quickly, unless you also develop sensible eating habits, you will just put the weight back on.

FACTS OF DIETING

There is no mystery about weight gain and loss. The energy you take in as food must be burned up through physical activity or heat. If you expend more energy than you take in, you lose weight; if you burn less than you consume, your body stores surplus food energy as fat. Recognising the link between energy supplied by the food you eat and the energy burned up during physical activity is at the heart of any weight-loss programme.

Kilojoules or kJ (in the metric system) and calories (in the imperial system) are simply measures of energy. Your body burns up energy just by keeping up your metabolic processes – heart beat, temperature, breathing and so on. This is known as your basal metabolic rate (BMR) and varies from time to time depending on your age, weight and

Yo-yo dieting

More than 95 per cent of crash dieters regain all the weight they have shed within a few years, if not months or weeks, only to go on another crash diet. This cycle of rapid weight loss followed by weight gain is called yo-yo dieting.

In some cases, yo-yo dieters put on more weight between diets than they had previously lost. One reason for this is that dieters tend to binge on fatty foods when they stop dieting, leading to accelerated weight gain. The answer is to avoid crash diets, develop sustainable diet habits, and choose starchy foods instead of high-fat products.

activity level. A sedentary woman, for example, who is 162 cm (5 ft 4 in) tall and weighs 65 kg (145 lb), will burn up around 7500 kJ (1800 calories) in 24 hours. If this woman consumes more than this, she will put on weight. It may seem logical that if she went on a crash diet and cut her daily intake to, say, under 6000 kJ (1400 calories) per day, her body would be forced to burn up 1700 kJ (400 calories) of stored fat and she would lose weight.

However, this is not necessarily the case. Your body reacts to a sudden and dramatic reduction in food as it would to starvation, lowering your BMR to match your reduced intake. As a result, crash diets leave you feeling permanently hungry, without, in the short term, an appreciable loss of weight. In many cases, this fact alone is enough to destroy the willpower of dieters and they soon return to former eating patterns.

This does not, of course, mean that there is no point in trying to lose weight. But it does mean you achieve nothing by starving yourself. The method of weight control and reduction that has proved consistently successful is to equalise kilojoule (calorie) intake and output at a level you can sustain. This means raising your energy output, by increasing your daily activity as much as possible, and reducing your food intake (if necessary) to match this figure.

On average, approximately 65–70 per cent of the energy you derive from food is used to maintain body temperature and keep vital organs and tissues functioning. Around 10–15 per cent is used during digestion, and 15–20 per cent fuels the muscles during

ARE YOU A HEALTHY WEIGHT?

The body mass index (BMI) is a standard way of working out whether you are a healthy weight for your height. Look at the chart on the right to work out your BMI.

▶ A BMI of under 20 is considered underweight. You should plan to steadily gain weight.

▶ You are a healthy weight if your BMI is between 20 and 25.

▶ A BMI over 25 is considered overweight, and you should try to lose weight gradually until you fall below 25.

▶ A BMI over 30 is clinically obese. You should start a serious weight-loss programme immediately. Consult your doctor or nutritionist for professional advice.

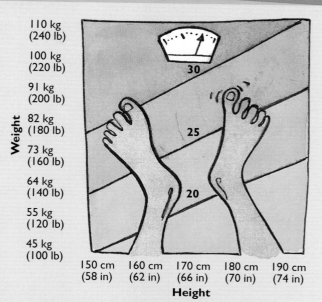

Look at the chart. Find your height along the bottom line and your weight along the side. Using rulers, find the point where the two lines intersect. This is your BMI number.

---

physical activity. What is not used is stored as fat. By increasing your activity, you raise your energy output in two ways. First, you burn up extra energy while doing the activity. Aerobic exercises, in particular, are fuelled by fat and so help you lose weight. Second, regular physical activity raises your BMR by increasing the amount of muscle in your body – muscle is metabolically active, so it burns up energy even when resting (see Chapter 1, pages 14–40, for exercise ideas).

REDUCING ENERGY INTAKE

There are no quick-fix methods of weight control that will provide lasting benefits. The best method is to eat a variety of foods that contain all the nutrients you need to keep healthy and yet are relatively low in kilojoules (calories). This means cutting down on high-fat, high-sugar foods and eating more high-fibre, starchy foods, plus fruit and vegetables. These will fill you up but have far fewer kilojoules (calories). Speciality breads containing olives, sun-dried tomatoes, nuts

and seeds taste good in their own right and can reduce the desire for butter, margarine or other high-fat spreads on bread.

WATCH YOUR FAT INTAKE

The prime cause of becoming overweight is a diet high in fat (and, to a lesser extent, refined sugar).

The typical Western diet contains around 38 per cent fat, compared with an average of 30 per cent in the developing world.

You should consider this significant difference and take steps to cut your own fat intake, especially of saturated fats. Surprisingly, the percentage of fat consumed in the West has not changed significantly in the last 100 years. The difference now is that people now lead much more sedentary lives – using labour-saving domestic appliances, travelling mainly by car, working in fully automated or desk-bound jobs, and watching television instead of going out for entertainment. As a consequence, much of the fat people eat is surplus to their energy requirements, and they gain unwanted weight.

All food is potentially fattening, in that it will be stored as fat if it is not used to provide energy or heat for the body's needs. But fat is more fattening than other foods, for two reasons. Gram for gram, it contains more than double the kilojoules (calories) of other foodstuffs (1 gram of fat contains 38 kJ [9 calories], compared with 15.7 kJ [3.75 calories] for carbohydrate and 17 kJ [4 calories] for protein). This means you have to more than double your energy output to burn up fat, compared with the same quantity of another foodstuff. Second, it has been established that people tend to overeat fatty foods. This is partially because these foods taste good and do not fill you up as readily as a similar quantity of carbohydrate or protein foods.

TOO SWEET

According to nutrition experts and health organisations, the average Westerner eats around 1.4 kg (3 lb) of sugar each week. This figure has been rising over the years and is now approximately double the average sugar intake of 100 years ago.

The World Health Organization recommends no more than 12 teaspoons of sugar per day (less than 10 per cent of your diet). It is not enough just to go without sugar in your coffee and tea; you should also cut back on cola drinks, condiments, chocolate bars and many prepared foods. Cutting down on convenience foods and eating fresh produce instead is a good way of reducing your total sugar consumption and obtaining more nutrients.

To help reduce your intake of sugars, take the time to study food labels to keep a check on how much sugar you are eating. Many manufactured foods contain large amounts of added sugar.

Manufacturers use a wide variety of simple sugars as flavour-enhancers in processed foods – both sweet and savoury. As well as sucrose, manufacturers may add corn syrup, dextrose, fructose, invert sugar, honey, lactose, maltose and molasses.

Some of these sugars, such as lactose and fructose, are actually good for you when consumed in their natural form – in milk, and in fruit and vegetables. This is because these foods also contain important dietary components such as vitamins, minerals and, in the case of fruit and vegetables, fibre. During processing, many foods tend to lose most of their nutrients as a result of overcooking and refining. You should make a real effort to reduce your intake of processed foods that

HEALTHY ALTERNATIVES

If you want to lose some weight, swap some of the high-fat foods you eat regularly with tasty, low-fat alternatives. When you start looking, you will find it easy to cut back on fat.

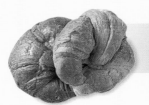

Saves 20 grams of fat

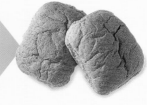

2 croissants
22 g fat, 1675 kJ (400 calories)

2 whole-wheat bread rolls
2 g fat, 586 kJ (140 calories)

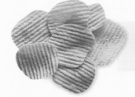

Saves 11 grams of fat

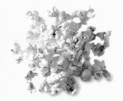

25 g (1 oz) crisps
12 g fat, 710 kJ (170 calories)

25 g (1 oz) unbuttered popcorn
1 g fat, 418 kJ (100 calories)

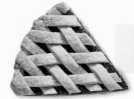

Saves 8 grams of fat

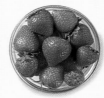

50 g (2 oz) fruit tart
9 g fat, 710 kJ (170 calories)

2 cups fresh strawberries
1 g fat, 385 kJ (92 calories)

Healthy cooking tips

The right choice of ingredients and cooking methods will help you easily reduce kilojoules (calories) and promote good health:

Choose lean cuts When shopping, pick leaner cuts of meat and trim off surplus fat before cooking or serving.

Use low-fat milk Replace whole milk with fat-free (skimmed) or low-fat (2 per cent) milk.

Replace cream Use lower-fat alternatives, such as low-fat yoghurt or crème fraîche.

Cook with vegetable oils Use olive, sunflower, safflower, corn or soya bean oils and margarine instead of butter or lard, which contain saturated fats.

Dry roast or broil Allow fat to drain away by placing meats on a rack during and after cooking. Avoid basting with or adding extra fat.

Steam food Cook food in its natural juices by steaming or wrap in foil and bake in the oven.

Avoid conventional frying Stir-fry food quickly in a little olive oil or use a non-stick frying pan and reduce oil usage.

Avoid burnt food Do not overbrown meat before adding to stews or casseroles; there are some concerns about burnt food and cancer.

Remove skin The skin on poultry, particularly duck, is high in saturated fats. Remove the skin before cooking or serving.

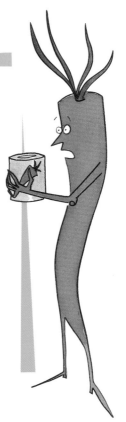

contain refined sugars or, ideally, simply cut them out of your diet altogether and replace them with fresh, unprocessed ingredients.

ARE YOU A HEALTHY WEIGHT?

Before starting a diet, you should know whether you are a healthy weight now or, if not, how much weight you should lose or gain to achieve that weight. There are many ways of judging whether you are in a healthy range. One of the most common is the body mass index (BMI – see page 61), which your doctor or nutritionist will use to see if you are a reasonable weight for your height. According to the most recent studies (in 1998), a healthy range for your BMI is between 20 and 25. Anything between 25 and 30 is considered unhealthily overweight and over 30 is obese. If your BMI is under 20, you are considered to be unhealthily underweight.

WEIGHT CONTROL

Keep a weekly diary of all the foods you eat and when, and try to identify problem foods, such as high-fat, high-sugar snacks, and problem times, such as late evening. Then, replace these with healthier foods. If you snack on crisps when you are watching

SIMPLE WEIGHT-LOSS PROGRAMME

Cut down on fried foods and foods high in fat, such as cakes, pastries and full-fat dairy products.

Limit alcohol to no more than 125 ml of wine, 30 ml of spirits or 285 ml of beer a day.

Eat plenty of rice, sweet corn, potatoes, cereals, peas, beans, lentils, fruit and vegetables.

television, for example, switch to low-salt pretzels or plain popcorn. Be honest with yourself – pretending that you eat fewer fattening foods than you do won't get you anywhere.

Eat mainly high-carbohydrate foods that are also high in fibre, such as whole-grain toast, as these are filling. Take smaller mouthfuls, chew your food thoroughly and finish each mouthful before taking another. Drink plenty of water with meals to fill you up, so that you feel satisfied with less food.

If tempted to have seconds, wait a while before serving yourself. There is a time delay before the satiety signals that indicate you are full actually reach the brain. Because of this delay, people tend to overeat and feel bloated after meals. Leave the table wanting just a little more; you will find that this feeling soon passes. Make a point of sitting down at a table to eat, and make your meals special occasions to be enjoyed with family or friends. You are more likely to overindulge if you eat on your own, when you tend to fill up on high-fat snacks or prepare too much food.

Serve meals on smaller plates to avoid overfilling your plate and store surplus food in the fridge or freezer.

Plan your weekly meals to include occasional treats and accept that you're only

Over-the-counter supplements work on the digestive tract or brain to curb hunger and prevent weight gain. But benefits are often transitory because diet aids do not encourage people to develop healthy long-term eating habits. They may interfere with the absorption of nutrients.

Diet aids

There is a growing market for diet aids, which come in the form of pills, drinks and snack bars. However, some products contain ingredients that are potentially harmful, and they are not effective for long-term weight loss.

In the case of non-prescription diet aids, hunger is suppressed usually by bran or another expanding ingredient that fills your stomach. This process is relatively harmless if used carefully, but many diet aids also contain drugs that are potentially harmful.

Stimulants, such as caffeine, are used to speed up the metabolism – burning kilojoules (calories) faster and reducing appetite, but increasing stress and blood pressure and preventing proper nutrient absorption.

Some products also contain mild antidepressants or tranquillisers to ease the dieting blues. Others include laxatives to stimulate the fast removal of food from the body, thus limiting nutrient absorption in the digestive system. These are not effective weight-management tools, and you must check the ingredients of any product that you use. Diet aids may help you to lose weight, but are they safe – and can you keep the weight off after you stop taking the pills?

human and will overindulge occasionally. If you set yourself unrealistic rules – such as, say, never having chocolate – you'll feel that you're a failure if you succumb, and may abandon your efforts altogether.

Eat frequent but smaller meals. In addition to breakfast, lunch and dinner, eat healthy snacks when you feel hungry between meals. This is effective in several ways. By eating smaller meals you train your stomach to expect smaller portions. You are also less likely to overeat and feel bloated and guilty after a meal.

By eating more frequently, your digestive system burns up more energy processing the food, so less is stored as fat. By having regular meals throughout the day, you do not get as ravenously hungry and so are not tempted to binge. Having one great big meal in the evening is the worst habit you can get into. Firstly, you do not have enough time before you go to bed to digest the food properly or make use of the energy derived from the food – it is more likely to be stored as fat. Secondly, you expand your stomach by eating a lot at the same time. This will make you hungry in the morning and throughout the daytime, encouraging you to eat more. Keeping meals small – just enough to satisfy you – is the key to weight loss.

Plan ahead for an attack of the munchies by stocking up on healthy snacks, such as fruit, breadsticks or plain popcorn, that you can have at home or take when you go out.

COMFORT EATING

Sweet and carbohydrate foods stimulate parts of the brain that produce mood-enhancing chemicals, which make you want to eat more of them. Such comfort eating is most likely to appeal when you are depressed or have a low self-image and want to cheer yourself up. It only provides temporary relief, however, and if it becomes a habit, it could lead to a weight problem, which can contribute further to a negative self-image.

A better approach is to find ways to cheer yourself up that do not involve food. A warm bath scented with aromatherapy oils, for

FAT ON FOOD LABELS

The fat content of many foods is shown on the packaging. Food labels often list the total number of grams of fat present, the percentage of fat in the product and the number of kilojoules (calories) from fat. They sometimes also show the different types of fat present (such as saturated and poly-/monounsaturated fats). If the label does not tell you whether the fats are saturated or not, you can often guess by using a simple rule: unsaturated fats, such as olive oil and vegetable oil, are liquid at room temperature, whereas saturated fats, such as butter and lard, are solid.

Check if the product contains trans-fatty acids, which are as harmful as saturated fats, by looking for the words partially hydrogenated or partially hydrogenised. You should also watch out for palm oil and coconut oil, which are saturated fats but may be listed as vegetable oils.

Health claims printed on many food packages can be misleading – check the Nutrition Facts panel, which describes the ingredients fully.

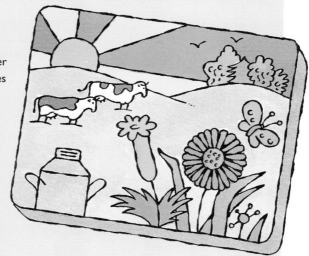

▶ **Low-fat** Under 3 g per regular serving.

▶ **Fat-free** Under 0.5 g of fat per regular serving.

▶ **Reduced/less fat** 25 per cent less fat than the full-fat version.

▶ **Light** Could mean any of the above.

---

example, is soothing and mood-enhancing and so, too, is a professional massage. Phone a friend or go for a walk, rent a comedy video or read a good book.

You could also engage in a hobby that keeps you occupied and takes your mind off food, or find a challenge to channel your energies in a more healthy direction.

A few more helpful hints for sensible and successful weight loss include:

▶ **Easy does it** Change your diet gradually. This is easier than trying to alter your eating pattern overnight.

▶ **Friendly support** Let people know you're watching your weight so they aren't tempted to ply you with fatty foods.

▶ **Fill up on H$_2$O** Drink more water with your meals. Water is filling and also aids the digestive process.

▶ **Varied diet** There is no reason why your meals have to be monotonous and boring.

▶ **Forward planning** Never shop when you are hungry. You will tend to buy more food than you really need and are more likely to choose high-fat foods.

▶ **Sensible snacking** Choose toast, bagels, pretzels (without high-fat toppings), fruit and low-fat yoghurt to stave off hunger.

▶ **Regular meals** Don't skip meals. This lowers your metabolic rate without leading to weight loss. You also get too hungry, and are more likely to overeat at your next meal.

▶ **Low-fat options** Avoid eating too many fatty foods because fats and oils contain more than twice the kilojoules of other foods. Eat healthy snacks instead of biscuits, crisps or ice-cream. Don't cut out all dairy foods; choose low-fat or fat-free versions.

▶ **Occasional treats** You don't need to avoid all your favourite foods. Include them as a treat – say, once or twice a week.

12 ways to **manage your weight**

**Here are a few pointers to help strengthen your resolve –
and enjoyment – so that you are more likely to stick to a
weight-control programme.**

Cook the low-fat way

1

Choose cooking techniques that keep fat low and flavour high.
► Use cornflour to thicken sauces (add towards the end of the cooking time) instead of flour.
► Top pot pies with mashed potato instead of pastry.
► If using minced meat, choose lean cuts. Heat the meat and drain off the fat before adding to casseroles and stews. Alternatively, use vegetables, pulses or soya protein.

PLAN YOUR SHOPPING

2

Write out a shopping list before you go to the store, including mostly healthy items that are low in fat and refined sugar – but a few treats as well. Don't deviate from it. This way you are less likely to buy fattening foods on impulse. Eat before you go – never shop when you are hungry, or you'll end up buying more than you need.

DRINK COLD WATER

4

Water is filling in itself and also adds bulk to your food, especially if you eat plenty of fibre (which absorbs water). Cold water actually uses up energy because the body burns it up in raising the temperature of the water once it is inside your body. Drinking five glasses of cold water throughout the day is equivalent – in energy terms – to forgoing a slice of bread.

Make healthy swaps

3

Replace some of your favourite high-fat foods with lower-fat alternatives. Here are a few examples:
► Swap mayonnaise-based dressings for low-fat versions.
► Instead of a bacon-and-egg breakfast, choose fruit and wheat toast.
► Replace ice-cream with frozen yoghurt, and an iced cake with a light sponge cake topped with puréed fruit.
► Instead of butter and sour cream, top baked potatoes with low-fat fillings, such as yoghurt, cottage cheese or beans.

GIVE YOURSELF A (NON-FOOD) TREAT

5

Instead of indulging yourself with chocolates or pastries, spoil yourself with inedibles such as a bunch of flowers, a music CD, a book or magazine, a beauty product or a night at the cinema.

Make a fuss of yourself

6

Developing a positive self-image can help you keep to a healthy diet. Don't wait until you have shed surplus weight before taking pride in your appearance; start creating the new you now. Indulge yourself with some new clothes or a new hairstyle. Have a makeover or seek advice from a colour or clothes consultant.

Discover new foods

Don't just cut foods from your diet – add new ones as well. There is a whole world of exciting dishes for you to try, including exotic new fruits and vegetables, and meat alternatives, such as tofu. Try out recipes that incorporate these foods, and experiment with ethnic cuisine – Indian Tandoori dishes, Italian polenta-based meals and Mexican pancakes and beans are delicious yet relatively low in fat.

7

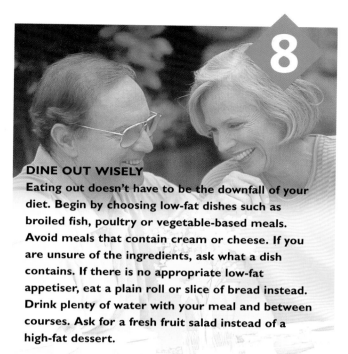

DINE OUT WISELY

Eating out doesn't have to be the downfall of your diet. Begin by choosing low-fat dishes such as broiled fish, poultry or vegetable-based meals. Avoid meals that contain cream or cheese. If you are unsure of the ingredients, ask what a dish contains. If there is no appropriate low-fat appetiser, eat a plain roll or slice of bread instead. Drink plenty of water with your meal and between courses. Ask for a fresh fruit salad instead of a high-fat dessert.

8

KEEP BUSY

9

If you have too much free time you may become preoccupied with your diet and will be more likely to weaken and binge on inappropriate foods. There are plenty of things you can do to keep busy, such as catching up with telephone calls and letter writing, tidying up drawers, cleaning out cupboards or arranging a new photo album. Surfing the Net, catching up on your reading or doing a jigsaw are all worthwhile activities. Longer-term measures include joining a health club, taking up a hobby or registering for a class.

KEEP ACTIVE

A good weight-loss diet is one that combines kilojoule (calorie) control with a raised level of aerobic activity. Go for a stroll at lunchtime – whether at home or at work – no matter how busy you are. Do something even more energetic before your evening meal, such as a brisk 30-minute walk, jog or cycle, a session on a rowing or skiing machine or treadmill, or a workout in the gym. At other times, find different ways to be more active (see pages 38–39 for other ideas). Collectively, taking these opportunities will burn up fat and boost your metabolism.

10

SPICE UP YOUR MEALS

11

Add flavour to your meals with peppers, chillies, mustard and other spices instead of salt, which can lead to fluid retention. Spicy foods also raise your temperature, increasing your metabolism by as much as 25 per cent for several hours after eating them.

HAVE HEALTHY SNACKS ON HAND

12

You are bound to get hungry when you are out and about, so don't risk giving in to temptation. Dried or fresh fruit, bagels, plain popcorn, cut-up vegetables and breadsticks are all easily portable. Nibble them when you get hungry, particularly at danger times, such as during a film or a football match, when you may be tempted to eat sweets, ice-cream or burgers.

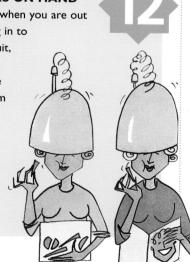

BASIC GUIDE TO
health spas

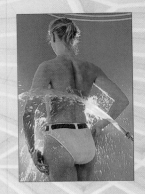

Over the last decade health spas have boomed in popularity. Health spas are located close to home as well as at exotic locations, so you can spend a day, a weekend or a week at the venue of your choice. Many are set among beautiful scenery – mountain retreats, water-side sites or rolling green fields – so that just staying at one can be an uplifting experience. The services can vary widely, so decide exactly what it is you want from your stay before you commit yourself to a particular spa. For example, do you want to lose a little weight, improve skin condition, tone up muscles, or rid yourself of the aches, pains and tensions of a stressful job? Or do you want to get physically fit, get in touch with your spiritual side, or learn yoga positions you can use back at home?

You can have more than one aim, but try to be realistic. If you expect to achieve too much during your visit – particularly if it's short – you are likely to be disappointed. On the other hand, without setting clear goals, you might spend a lot of money on what is no more than a holiday – albeit an enjoyable one. The next step is to contact spas in your price range to find out what they have to offer.

There are basic services you should expect from any good spa. When you arrive you will get a check-up from a qualified nurse who will help you to plan your stay. Healthful meals are a feature of many spas, so the nurse will need to know about any dietary requirements, allergies or sensitivities you might have. Gym equipment should include resistance apparatus, cycling and rowing machines, and treadmills. Instructors are usually available to devise a fitness programme that is specially tailored to your needs.

Health spa treatments

In addition to fitness programmes, dietary regimes, skin-care treatments and stress relief, many spas also teach disciplines based on Eastern philosophies that are designed to help visitors to achieve physical and mental health and inner peace.

Flotation is mainly intended for stress relief, and involves partial submersion in a sound- and light-proof water tank. The water in the tank contains a mixture of mineral salts for effortless floating. It is based on the theory that by removing all external sensations you will find it easier to relax and meditate.

A herbal wrap is a detoxification and relaxation technique in which the body is wrapped in hot linens, plastic sheets or blankets to enable heat, moisture and herbal essences to penetrate the skin.

Hydrotherapy is one of the oldest spa treatments. It includes water massage, hot and cold showers and compresses. Some health spas are based near natural hot springs where clients benefit from the minerals and heat.

Massage is a form of therapy usually involving stroking, kneading and pummelling to manipulate the soft tissues. The most common form is Swedish massage, but others include Thai massage and shiatsu.

Naturopathy is based on the principle of 'allowing the body to heal itself'. It can include exercise, massage and relaxation, and involves a diet rich in raw fruit, vegetables, juices and water to flush out toxins and boost nutrient levels. Many spas offer naturopathy in weight-reduction and toning programmes.

Polarity therapy is a combination of meditation, massage, exercise and diet to balance energy levels.

Chapter 3

Looking good

Skin care

Skin is your external wrapping – the first part of you that others see, and a reflection of your age, health and lifestyle. Keep your skin healthy with good care, a nutritious diet and exercise.

Your skin provides a barrier between your bodily tissues and the environment; it is under constant threat from within and without. On the inside, it is attacked by toxins in the food you eat and the rogue molecules called free radicals that can damage cells. On the outside, it is under threat from the wind, ultraviolet (UV) radiation from the sun, cigarette smoke, traffic fumes and many other environmental factors, including all the soot, dirt and dust compounds that are present in the air. So basic skin care involves two main approaches – consuming the nutrients that the skin needs to stay strong and healthy, and protecting the skin from damage and feeding it moisture to help retain its elasticity.

As you get older, the skin becomes more fragile and prone to damage – but some signs of wear can be combated. Your genetic make-up plays the most important part in the way your skin looks, behaves and ages.

Getting to know your skin and how it works and reacts to external factors can help you to look after it and adapt your lifestyle to keep it looking healthy.

LIFESTYLE FACTORS

Where skin care is concerned, the philosophy is quite simple: you can apply all the expensive creams you like, but without a balanced diet and exercise you will not achieve a healthy complexion. Exercise is crucial for pumping oxygenated blood around your body – 7 per cent of the oxygen you take into your lungs is used by the skin. As you get older, you tend to take smaller, shallower breaths,

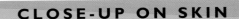

CLOSE-UP ON SKIN

Your skin is a working miracle: it's waterproof, it helps regulate body temperature, intercepts and destroys harmful bacteria, grows hairs, expels liquids and salts, has an amazing sense of touch and provides a protective mantle. Your skin works hard for you, so

Removing dead cells allows the pores to breathe healthily.

take special care of it to keep it healthy throughout your life. The skin is made from two main types of fibre – collagen and elastin. Collagen fibres create the underlying framework while elastin fibres provide elasticity. Over the top is a protective layer of dead skin cells that are constantly being worn away and replenished with newer cells. Pores are the tiny openings through which fluids, such as sweat, are released. They tend to become larger in warmer climates, due to the greater output of sweat glands, and also as you age. Keeping skin clean and moisturised prevents the build-up of toxins, which can destroy the skin's structure, leading to wrinkles, sagging and a poor complexion.

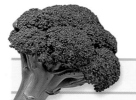

Healthy diet – healthy skin

The food that you eat feeds every system in your body – including your skin – and each nutrient plays a crucial role in body functioning. Your skin shows the signs of a good diet, particularly if it incorporates the nutrients listed below.

NUTRIENT	BENEFITS AND SOURCES
Vitamin A	This is useful if you suffer from acne, dry or scaly skin, sore eyelids or dry hands. Sources include yellow and orange fruit and vegetables, such as apricots and carrots.
B vitamins	These are helpful for menopausal symptoms, skin cracks or mouth problems, as well as lack of energy, anaemia and some skin conditions. Food sources include liver, eggs and whole-grain cereals. If you suffer from skin disorders, a B complex supplement may help.
Vitamin C	This is good for wound healing, the formation of collagen and the repair of broken veins. Food sources include most fresh fruit and vegetables, especially citrus fruits, tomatoes, potatoes, green vegetables and strawberries.
Vitamin E	As well as being a powerful antioxidant, this vitamin prolongs cell life, improves skin quality and hastens wound healing. Sources include vegetable oils, green leafy vegetables and whole-grain cereals.
Essential fatty acids	These are good for muscle tone and maintaining healthy skin. Main food sources include fish oils and linseed oil. Supplement sources include gamma-linoleic acids (GLAs) from starflower and evening primrose oils.

taking less oxygen in and expelling waste products less efficiently – leading to a toxin build-up, which ages the skin.

It is vital for the skin that you incorporate some exercise into your daily routine.

Regular exercise improves the absorption of nutrients and enables cells to be replaced more quickly, leading to more resilient, radiant skin. It aids the digestive system and speeds up the metabolism, helping to eliminate toxins and giving an instant glow to your complexion. Exercise is also needed for a healthy lymphatic system – the network of channels containing lymph that bathes the cells with nutrients and removes wastes. Exercise promotes lymph circulation, which ultimately drains into the bloodstream, taking toxins with it. It also alleviates stress, which contributes to premature skin aging.

Regularly spend time outside, as fresh air gives a radiance and bloom to your skin – although you must avoid exposing your skin to too much sun. A dry atmosphere, caused by heating and air conditioning systems, dehydrates the skin. To increase the moisture content of air, use humidifiers or place a few bowls of water next to radiators or heat vents.

What you eat is reflected in the appearance of your skin. Plenty of fresh fruit and vegetables should feature in your diet, especially green and orange varieties. These are rich in antioxidant vitamins, which can combat the effect of free radicals – a major cause of premature skin aging. Smoking promotes free radicals and so stopping should show visible results in your skin's health.

Adequate fluid consumption is essential; drink plenty of water every day to hydrate your body and keep your skin fresh looking.

6 ways to **younger-looking skin**

Give your skin a treat every week with a deep massage, sauna or Turkish bath. Or simply spend an evening at home relaxing in a warm tub and paying your skin a little extra attention to keep it clean and moist.

BATHE WITH ADDED MOISTURE

1 Use moisturising products as part of your daily cleansing routine. Applying a moisturiser or oil to damp skin after a bath or shower will seal in moisture and keep skin soft and supple.

TURKISH BATH

2 The humid warmth of a Turkish bath is the perfect way to cleanse your skin thoroughly. Simply spend an hour or so letting the gentle steam penetrate your whole body. The steam works by increasing sweat production and water moisture in the air, removing all the dirt from your skin. You may also find the relaxing bath helps to relieve stress, leaving you feeling cleansed and refreshed.

KEEP TRIM AND FIT

3 Many skin problems can be countered simply by watching your weight and exercising regularly. Blotches or raised bumps on the skin are commonly caused by the failure of fluids to drain properly or poor blood flow and functioning. These can be helped with a little exercise a few times a week. If you are overweight, this problem is compounded, and you may be increasing the risk of sagging. Climbing the stairs instead of using the lift, and taking other easy chances to exercise, will contribute to the health of your skin.

REGULAR MASSAGE

4 Treat yourself to a professional massage or you could massage yourself. Using gentle circular motions with either your fingers or your whole hand, a daily or weekly self-massage improves the lymph and blood circulation, speeding the removal of wastes and pollutants and bringing new nutrients to the skin.

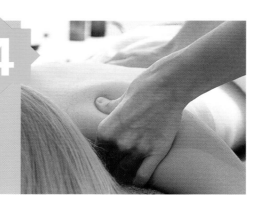

Give up smoking
....

5 If you smoke, stopping is probably the single best thing you can do for your skin. When you smoke, your blood, and therefore your skin, receives less oxygen and more pollutants.

DRINK UP

6 Drink more fluids, especially water, which speeds the cleansing of your skin. Fruit and vegetable juices contain antioxidant vitamins, minerals and phytochemicals that help to nourish and renew the skin and counteract the damage caused by pollutants.

Too little sleep shows clearly in the appearance of the skin, leading to a dull complexion and dark circles under the eyes.

Night is an important time for the skin, as this is when skin cells regenerate collagen, and keratin production steps up.

Aim to get seven or eight hours of quality sleep every night. As you get older, you may feel you need less. If you find getting to sleep difficult, see pages 149–150 for tips on encouraging sleep or combating insomnia.

Hormonal changes also affect your skin. A woman's natural oestrogen keeps her skin supple, but at menopause oestrogen levels decline drastically. Taking hormone replacement therapy (HRT, see pages 137–139) can put a glow back into your skin. Because hormone function is greatly dependent on nutrition, making sure you have a well-balanced diet is vital.

Many links have been made between stress and skin conditions such as dermatitis and eczema.

If you have a skin disorder that seems to flare up following times of stress, consider the possibility that it may be stress-related. Ideally, you should try to reduce the stress in your life and see if your skin clears up. However, this is often easier said than done. Using relaxation and visualisation techniques to calm yourself down might help you to relieve or alleviate a stress-related skin disorder.

EXTERNAL FACTORS

The weather can have many unwanted effects on your skin – especially weather extremes. It's not only the sun that can damage your skin – windy, cold and dry weather all take their toll.

The perfect forecast for your complexion, unfortunately, is a mild, moist, windless day with no sunshine at all!

The sun is your skin's worst enemy, leading to premature aging and, in some cases, skin cancer (see page 113). It causes skin to thin and sag, accounting for over 90 per cent of wrinkles. Your body needs a certain amount of sun – it's essential for vitamin D production – but overexposure should be avoided.

A suntan may look healthy, but it actually indicates that damage has occurred.

Together with strong winds and cold, the sun can also lead to tiny broken veins in the skin

To tan or not to tan?

If you must get a tan, do keep these guidelines in mind:

Sunblocks Containing mineral particles such as titanium dioxide and zinc oxide, sunblocks form a protective coating on the skin that reflects all UVA and UVB rays so the sun can't burn the skin.

Sunscreens These bind onto proteins in the top layer of skin, where they absorb some of the UVB and some UVA radiation. The sun protection factor (SPF) number multiplied by 20 minutes indicates the amount of time an average person can stay in the sun without burning. For example, SPF10 will protect you for 200 minutes (3 hr 20 min). You should reapply sunscreen hourly, and after swimming and perspiring, for adequate protection.

Self-tanning lotions These interact with your skin to turn it a natural-looking golden-brown colour – the safe 'tan' without the dangerous UV rays. The tan gradually fades over a week as the top layer of skin is shed. Apply evenly and allow a few hours for the colour to develop; don't wear clothes during this time. Self-tanning lotions contain only a weak sunscreen, so you will need to apply extra sunscreen if you go out in strong sunshine.

Sunbeds The radiation from sunbeds is as dangerous as the sun, and a base tan is no protection. Always use a sunscreen and moderate your sunbed usage to one hour a week at the very most.

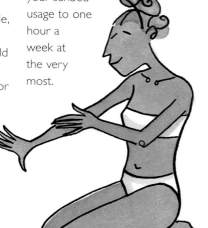

– an increasing problem as you get older – and leave your skin looking weather-beaten and leathery.

The sun's assault weapon is the UV radiation that bombards the Earth during the day. The three main forms of UV radiation are:

▶ **UVA** Most UVA rays reach ground level and, along with UVB, are responsible for the tanning and burning effects of the sun. UVA rays penetrate deep into the skin and cause a breakdown of the skin's underlying structure, resulting in premature wrinkling and aging. It is this type of UV that is needed for the production of vitamin D.

▶ **UVB** The most damaging UV radiation, UVB is partly screened by the ozone layer. Some UVB rays do get through, however, and can damage cell membranes and DNA, and contribute to skin cancer. UVB rays are strongest during the summer months.

▶ **UVC** UVC rays are potentially harmful but they rarely reach the Earth as they are absorbed by ozone in the upper atmosphere. Most sunscreens are formulated to block out UVB, although many broad-spectrum sunscreens, which block both UVA and UVB, are now widely available.

Although you cannot avoid the sun completely, take steps to prevent sun damage. In strong sunshine, apply a sunscreen of SPF15 or higher, which gives adequate protection for short periods – though some countries, such as Australia, are now recommending the use of SPF 30+. Reapply your sunscreen every one to two hours, or more often if you are perspiring heavily or are in and out of water, even if it is a waterproof variety.

You can also get sunburned on a cloudy day – over 80 per cent of the sun's UV rays that pass through the upper atmosphere can also penetrate clouds.

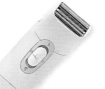

Unwanted-hair treatments

TREATMENT	DESCRIPTION	PROS AND CONS
Shaving	A variety of razors are on the market, from electric shavers to throw-away plastic razors.	It is a myth that shaved hair grows back thicker, but it does appear thicker as the hair is clipped at the thick stem rather than at the root. Regrowth occurs quickly.
Bleaching	Specially gentle dyeing creams are used to bleach darker hairs and blend them with the complexion.	Lasts for approximately one week, but does not remove hair and is therefore inappropriate for thick hair growth. It is relatively inexpensive, although it takes practice to do effectively at home.
Depilatory creams	Gentle creams dissolve the hair at the root.	Lasts for a week or two. May irritate the skin. Cheap and easy to use at home.
Waxing	Wax strips are placed on the hair, left to stiffen and then pulled off, wrenching the hairs from the root.	Lasts for a week or two. Cheap and easy to use at home, but can be painful and irritating to the skin. Strips are often easier to use than liquids, and are better for the skin.
Electric spring rotators	A taut spring is vibrated next to the skin, catching and pulling each hair out.	Lasts for a week or two and easy to use. Can be painful and cause irritation if the hair is coarse.
Electrolysis	Small electrical charges are sent through each hair, destroying it and weakening regrowth.	Lasting for up to a month, this must be done professionally and is therefore expensive. The hair does stop growing back eventually, although this may take a number of years for coarser hair.
Short-wave diathermy	Short-wave charges destroy each hair and prevent regrowth.	Lasts for up to two months, but this is an expensive and lengthy professional process. Regrowth thins out relatively quickly.

CELLULITE WORKOUT

Cellulite is the fat just under the surface of the skin that gives it a blotchy, 'orange-peel' look. It affects 80 per cent of women, mainly around the thighs and buttocks. It can be caused by high levels of the female hormone oestrogen and is linked to poor circulation, water retention, and toxins in the bloodstream.

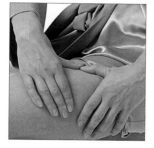

1 Massage the area deeply with a rough massage mitt, using a circular rubbing action. Press firmly to achieve good results.

2 Using your fingertips, work into the skin surface and cellulite. Use a rotating action, applying varying pressure. Perform this routine for 10 minutes every day.

Clothing can also protect you from the sun. Tightly woven fabrics such as denim offer more sun protection than the loosely woven cotton of a T-shirt, for example, which provides a protection of SPF7 when dry and only SPF5 when wet. Specialised synthetic fabrics can provide SPF30+.

Also, remember to take care to protect your skin in cold and dry weather. Use vaseline on lips to prevent chapping and an extra-rich cream on exposed skin.

Air-borne particles caused by industrial pollution, exhaust fumes and cigarette smoke can clog skin pores. They may also contain damaging free radicals. Using cleansing and moisturising products that contain antioxidants help limit damage from such particles.

HAIR REMOVAL

Men and women in Western countries spend countless hours plucking, shaving and waxing unwanted hair. There are no techniques to actually prevent the hair from

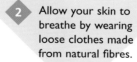

3 TIPS FOR HEALTHY SKIN

1 Avoid irritants, such as abrasives, strong detergents and extreme temperatures.

2 Allow your skin to breathe by wearing loose clothes made from natural fibres.

3 Keep your skin clean by washing or cleansing daily, but avoid drying soaps.

growing back, although electrolysis and diathermy weaken regrowth – hair growth may cease after years of regular treatment.

For most people, hair removal means an at-home treatment with a razor, wax or depilatory cream. After using any of these products it is important to moisturise the area thoroughly with a mild cream. Do not use deodorants or other irritants on your skin after shaving or waxing. If you are using a depilatory cream always follow the instructions on the packaging.

SKIN DISORDERS

Dermatitis is a dry, blotchy skin condition caused by irritants in soaps, detergents, solvents and oils, which remove the protective oil from the skin surface. Allergic dermatitis can be caused by a reaction to jewellery, perfume, plasters or glue. If you can identify the cause, you'll know what to avoid. Switching to chemical-free cosmetics, soaps and detergents can often help.

Psoriasis is the name given to patches of inflamed, red skin covered with silvery scales, which usually form on the upper body. It occurs when the skin replaces itself too quickly. It can be caused by tiredness, stress, illness or physical trauma and is treated with rest, stress management and, in severe cases, prescription creams or corticosteroid drugs.

Eczema, which appears to run in families, is characterised by red, itchy patches that may have small blisters. If your family has a history of eczema, asthma or hayfever, you are more likely to contract eczema, although some forms appear to be related to stress and skin yeast infections. Many over-the-counter treatments are available, but you should consult your doctor if symptoms persist.

Urticaria, also known as hives, is a raised, blotchy rash that can affect any part of the body. It can be triggered by eating nuts, berries or shellfish, by a bee sting, or by stroking an animal you are allergic to. Simple anti-itching creams can be useful for minor flare-ups, but visit your doctor for persistent rashes. If a rash causes the lips, tongue or throat to swell, seek immediate medical help.

Face care

Your face is your most expressive physical feature, reflecting your health, mood and feelings. Health and contentment are the greatest beauty aids – but it also pays to take care of your skin.

The state of your skin is often a reflection of your lifestyle – your diet, health, fitness, environment, personality, workload, emotional state and sleep pattern. It's well worth taking care of your skin.

Simple measures you can take to safeguard your complexion include cleansing, to remove impurities that can clog the skin pores, and moisturising, to counteract the drying effect of the sun and of heated and air-conditioned environments.

The hormonal changes that occur as you get older take their toll on your skin. The skin's production of natural oils diminishes, making skin drier and less elastic, and slowing cell renewal. Also, the number of collagen and elastin fibres in the skin declines, which accelerates the sagging and drooping caused by gravity and years of facial movements. Other factors also contribute to dry skin, such as tobacco smoke and daily washing with soap-based products. Avoid using harsh cleansers or toners that strip the skin of essential moisture. To help keep the skin hydrated, use a good moisturiser. It won't actually add moisture, but will prevent moisture loss and help protect your skin against the effects of wind and dry conditions. Choose one that also provides UV protection.

Other measures often recommended for healthy, supple skin include facial exercises and massage. If done regularly, facial massage can be effective – it improves blood circulation and speeds up the flow of lymph, so that nutrients reach the skin more easily and waste products are expelled.

Wrinkles occur as a result of sun damage and years of facial muscle movements, such as smiling, squinting and frowning. Look at your wrinkles fondly and remember the expressiveness that accounts for many of them. Beware of some anti-wrinkle products – price is no indication of their effectiveness. A number of studies have shown that inexpensive moisturisers often do as good a job – or even better – than many higher-priced products (see page 78).

The wonder products

What do all the new miracle ingredients really mean, and how well do they work?

Alpha- and beta-hydroxy acids (AHAs and BHAs) Also called fruit acids, these are commonly used as exfoliants to remove dead skin and speed up the process of cell renewal. Derived from natural products such as apples, milk, sugar cane and papaya (pawpaw), they work by dissolving the natural adhesive that attaches dead skin cells to the epidermis, accelerating cell production. Both AHAs and BHAs can be harsh on dry or sensitive skin, and concentrations of about 4 per cent are considered safe.

They may also enhance older skin (over the age of about 35), particularly if damaged by years of sun exposure.

Antioxidants These come in the form of vitamins A (see page 79), C and E. They protect the skin from the damaging effect of free radicals, resulting from exposure to the sun, tobacco smoke and other factors. A recent French study suggests that antioxidants in skin-care products may also repair skin damage.

Ceramides Helping to stabilise skin structure by bonding cells, ceramide creams are believed to be beneficial for older or sun-damaged skin.

QUICK & EASY
facial workout

Good news in the beauty world: exercising your facial muscles may provide long-term benefits that can compete with cosmetic surgery. Toning the muscles in your face and neck tightens loose skin and breaks down fat, giving your face a better and younger shape. Areas that respond well include the jawline, notably combating a double chin and the jowls around the mouth and nose.

If you do the exercises at least once a day, really working your facial muscles, you should soon see great results. Aim to repeat each exercise 10 times, which will take about 10 minutes.

FIRMING YOUR JOWLS

1 Push your lower lip over your upper lip, jutting your bottom jaw outwards. Stretch your chin forwards and upwards so the skin is taut.

2 Smile your lips upwards and outwards for the count of 5. Hold the position for the count of 5 and then slowly relax. Repeat.

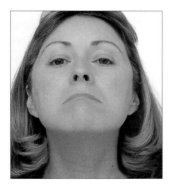

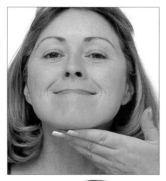

DOUBLE-CHIN WORKOUT

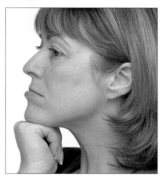

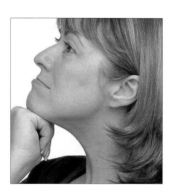

1 Lean on a table with your chin resting on your fist. Pull your lower lip over your top lip, jutting your bottom jaw outwards.

2 Press your tongue against the roof of your mouth behind your front teeth and feel the muscle pulling under your jaw. Relax and repeat.

IMPROVING UPPER EYELIDS

1 Looking ahead, place your index fingers along the bottom of your eyebrows. Push your fingers up firmly against your forehead.

2 Close your eyelids slowly and hold closed. Count to 5, slowly relax and open your eyes, then repeat.

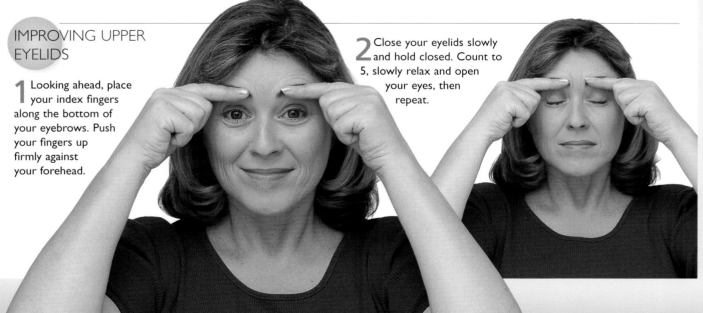

Research and development in the field of enzyme technology have resulted in a new generation of beauty products. These new skin treatments aim to use enzymes to promote healthier, younger-looking skin.

Enzyme technology

Within your skin, a number of chemical reactions take place, brought about by communication between enzymes. Some reactions boost skin cell production and growth, promoting a healthy, firm complexion. Other enzymes are destructive, and these may become overactive in old age or as a result of pollution and sun damage. Another group of enzymes encourages skin cleansing by dissolving proteins and fats, making excellent exfoliants.

Extracts from natural substances are used to control the enzymes. For example, pineapple and papaya (pawpaw) extracts are used in many moisturising formulas, and honey and heather are particularly good for firming creams.

New research into how enzymes communicate with one another may take enzyme technology a step further. It is thought that if we know how they interact we can improve the efficiency of other products. However, research is in its infancy and major advances may take some time.

The new generation of skin-care products claims to harness the beneficial effects of plant enzymes to create a cream capable of improving skin health and keeping skin youthful.

Moisturising your skin – whatever the weather – protects your face from dirt and pollution and helps to keep it supple.

Your choice of moisturiser will be determined by your skin type. Unless you have extremely dry skin, avoid creams with a high oil content as these can make your skin look droopy. You should also apply a light moisturiser or special eye cream to the delicate skin around the eyes two or three times a week – avoid heavy ones, which can promote wrinkles. Try not to stretch the skin, by applying eye creams with a light dotting movement; the moisturiser quickly soaks into the skin so there is no need to rub this delicate area. The lips should also be regularly moisturised.

Since the neck is prone to dryness and wrinkling, it is advisable to apply a specially enriched neck cream every evening.

In cold winter climates, you may need a slightly heavier moisturiser as an additional layer. You can help protect the skin from extremes of indoor heat and outdoor cold by moisturising throughout the day.

Most of the skin's repair and regeneration take place while you sleep. Although sleep itself is the major factor in allowing skin renewal, some people feel that they also require a rich night cream to feed and moisturise the skin. Some night creams contain antioxidant vitamins A and E, which counteract free radicals and other toxic molecules.

Many people say their skin feels tight and taut unless they apply cream at night, while some experts believe moisturising your face overnight keeps the skin from breathing while you sleep. Your skin type will determine the best skin-care routine for you.

Air-borne pollutants should also be avoided, including exhaust fumes, dust and, of course, cigarette smoke. Give up smoking; it prevents your blood from transporting nutrients and starves the cells in your body of oxygen.

SKIN-CARE ROUTINE

A basic routine can take as little as five minutes, with visible results within a few weeks. If you find your skin drying or showing damage as a result of your new routine, you may need to change your cleanser or toner. Always be gentle and use light motions when applying cream around the eye area, and don't use toner here.

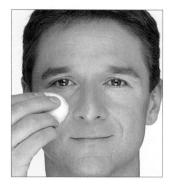

1 Pour a small amount of cleanser on to a cotton ball and gently wipe your face. Take a clean cotton ball and wipe off any excess cleanser.

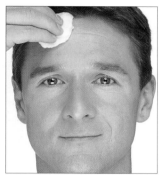

2 Using a toner suitable for your skin type, pour a little on to a cotton ball and smooth over your skin. You will feel the astringent effect.

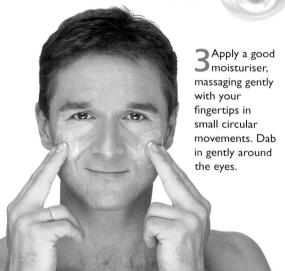

3 Apply a good moisturiser, massaging gently with your fingertips in small circular movements. Dab in gently around the eyes.

Eat healthily, with plenty of antioxidant-rich fruit and vegetables (see page 47–48), and drink plenty of water to spring-clean your system. Keeping your weight steady prevents the skin sagging and the occurrence of stretch marks.

OTHER SKIN-CARE TREATMENTS

Exfoliation is the process of removing layers of dead skin – making your face feel clean and refreshed. The most widely used exfoliants contain tiny granular elements and chemicals such as plant enzymes to slough off dead skin, draw out impurities from the pores, and cleanse and tighten the skin (see page 78). Give your skin a weekly exfoliation treatment at home with one of the many exfoliants available from chemists.

Combination beauty treatments, including facials, can enhance the complexion, although they are unlikely to eradicate lines and wrinkles. They can aid deep cleansing and enhance circulation, encouraging better

skin health and helping to prevent further damage. By promoting relaxation, they can alleviate stress – a major contributor to skin aging.

REVOLUTIONARY WRINKLE REPAIR

Recent research into the anti-aging effects of vitamin A has resulted in a skin-care product that is now available over the counter.

An earlier product, Retin A, which contains retinoic acid – vitamin A in its most powerful form – has been available on prescription since the 1970s and was hailed as a remarkably effective treatment for acne. Users of the product also reported that fine lines and wrinkles disappeared and their complexions were smoother. It has taken years for vitamin A to be refined into a form mild enough to be incorporated into beauty creams sold over the counter. Look out for facial beauty products containing 'retinol'. This mild vitamin A derivative stimulates the renewal of skin cells and generates collagen production, ironing out fine lines and tightening the skin, making it appear younger.

MAKE-UP TIPS FOR OLDER WOMEN

For some it provides a great confidence boost, for others it adds a theatrical touch to their lives; make-up offers a fun, creative and practical way to enhance your appearance. Make-up artists can create many different looks – from the natural to the outrageous – but there are no hard and fast rules. Make-up is an art form and finding your own style can be an exciting challenge.

As you get older, your make-up should be adapted to your skin and personality changes. Take a critical look at your make-up. Have you always worn your make-up this way? What kind of overall effect are you trying to achieve? Do you like the classic 1950s chic appearance, with carefully coiffured hair, sharp, strong lipstick and subtle browns around your eyes? The creative, earthy look with greens, golds and browns? Or do you prefer no-nonsense shades that blend with your complexion? Glamour calls for dark eye make-up and bold lipstick, but this may be

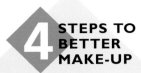

4 STEPS TO BETTER MAKE-UP

1 Stick to natural-looking colours.

2 Avoid making harsh or bold lines.

3 Blend blushers and shadows with the surrounding area.

4 Use a light touch with foundation and concealer.

too harsh a look for older women. Use blue, mauve and pink eye shadows for a softer, more feminine style, painting the lips a natural-looking pink. Always make sure that your style complements your personality.

Concealers come in several forms, from the simple and portable stick blemish concealers to liquid types that are designed to cover large areas. Some products have light-reflective crystals that help disguise harsh lines and blemishes such as small thread veins around the nose. Whatever your choice, make sure it blends with your foundation – if it is too light, you will highlight your blemishes! You may also want to use a primer – a tinted cream that is used to add colour to your face – or a tinted foundation to rebalance or even out colour. Green foundation is used to tone down a rosy complexion, mauve lifts sallow, olive skin and peach gives pasty skin warmth. White is sometimes used for a clear-looking, porcelain effect but it can be too dramatic for an older face.

FOUNDATION

Make-up is a great way to accentuate your good points and create a certain style; it can also hide any blemishes, such as shadows, spots or broken veins. Finding the right look for you can take practice and you need to decide what impression you are trying to create before you start.

3 Use a brush or a powder puff to lightly coat your face evenly with translucent powder. Using a tissue, gently wipe off any excess and smooth the finish.

4 Subtly brush blusher on to your cheeks, using a shade darker than your foundation. Use highlighter above the cheekbones.

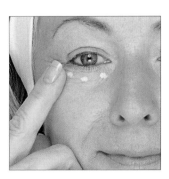

1 Use concealer to cover any blemishes or dark patches on the skin, such as scars or shadows beneath the eyes. Apply lightly with a dotting action.

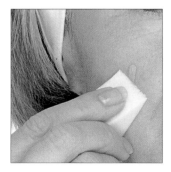

2 Apply foundation gently with a slightly damp make-up sponge. Choose a shade close to your natural colouring. Blend it from your face into your neck.

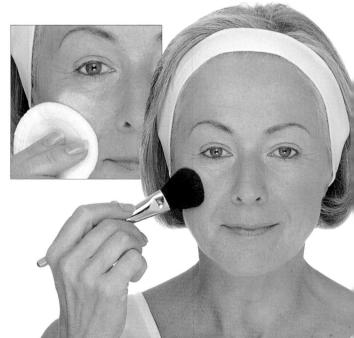

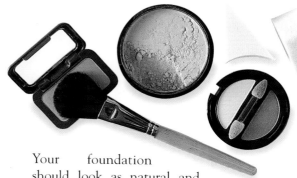

Your foundation should look as natural and invisible as possible. Heavy foundations will cover a poor complexion, but they contain large amounts of powder and can appear cakey. A temptation for many older women is to pile on the foundation in an effort to conceal wrinkles and mask uneven skin tone. This is the worst thing to do, however, since the foundation will simply clog wrinkles and end up highlighting them. The best approach is to use a medium-cover formula that covers the skin evenly but lightly and lasts longer. Apply sparingly, as a light touch will flatter older skin. Look for foundations containing light-reflecting particles that give the skin a dewy finish. If you have oily skin, use an oil-free base, and a moisture cream formula for dry skin.

Use a loose translucent powder, which provides a natural-looking finish. Avoid heavy, dark-looking powders that can fill up even small creases in the skin, making it look older.

Blusher enhances your bone structure, acting like a shadow. Take a good look at your face and decide what you want to accentuate and what you would rather downplay. Most people find that using a subtle blusher under the cheekbones helps to give their face the best contours.

Try to create an impression rather than a strip of colour – the blusher is there to accentuate the natural shape of your face in a subtle way.

Others use it on the sides of the forehead and chin, and you may want to experiment with these areas to see what effect they have. For an older complexion, muted tones of blusher are the most flattering – avoid vibrant pinks and reds. Apply lightly so that just a hint of natural-looking colour is evident.

EYES

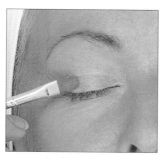

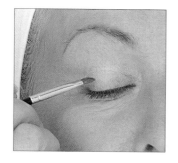

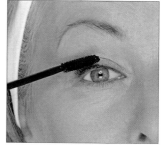

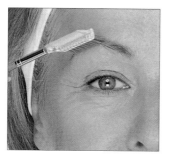

5 Apply eye shadow a little at a time to test the results. Darker shades in certain areas will have different effects on your look, so try a few variations before deciding on a final result. A dark colour on the eyelid with a lighter shade below the brow will make the eyes look larger. A darker shade along the socket area with a very light colour on the lid will brighten the eyes.

6 Eyeliner defines the outside of the eye, making the eyes look larger. Using a pencil or an eyeliner brush, make one continuous sweeping movement to apply the liner directly under the eye and above your upper eyelash. Don't overdo it – and wipe any mistakes off carefully with a cotton bud.

7 Before you put on mascara, carefully comb out your eyelashes to separate them and prevent the mascara from clogging. Avoid using thick mascara and apply sparingly. If your eyelashes stick out straight, use an eyelash curler to give them extra shape.

8 Use a damp toothbrush to comb your eyebrows. Pluck any wayward hairs with a pair of tweezers. You can also use tweezers to shape or thin your eyebrows. Pluck hairs below the brow, following their natural shape. Colour with a black or brown eyebrow pencil for definition.

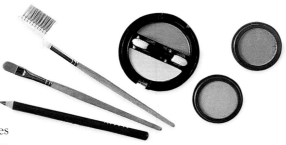

Microfine powder blushers are best for a light, subtle blush that you can build up or tone down easily. Creams eventually dry and lose that fresh look. Be wary of blusher gels, they dry quickly, which makes them difficult to blend properly. New powder–cream blush formulas combine a lasting matt finish with excellent colour.

Eyebrows may be enhanced using an eyebrow pencil, but use the colour most similar to your own and apply lightly. Remove stray hairs, but don't overpluck your eyebrows or use heavy eyebrow make-up.

Mascara should be worn very lightly and in a colour close to your own eyelashes. Make sure that your mascara wand is not clogged, or your eyelashes might get stuck together. You can curl your eyelashes with an eyelash curler, which will open up the eyes and make the eyelashes appear longer. Remove any smudges from around your eye with a cotton

bud. Mascara can be waterproof, smudge-proof, long-lasting, lash-lengthening or lash-thickening. Select the variety that is most suitable to your lifestyle and try it out.

Eye shadow and eyeliner can really bring your whole face to life. Eye shadow comes in a host of colours and can create many different effects, but make sure you use shades that will enhance your natural colouring. Eyeliners are available in pencil and liquid form and can be worn alone or in conjunction with eye shadow. See page 81 for some tips on applying eye make-up.

Using a kohl eyeliner pencil or a liquid eyeliner brush, carefully draw a line over the

LIPS

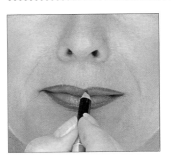

9 Carefully outline your lips with a lip pencil to help prevent lipstick from running into the surrounding skin. Follow the natural line of your lips with a sweeping motion.

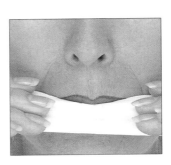

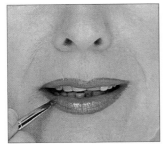

10 Paint your lips with a lip brush or lipstick. Colour up to the lip line, but do not cover it. Ideally your lipstick should be slightly lighter than the lip pencil.

11 Use a clean tissue to remove any excess lipstick from your lips. Do this by folding the tissue and placing between your lips and holding them closed for a few seconds. Do not rub them together.

The end result is the best measure of your make-up skills. Take a critical look at yourself in a well-lit mirror and judge the colours you are using and the way you have applied them. Try out different techniques until you find a look you like. Bear in mind that this will probably change over time. Rework your make-up style every six months or so to keep up with your changing appearance.

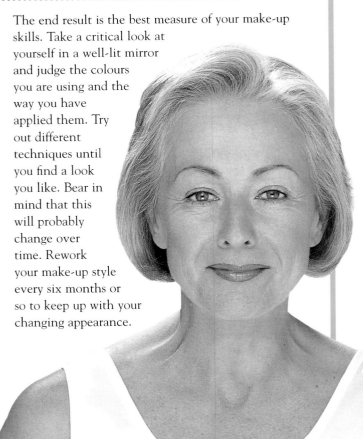

upper lid from the inner to the outer corner, just above the base of the eyelash. A slow, sweeping motion suits most people, although you may find your own method easier. Opening your eye, you can draw a line on the bottom inner rim, taking it into the corners of the eye. The corners of the eye can be emphasised with eyeliner to lengthen the eye, although you must apply the eyeliner thinly for a subtle effect.

Consider the eye shadow colour that you most frequently wear and the reasons why you wear it. Try out a few other colours and note the different effects that they create. The artistry of make-up is as much about experimentation and change as it is about knowledge and experience.

When applying eye shadow, particularly dark colours, place a square of tissue paper under the eye to catch any stray particles of powder that may fall and become lodged in the fine wrinkles beneath the eyes.

Lipstick is the final touch; in fact, many women wear lipstick alone regularly, bringing colour, light and life to their faces. Only you know the colour that looks right and feels good, although there are some considerations. Matt lipstick is usually preferable to gloss or shimmering lipstick for the older woman as it appears more subtle and natural. A strong colour, such as burgundy, can look most effective with pale eye make-up. Play down your eye shadow and embolden your lips for a dramatic look.

Lipsticks are now made to be long-lasting and smudge-proof, using a base of polymer and silicone. They also seal moisturising ingredients into the lips, providing a demi-matt finish and moisturising from within.

Lip liners, either pencils or liquids, give a solid durable colour that can be used for defining the shape of the lips. They also seal in lipstick, preventing it from bleeding outside the natural border of your lips – a problem many older women encounter. Lip gloss can be added over lipstick and liners, to give a subtle shine, but use it sparingly, since it may destabilise and smudge lipstick if applied too liberally.

Special effects for special problems

Different make-up combinations can balance an uneven face or cover up problems:

Shapeless lips Use a lip liner or lip pencil to subtly exaggerate the shape of the lips, especially the 'm' shape at the top.

Thin lips With a lip liner or pencil, draw a line just outside, or on the outside edge of, your lips. Fill in as usual.

Deep-set eyes Use a pale colour on the eyelid and a slightly darker shade above the eyelid and below the eyebrow. Use mascara sparingly.

Small eyes Circle the entire eye with a smudged brown or grey shadow and use eyeliner above the top eyelash. Highlight the area just below the eyebrow with a pale shade of the same colour.

Long face Shade the jawline and around the top of the forehead with darker foundation.

Round face Use a darker foundation under the cheekbones to give your face more shape, and highlight on top of the cheekbones and a little in the centre of the chin.

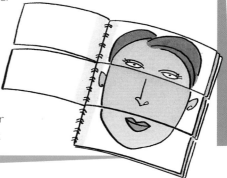

Remove your make-up properly before you go to bed. If you leave it on while you sleep, it will be absorbed into the pores, clogging them and causing blemishes and skin damage. It will also dry out the skin and be more difficult to remove in the morning. There are many make-up removal products that enable you to take off even the heaviest make-up. Some, however, can be very greasy and it may be necessary to cleanse or wash your face afterwards.

Don't be afraid to experiment with colour and style, but be wary of overusing make-up in an effort to turn back the clock. Remember that accepting the changes in your looks and subtly using make-up as a tool for making the most of your appearance are far more effective and flattering than trying to look like something you're not.

Cosmetic surgery promises a quick-fix approach to aging skin, but the high cost and potential risks lead many to seek alternatives. Natural treatments can give cheaper and less artificial-looking results with just a little effort.

BEFORE MEDICAL FACELIFT

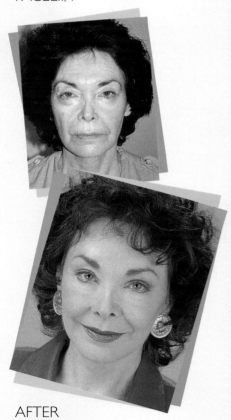

AFTER MEDICAL FACELIFT

NATURAL AND
medical facelifts

Some people undergo cosmetic surgery to remove wrinkles and other signs of aging. But most prefer the natural approach to the quest for youthful looks – using skin-care concepts, exercise and special complementary remedies to counter or conceal problems.

There is no question that cosmetic surgery has a more dramatic effect on your facial appearance. No natural treatment can lift the face and smooth the complexion as effectively. Cosmetic surgery is also fast and easy, requiring no strenuous exercise or daily care routine.

A facelift raises your profile, brightening your expression and giving your skin a firm and youthful look. It eliminates the lines, wrinkles and sagging acquired with age that make you look tired. Many people describe feeling younger and vastly more confident after cosmetic surgery. However, a facelift won't remove superficial lines around the lips and eyes, and the effect on nose to mouth furrows may be minimal.

Also, there are significant drawbacks to cosmetic surgery. One main factor is the expense. A basic facelift costs as much as a luxury cruise – for most people it is simply not an option.

Furthermore, although the surgery itself is usually quick and easy, it may be months before the final result can be seen. Minor facial surgery, such as a brow lift, takes around 10 to 14 days for recovery, but it can take up to six months for full facelifts to settle and for swelling to subside. Following a facelift, most people have painful swelling and serious bruising and have to stay at home for a couple of weeks. Bruising often continues into the second month of recovery, although, at this stage, make-up can disguise it. Loss of sensation and numbness in the skin can remain for six months or more.

Computer imaging techniques can provide a preview of the 'new' you but there is no guarantee that the end result will be exactly as you anticipated. Most facial surgery is irreversible, so be sure that you can live with the final effect.

Serious physical risks include nerve damage, visible scarring, infection, areas of permanent numbness, loss of natural movement and facial unevenness.

There is also a chance that the beneficial effects of the surgery will not last – scarring can swell and make the skin age faster; damage to the skin and muscles can lead to skin sagging; or the ears may pull down and distort the skin. If you are considering cosmetic surgery, contact a reputable surgeon, preferably through recommendation by a former patient.

There are many natural ways that you can keep yourself looking young without surgical treatment. The effects are not as drastic or far-reaching, but neither are the costs so great or the risks so high.

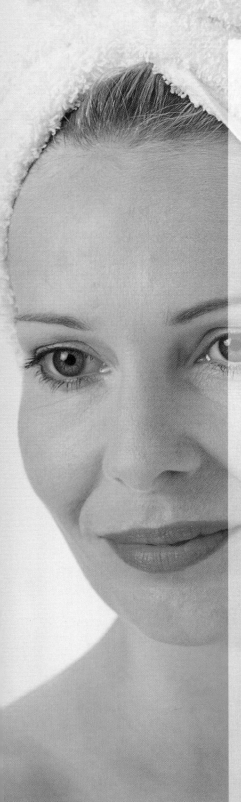

COSMETIC SURGERY

Frown lines It is possible to improve frown lines with surgical injections of collagen, although the results are only temporary. Botox – botulism toxin – injections are highly effective. The toxin paralyses the muscles in the forehead that make you frown. An alternative measure is a surgical brow lift.

Eye bags Techniques such as upper or lower blepharoplasty are used to reduce sagging around the eyes. Fat is permanently removed and the skin and muscles around the eyes are tightened.

Dark circles Darkness around the eyes can be improved with laser treatment. Some dark circles are shadows from bags, in which case blepharoplasty (see above) is useful.

Spider veins Surgeons can remove these veins with a hyfrecator – an electrical device that uses intense heat (cauterisation) to seal the blood vessels below the skin's surface.

Lip lines The injection of collagen (lasting around six months) or silicone can reduce the lines around the lips and also make lips appear much fuller. A newer, and more expensive, technique involves Gore-tex thread, which is inserted into the skin around the lips to create a padded effect.

Double chins and jowls These can be eliminated with a total facelift. Surgeons make an incision behind the ears and literally pull the skin up to achieve the desired effect. Liposuction is another option.

Age spots Laser resurfacing or a chemical peel will treat liver spots by removing the top layer of skin. Liquid nitrogen, electrocoagulation or frozen carbon dioxide are other treatments.

NATURAL TREATMENTS

Frown lines To improve a furrowed brow, use a good antiwrinkle cream. Products containing 'retinol' are considered most effective (see page 79). Facial massage and exercises promote blood flow and good muscle tone, which both help tighten the skin.

Eye bags Soothing eye gels and eye masks can gently tighten the skin – as can placing a couple of cool, damp camomile tea bags over your eyes and resting for ten minutes.

Dark circles Shadows under the eyes are not necessarily caused by tiredness, although they are exacerbated by it. Try to get plenty of exercise during the day so you sleep properly at night. Applying a light artificial tanning lotion to the face will even out dark areas.

Red patches and rosacea By taking vitamins B_1, B_2 and C and the mineral zinc you can improve skin condition. A vitamin A supplement may also help restore and maintain clear skin, but taking too much can be dangerous.

Lip lines A bi-weekly application of a rich face cream to the skin can reduce wrinkles around the mouth. Afterwards, dab a bandage or strong tissue, with peanut oil, stretch over the area and leave for ten minutes.

Double chins and jowls Use facial exercises (see page 77) and massage techniques to reduce sagging in the chin and jowl area. These exercises also tone the muscles and strengthen the skin's underlying collagen.

Age spots A self-tanning lotion will conceal the dark pigmentation of liver spots and even out skin tone. Or, apply a little lemon juice to the area – it has a slight bleaching effect.

Body care

Your overall appearance results from a combination of factors, including your bone structure, posture, musculature and body fat. Many of these are inherited, but you can still enhance the way your body looks.

Your body shape is determined by two main factors: your genetic make-up and your lifestyle. In other words, you can't change your basic build, but you can make the most of your body shape by taking steps to keep yourself fit and healthy.

Your genes determine your skeletal framework, including your height and the shape and size of your bones in proportion to each other. Consider your own genetic shape – once you get to know it, you can start to make the most of it – accepting your faults and capitalising on your assets.

SHAPING UP YOUR LIFE

The amount of fat on your body, and where it is stored, greatly affects your appearance. Factors that dictate fat storage include exercise, diet, your digestive system and your metabolism. Stress, sleep patterns, hormonal fluctuations, and the use of stimulants and other drugs, prescribed or recreational, also play a part. There is little you can do to influence where your body stores fat, but you can control the quantity of fat you carry. See Chapter 1 for ways to increase your metabolism and Chapter 2 for ways to lose weight.

WHAT DOES YOUR POSTURE REVEAL?

Your posture and body profile probably say more about you than you know! The way that you stand shows others how you view yourself and the world around you, be it defensively or enthusiastically. Stop to think about what your posture says about you. Here are a few common patterns that people slip into and how other people are likely to interpret them.

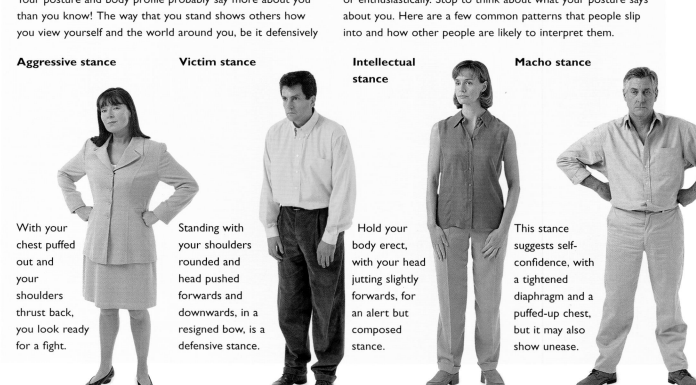

Aggressive stance

With your chest puffed out and your shoulders thrust back, you look ready for a fight.

Victim stance

Standing with your shoulders rounded and head pushed forwards and downwards, in a resigned bow, is a defensive stance.

Intellectual stance

Hold your body erect, with your head jutting slightly forwards, for an alert but composed stance.

Macho stance

This stance suggests self-confidence, with a tightened diaphragm and a puffed-up chest, but it may also show unease.

QUICK & EASY MANICURE

Your hands are on show all the time and in use most of the time. Spending a few minutes every week on a simple manicure is sure to be a good investment.

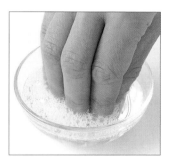

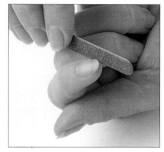

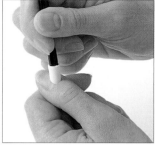

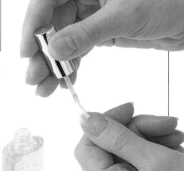

1 Soak your fingers in a bowl of warm, soapy water for a few minutes. Use a nail brush to get your nails really clean. Rinse and then dry thoroughly.

2 File your nails with an emery board, using long, sweeping movements. Cut them first if necessary. Rinse again and dry carefully.

3 Use some cuticle cream on each nail and gently ease back the cuticles.

4 Use a buffer to build up a natural-looking shine. You may want to paint your nails. If so, apply a couple of coats to prevent chipping.

Many people gain weight as they approach middle age. They often find that keeping in trim is not as easy as it was when they were younger, and it becomes something that must be concentrated upon and actively worked at (see Chapter 1 for inspiration).

A much neglected part of good shape is good posture – the way that you hold yourself not only influences your skeletal form, but also speaks volumes for the kind of person you are.

Consider your posture by standing in front of a mirror in a balanced and upright position, and then in your usual stance. You may need to do this several times before you pick up all the nuances of your particular posture. The difference between the two poses will help you to identify your posture problem areas.

The shoulders tend to store stress and tension, particularly in relation to responsibility and work. Tension in the shoulders and neck often causes people to slouch or, less commonly, to hold their shoulders up or back stiffly and unnaturally.

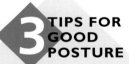

3 TIPS FOR GOOD POSTURE

1 Imagine that someone is suspending you from a thread at the top of your head.

2 Distribute your weight evenly over both feet.

3 Keep your shoulders square and upright. Do not slouch.

Slumping the abdomen forwards is another common problem. Tension or change in the natural line of the abdomen and pelvis is thought to reflect attitudes to sexuality, pleasure and relationships – many actresses develop the habit of sticking their backsides out to accentuate their sexuality. On the other hand, a fat stomach or pregnancy can also make you arch your back and stick out your bottom as you attempt to compensate for the weight in front.

The way that you hold your head and the posture of your neck are also important, especially if you jut your chin out or forwards, which can make you seem aggressive.

Maintaining good posture actually takes less energy in the long run than slumping or slouching because of the imbalance created by a poor stance and the effort needed to compensate for it. Improving your posture is also good for your health, easing muscle tension and improving circulation.

Many of the back and neck problems suffered by older people are the result of poor posture. It is well worth making the effort to correct bad posture habits and prevent or alleviate any discomfort.

TROUBLE AREAS

Lack of muscle tone in the arms is a common problem for older women. This causes sagging flesh and pallid, listless skin, and results in poor circulation. Many everyday tasks can keep the arm muscles active and toned, including kneading bread, gardening, household cleaning and washing the car. Swinging your arms while walking will also help. Putting extra vigour into these activities will make a difference, or you can do specific exercises to tone your arms.

The stomach is a problem area for many older people – particularly men. Many men find that although their legs and arms can be quite toned and shapely, fat settles in the stomach area, giving them a bloated appearance incongruous with the rest of their body. Cutting down on fatty foods and alcohol is important but not always fully effective. Regularly performing exercises that specifically target the abdominal muscles is the best way to flatten the stomach and improve posture, as it supports your spine. See page 29 for examples of abdominal exercises and ways to improve general muscle tone.

Other weak spots for older women are the thighs and buttocks. In women, fat deposits usually settle in these areas and tone and contour are easily lost. Walking is great for targeting these areas. Walk briskly so you can really feel these muscles working – whether you are walking to a shop or going to the park. For concentrated exercises for the thighs and buttocks, see page 33.

Varicose veins can be caused by many factors, although poor diet and inactivity are particular culprits as they impede the blood flow to and from the legs. Pregnancy and circulatory disorders can also lead to varicose veins. If you have any problems with veins, such as discoloration or swelling, you should see your doctor. To help prevent varicose veins developing, avoid standing for long periods and keep your weight at a healthy level. To prevent or alleviate varicose veins, walk regularly and wear support tights. If they are particularly troublesome, ask your doctor to refer you to a surgeon for complete removal.

FOOT CARE

Giving your feet a good pedicure and massage is a real luxury—people often simply don't have time for their feet. Take a few minutes every week to pay a little attention to the feet that carry you around.

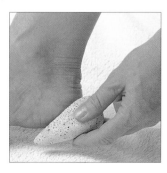

1 After soaking your feet in warm, soapy water, use a pumice stone to remove any hard or dead skin from the bottom of the foot.

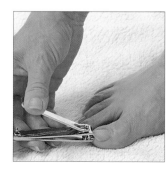

2 Cut and file the nails. To prevent ingrowing toenails, cut the nails straight across, and file the corners smooth.

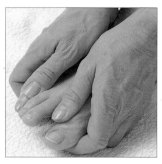

3 Rinse again and dry the feet well, especially between the toes. Apply moisturiser or foot cream.

4 Apply cuticle cream and gently push back your cuticles, particularly if you plan to paint your toenails.

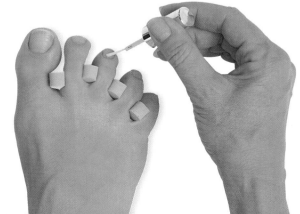

COSMETIC
body surgery

Some people – men as well as women – turn to cosmetic body surgery, either to enhance what heredity has bequeathed or to repair the ravages caused by time, lifestyle, illness or pregnancy. As with all operations, there are risks of complications. Some forms of cosmetic surgery may result in scarring, and particularly where fat removal is concerned, any improvement may only be temporary. In addition, surgery is expensive and success is not guaranteed. Choose clinics and surgeons that are accredited by a reputable organisation and seek a referral from your doctor, or, preferably, ask friends who have undergone similar treatment to recommend one. Discuss the procedure, risks and possible side effects with the practitioner so you know what to expect. Don't commit yourself until you have given all aspects serious consideration.

HANDS AND ARMS

Hand surgery Bony hands can be filled with fat drawn by liposuction from other body areas.

Underarm lift This operation removes the excess flesh that causes sagging. It can leave a large scar.

BREASTS AND CHEST

Chest reduction/augmentation Men who have excess fat around the chest area can have it removed by liposuction. Augmentation involves inserting an implant under the pectoral (chest) muscles to create a more muscular look. The procedure leaves thin scars under the arms, which may fade with time.

Mastoplexy This is surgery to lift and reshape the breasts. It involves removing excess tissue, tightening the breast and repositioning the nipple. A similar procedure is used to reduce overlarge breasts.

Breast augmentation Implants may be inserted for enlargement or improved shaping. Because of concerns over the safety of silicone, many implants now contain saline or soya oil. The procedure leaves a thin scar at the base of the breasts.

ABDOMEN

Abdominoplasty (tummy tuck) Involving major surgery, this technique is used to remove excess fat and skin, leaving thin scars.

HIPS AND THIGHS

Fat transposition Fat is removed from area where there is an excess, such as the abdomen, and injected into other areas to even out lumps.

Ultrasound body sculpting A chemical is injected under the skin and then high-frequency sound waves are used to liquefy the fat layer, which is then suctioned out.

Cellulolypolysis This procedure removes cellulite ('orange-peel' type of fat under the skin). Fine-needle electrodes are inserted under the skin to heat the tissues and melt the fat so that it can drain away. Patients control the current through the electrodes.

Thigh lift Cuts are made in the groin area and excess skin removed to tighten flabby inner thighs. The patient must stay immobile for extended periods for proper healing.

LOWER LEGS

Sclerotherapy Here varicose veins or spidery thread veins are surgically removed. Sometimes, glycerine, or another chemical with similar properties, is injected into the blood vessels to seal them.

Calf implants In this procedure, fat is removed by liposuction from elsewhere in the body and inserted to give extra shape to spindly calves.

Style

Practical or chic, clothes can flavour your life with a special personal style, boosting your confidence and complementing your lifestyle. True style is about knowing what is right for you and when to wear it.

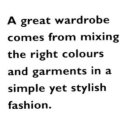

A great wardrobe comes from mixing the right colours and garments in a simple yet stylish fashion.

Clothes have always made a statement – from the pantaloons worn by dandies of pre-revolutionary France to the figure-enhancing dresses of the 19th century. Contemporary fashions seem quite tame by comparison.

The secret of stylish dressing is to develop your own style, based on your colouring and figure. Start by taking an objective and realistic look at your body and figure type. You need to assess your good points, identify the figure flaws you wish to downplay, and consider the practical requirements imposed by your work and your lifestyle.

YOUR PERSONAL STYLE

Do you have a favourite article of clothing? If so, what is it and why is it so precious to you? Many people like specific clothes because they say something about them – expressing particular aspects of their personality, views and beliefs.

Think about what you communicate through your clothes. Here are some of the fashion statements that people make at different times.

▶ *Classic* Making great use of black, navy, white and ivory, the classic look aims to add a subtle sense of the past. Always understated and appropriate, this timeless formula is easy to manage, includes up-to-date pieces and suits many people.

▶ *Outdoors* Healthy and bursting with energy, this practical look cares little for figure-enhancing styles – although many say that being fit means that you never need them! Tracksuit tops and bottoms, sneakers or walking shoes, anoraks, bright clean colours and a healthy glow are all you need.

▶ *Natural* Using plain, traditional styles, this look relies on natural fibres and colours to convey a feeling of earthiness. Designs are loose and fluid, and use plenty of layers.

▶ *Casual chic* A friendly and practical style, you can do almost anything in a stylish shirt or polo-neck, a pair of casual trousers and comfortable shoes. A black shirt and jeans, or a white T-shirt under a black leather jacket, create a clean, comfortable look.

▶ *Artistic* Brightly coloured scarves, beads and flowing shirts, often in ethnic prints, are the mainstay of an artsy wardrobe. Retro jackets and old hats can be the focus of an outfit, often worn with personality, charm and humour by creative types.

▶ *Glamorous* Figure-hugging, fitted dresses, tops and trousers are often worn to present a sleek, dramatic and well-groomed image. Bold, simple colours such as black, white, red and gold make the most effective statement – think Hollywood!

REVAMP YOUR WARDROBE

Give yourself a wardrobe workout: go through absolutely every item of clothing that you have in your wardrobe and consider the following questions – Do I wear this often? Does it look good (you may need to try it on)? Does it still fit properly? Is it looking worn or losing its shape? Is it looking a little dated? Do I still like it?

Decide which of the following four categories each item of clothing falls into, and put them into different piles.

▶ *Pass with flying colours* You wear this a lot and know that it suits your image.

▶ *Fail* These clothes are doing you no favours: you don't wear them or like them. Throw them out or give them away.

▶ *Have possibilities* You may be able to do something with these clothes if you can find the right items to team with them.

▶ *Need mending or altering* You obviously need to find time to get these done. Put them in order of priority and be realistic – will you really wear that pair of jeans if you make them into shorts?

Go through your belts, bags, shoes and other accessories and do the same, teaming them up with suitable outfits and throwing out anything that isn't of any use any more.

When you have your four piles of clothes in place, take a step back and look for gaps in your wardrobe. First, look at your 'pass' pile, putting outfits together in your mind and deciding if there is anything missing. See if the missing articles can be taken from the 'have possibilities' or the 'need mending' piles. If not, they go down on the shopping list. Patching up your wardrobe need not be expensive, and if you find yourself with a very long list, go through the procedure again with a less critical eye. Buying from bargain basements and second-hand shops or making your own clothes are cheaper options.

FASHION STATEMENTS

You can make your own fashion statement with the help of a few accessories and one or two specific items of clothing. A colourful scarf or a hat can add character to an outfit; a belt can lend you an air of style and polish.

Old-fashioned or traditional costumes add character and confidence. Consider your own personality and lifestyle and think about how you can use clothes and accessories to convey the image of your choice.

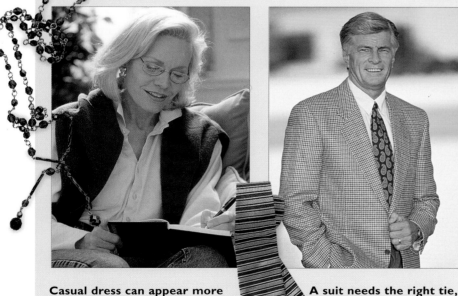

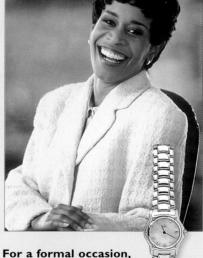

Casual dress can appear more sophisticated with a necklace, scarf or a bright jumper thrown over the shoulders.

A suit needs the right tie, shoes and wrist watch. Colour matching can bring it all together.

For a formal occasion, accessorise with simple elegance, such as pearl studs and a dress watch.

Shopping for clothes is an art in itself. Avoid always shopping in the same shops, it's easy to become bored with what you see. Try on each item before you buy it. Look at yourself critically in the mirror and answer these questions: Does it fit? Does the colour suit me? Does the style suit me? Does it go with the other things in my wardrobe? Will I get plenty of use out of it? Do I really like it? If the answer to all of these questions is yes, you can be sure you are buying the right clothes.

THE EFFECT OF STYLE AND SHAPE

Make the most of your shape with a style that enhances your best and hides your worst. The charts on pages 93 and 94 describe some of the ways to disguise common shape problems.

For larger figures, simple styles with a minimum of detail are the most flattering, so avoid frills and flounces, bows, gathered material and big patch pockets. Soft, fluid fabrics are best, since they skim the prominent parts of the body rather than clinging to them and emphasising them. If you are big, choose loose tops over skirts and trousers but avoid shapeless garments. Shop for longer-length tops rather than cropped styles that finish at the waist, and wear shirts and blouses untucked. Look for light materials such as sandwashed silk or microfibres, which tend not to crease and are easy to clean.

Are you a larger man? If you have a big belly, plain, single-coloured T-shirts will emphasise it. Jumpers that loosely cover your waist will hide it better, and a shirt with a slightly open neck draws attention up to the face and away from your midriff area.

Both men and women should make sure that they wear the right size in clothes; buying a size too small actually makes you look bigger, as does covering up in baggy clothes. Avoid tight trousers and dainty shoes, which will make your legs look larger.

SPECIFIC FIGURE CHALLENGES

As well as problems caused by overall shape, there are specific figure challenges that apply to both men and women.

Minimise unattractive features and accentuate your positive points with the following guidelines.

▶ **Double chin/short neck** To prevent the face and neck from appearing broader or thicker, wear V-neck tops or leave the top buttons of shirts or tops open to expose the neck. Avoid round or stand-up collars, polo-necks and padded shoulders, which make the neck appear shorter.

▶ **Heavy upper arms** Choose loose-fitting blouses and T-shirts, preferably with sleeves long enough to cover the upper arm. Layer blouses with an attractive vest to draw the eye away from the arms.

▶ **Large stomach** Wear comfortable waist-bands and long tops. For women, avoid waisted styles – choose dresses rather than skirts, for instance. Both sexes should avoid horizontal stripes and patterns that exaggerate fullness in the waist. Vertical striped blouses and shirts in plain colours are best. Make sure there is no strain over the girth. Where possible, wear your shirt loose and outside your trousers. If you prefer double-breasted suits, opt for the high-fastening, three- or four-buttoned style. Single-breasted jackets are a better option, however, since they can be worn undone and add less bulk to the stomach area.

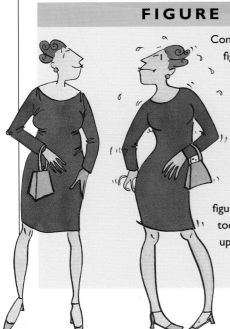

FIGURE SHAPING

Conceal your bulges and shape your figure with controlled underwear. For women, girdles remain a popular way of pulling in and supporting the lower belly. Newly developed tights can slim the legs, particularly the thighs. For men, stretch-fabric undergarments can hold in the stomach to give a more svelte appearance. But don't wear figure-enhancing underwear for too long – it can be uncomfortable and upset your proper body functioning!

Clothes solutions for female figure types

Be objective about your figure and dress accordingly. In general, aim to create a balanced look by highlighting your assets and drawing attention away from your figure flaws. It may help to try on different styles to determine what is the most flattering for you.

PEAR SHAPE

Figure: Small bust and torso, heavy thighs and large hips.

Good ideas: Make the most of the slim top half of the body with attractive, fitted tops, shoulder pads and detail at the bust or shoulder. Hide the hips with long jackets, tops or tunics, bias-cut skirts that skim the hips, and trousers that are loose and on the long side.

Bad ideas: Drawing attention to the hips and thighs with A-line skirts, figure-hugging trousers or skirts, and small shoes.

HOURGLASS

Figure: Full bust, small waist, full hips.

Good ideas: Accentuate the waist with dresses that follow the figure line, tailored jackets that nip in at the waist and hip-length jumpers. Hide the bulge of the hips with straight or tulip-shaped skirts. Shoulder pads and low necklines balance a large bust.

Bad ideas: Drawing attention to the large bust or hips with dresses with a dropped or no waistline, and full skirts.

TALL

Figure: Tall with narrow shoulders, slim hips and a relatively uncontoured body.

Good ideas: Broaden the upper body with shoulder pads, scarves and sweaters over the shoulders, pearls and long beads. Accentuate the hips with gathered skirts and trousers that bring in the waist.

Bad ideas: Anything that accentuates the length of the body, such as straight skirts, pinstriped trousers, dropped waistlines, tight or fitted trousers, and high-heeled shoes.

INVERTED TRIANGLE

Figure: Broad shoulders, a full bust, relatively narrow hips.

Good ideas: Accentuate the waist and lower half of the body with well-tailored trousers and skirts, details on dresses and skirts.

Bad ideas: Drawing attention to the top half of the body with boxed jackets, double-breasted jackets, pattern and detail on the bust or shoulder, and belted garments.

STRAIGHT

Figure: Square shoulders, smallish bust, little or no waist.

Good ideas: Make the most of shoulders with long single- or double-breasted jackets, layered outfits and long cardigan-style jackets. Accentuate the hips and legs with short skirts to the knee, classic tailored trousers, and dresses with a dropped or no waistline.

Bad ideas: Drawing attention to the waist with fitted tops and jackets, hipsters and fussy details around the waist.

PETITE

Figure: Small in height, with bust, waist and hips in proportion.

Good ideas: Lengthen the body with slim-fitting, tailored clothes, such as tapered trousers, straight skirts and dresses, (particularly above the knee), and solid colours. Knee-length boots lengthen the leg.

Bad ideas: Bulking the body with flowing skirts and dresses, wide trousers and baggy tops. Avoid fabrics with large or bold patterns.

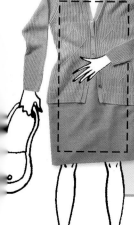

▶ **Large bust** Wear well-cut, fitted jackets, shirts and tops. Avoid short, boxy tops and jackets that come in at the waist as they can make you look plump all the way down. Padded shoulders draw attention away from a large bust. Make sure you wear a good, supportive bra that lifts your bust and prevents excessive movement.

PRACTICAL CLOTHES

The divide is eroding between casual clothes and clothes for practical activities, such as sports, leisure pursuits or even work.

Never before have practical clothes been so stylish, and the benefits are immense – you can now buy a jumper or fleece jacket that can be worn on a mountain, after a marathon or for shopping in your local supermarket.

As many people have more leisure time and are recognising the benefits of an active lifestyle, casual clothes are adapting to fit a more versatile market. A comfortable, quality pair of trainers can take you around a running track and then to a PTA meeting. The sporty look expresses enthusiasm and an energy for life and the ability to be ready for action at any time; it also suggests that the wearer has a busy lifestyle.

Casual clothes are making new headway into the world of work. Many companies realise that you don't need to wear a smart suit to write computer programmes or to analyse a spreadsheet. The workplace is gradually becoming more relaxed, and style and comfort – not formality – are the objectives. For this, a casual approach is best, using plain slacks and a tailored jacket. A tie may not be necessary for men, and often a smart polo-neck sweater strikes a sufficiently stylish but relaxed chord.

Basic male figure types

Think about balance when you are building your wardrobe. Use colour and form to broaden and shorten a tall thin stature and elongate and narrow a short, stocky one.

Try to draw attention away from your negative features. For example, if you are tall, you may need specially made trousers. Trousers that are too short will exaggerate your length.

TALL AND THIN

Figure: Long body, arms and legs, straight body with few curves, narrow shoulders.
Good ideas: Broaden the top part of the body with chunky knit jumpers and cardigans, polo-necks, three-quarter length wool, leather or cord jackets, double-breasted jackets with wide lapels, suits with matching waistcoat, blocks of colour or stripes running across the chest or shoulders, full-length winter coats.
Bad ideas: Elongating the body with jackets that end at the waist, slim-fitting tops and trousers, especially pinstriped suits.

APPLE SHAPE

Figure: Extra weight around the middle, and large neck, arms and legs.
Good ideas: Slim the figure with classic, generously cut clothes, such as trousers with pleated fronts. Bring the eye up towards the neck and shoulders with bold ties or necklines with ribbing or cuffs, V-necks and shoulder details.
Bad ideas: Drawing attention to the body with over-bright clothes, plain T-shirts, and double-breasted jackets.

SHORTER STATURE

Figure: Short body, arms and legs, although in proportion.
Good ideas: Elongate the body with the same solid colour trousers and jacket or shirt. Make use of slim-fitted and tailored clothes, single-breasted jackets, fitted shirts and V-neck tops.
Bad ideas: Wearing large or bulky clothes, such as trousers with turn-ups, full-length coats and double-breasted jackets. Don't break the outline with contrasting colours.

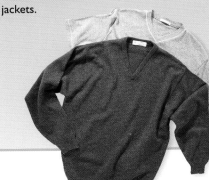

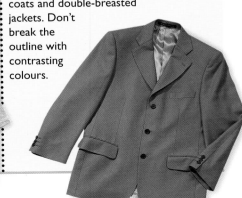

UNDERWEAR

When choosing underwear, you must first consider support and shape. There are a number of different types of bra available, each giving a different shape (see right) and varying degrees of support. If you are wearing a transparent top, you need to wear an attractive bra of a matching colour, or one matching your own skin colour. For sports, you will need a sports bra that provides extra support and restricts movement.

One problem most women identify with is the VPL (visible panty line) – or other unattractive lines and bulges created by underwear. To prevent panty lines, buy underpants that entirely cover the hips and backside, such as a full brief or teddy pants, or bypass the backside completely, as with a G-string. Eradicate hip bulges by wearing snug – but not tight – high-hipped pants. Sometimes, by finding specialised seamless underwear or by simply buying a larger size, you can eliminate these problems.

Bra lines are more difficult to smooth out because bras need to be well-fitting, and therefore often create bulges, especially under the arms and on the back. If this is a problem avoid very tight tops. Seamless bras prevent creases from cup seams, and if you are bulging out of the top of your bra, it is clear that you need a re-fit.

SWIMWEAR

Swimwear can't perform miracles, but it can help to make the best of your figure. Look for hidden extras such as underwiring, padded cups, structured cups and reinforced tops to provide uplift, hold or extra curves. To make a small bust seem larger, pick a swimsuit with ruching or detailing at the bustline. Choose high-cut legs, vertical stripes and dark panels at the sides to make your thighs look slimmer. For a smaller-looking waist, try a style with panels narrowing at the waist. A skirted style with downward-pointing chevron stripes will draw attention away from the waist and make the abdomen look flatter. Remember, however, to consider practicality and comfort as well as your appearance.

Special-purpose bras

A range of bras has been developed for particular purposes. In addition to those mentioned here, you can buy a seamless bra for a smooth bustline, a maternity bra for easy breast-feeding, and backless, strapless or halter bras for low-cut or sleeveless tops.

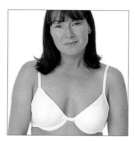

Underwired bra The underwire offers extra support, holding the bra in place and limiting excess movement of the breasts during day-to-day activities.

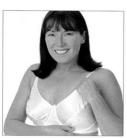

Uplift bra Padded and underwired, these bras push the breasts upwards, and often inwards, to create the appearance of a fuller, perter bust with a noticeable cleavage.

Size-reducing bra This is cleverly designed to spread the breasts over a larger area than a normal bra, to give the impression of a smaller, less prominent bust.

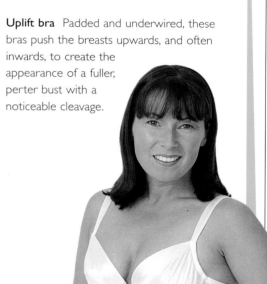

COLOUR

Some stylists believe colour is the most crucial element in personal fashion. Wearing the right colour, or range of colours for you, will complement your natural tones, making you look healthier, more attractive and younger. Professional colour consultants recommend the best colour combinations to enhance your natural skin tones and hair colour, and many customers have changed their whole wardrobes as a result of such advice, finding that their looks are greatly improved.

True colours

To find out which colours suit you, take scarves or fabric swatches one colour at a time and hold them under your chin. Determine which shades make your skin look warmer and are most flattering. These are the base shades for your clothes. Next, choose complementary colours to highlight the base colours. These guidelines may help.

YOUR COLOURING	CLOTHES	MAKE-UP
BLACK		
Hair: Black, very dark brown or silver **Complexion:** Black, brown, olive or dark beige **Eyes:** Black or deep brown	**Colour types:** Strong, bright and dramatic colours **Formal colours:** Charcoal or navy with turquoise accents **Evening colours:** Strong red, green or purple **Informal colours:** Pine green, hot pink and denim blue	**Lipstick:** Burgundy, plum or mahogany **Eye shadow:** Brown, purple or silver
BROWN		
Hair: Black, very dark brown or silver **Complexion:** Olive tan, golden brown or yellow brown **Eyes:** Black or deep brown	**Colour types:** Harmonious, clear colours, blues and pinks **Formal colours:** Grey, raspberry and taupe **Evening colours:** Royal or periwinkle blue and deep pink **Informal colours:** Blues and purple with grey and brown basics	**Lipstick:** Crimson red or bold red **Eye shadow:** Blue, grey or silver
AUBURN		
Hair: Auburn or golden blond **Complexion:** Warm beige, ivory, freckled **Eyes:** Topaz, hazel, green or teal	**Colour types:** Autumnal colours, browns, reds and yellows **Formal colours:** Bronze with orange-red highlights **Evening colours:** Teal green, soft purple or pewter **Informal colours:** Brown, camel, mustard and terracotta	**Lipstick:** Terracotta, cinnamon **Eye shadow:** Topaz, hazel or warm green
BLONDE		
Hair: Blond or blond–grey **Complexion:** Ivory to soft beige with peach tones **Eyes:** Blue, blue–green, aqua, light green	**Colour types:** Light and pastel colours **Formal colours:** Grey or blue with warm pastel highlights **Evening colours:** Warm pink, violet or emerald **Informal colours:** Beige, warm reds and blues	**Lipstick:** Peach, coral or clear **Eye shadow:** Brown, apricot or green
CHESTNUT		
Hair: Chestnut brown, medium brown or brown–grey **Complexion:** Porcelain, ivory, olive **Eyes:** Deep blue, hazel or hazel–brown	**Colour types:** Dark, rich colours and pale pastel shades **Formal colours:** Navy or rust with pastel highlights **Evening colours:** Black, emerald or violet **Informal colours:** Blues, greens, browns and reds	**Lipstick:** Red, strawberry pink **Eye shadow:** Grey and pink or violet
DARK BROWN		
Hair: Dark brown, dark chestnut brown or black **Complexion:** Olive or brown **Eyes:** Deep blue, hazel or hazel–brown	**Colour types:** Vivid, striking colours with warm undertones **Formal colours:** Olive, red or mustard **Evening colours:** Black, deep blues, greens and reds **Informal colours:** Rust, lime, terracotta with brown basics	**Lipstick:** Terracotta, red or cinnamon **Eye shadow:** Olive, green or purple
LIGHT BROWN		
Hair: Ash blonde, medium brown or ash **Complexion:** Ivory or beige **Eyes:** Soft teal, grey or hazel	**Colour types:** Dusty, well-blended, muted colours **Formal colours:** Green or brown with dusty pink accents **Evening colours:** Pewter, teal green or dusty purples **Informal colours:** Raspberry, dusty pink, blue and cocoa	**Lipstick:** Tan–pink, dusty rose, plum **Eye shadow:** Pink with cocoa

Consultants claim that developing a personal colour palette enables you to mix and match the clothes in your wardrobe more easily, cut down and consolidate the number of clothes you have, and greatly reduce the chance of making a bad purchase.

Answer the following questions honestly. If you answer yes to more than three of them, you may find it useful to get advice on your natural colour palette.

▶ Do you have many clothes in your wardrobe that you don't wear because you have nothing to go with them?
▶ Do you own blouses or shirts in both white and ivory or cream?
▶ Do you tend to wear the same lipstick all the time regardless of what you are wearing?
▶ When you open your wardrobe, do you see all the colours of the rainbow?
▶ Are some of your clothes electric or royal blue, while others are pale blue?
▶ Do you have different pairs of shoes in black, brown and navy?
▶ Can some colours that you wear make you feel pale and unhealthy?
▶ Do you follow trends in colours – regardless of how well they suit you – simply because they are popular?
A colour consultant will drape different colours over you to find the most flattering colour palette for your skin and hair. You only need one consultation, although your colouring does change over time and you may need an update every few years or so.

Colour your life with shades that enhance your natural glow and emphasise your individual tones.

The colour chart opposite is based on colour consulting techniques and you can use it to set up your own personal consultation at home. Find clothes, curtains or bedcovers in a range of different colours and sit in front of a full-length mirror (make sure that you are well lit, preferably with natural sunlight).

One by one, throw the clothes around your shoulders and consider the colour against your hair and face. You should soon become aware that certain colours look better on you than others. Make a note of them and put your newfound knowledge to the test.

As a general rule, black and white are popular because they lend a classic and often more expensive look than similar garments in different colours. Surprisingly, perhaps, their main advantage is that they are not memorable. This is why many women have a black dress which, by changing accessories, can be worn for years without looking dated. Black worn on the lower half of the body slims the legs and hips. If this is a consideration, opt for darker skirts and trousers.

Because patterned clothing and prints make a stronger statement than plain fabrics, they may be difficult to wear. Hold the pattern up to your face to see if it complements or overpowers your colouring. If a print incorporates several colours, determine which shade dominates and decide whether it ties in with the colours in your wardrobe.

SHOES
High-heeled shoes have gone in and out of fashion throughout the centuries for both men and women, adding height and elegance – but often torturing their wearers.

Today, many women like the elegant look of narrow, open-toed shoes, but unless they support the foot and ankle properly, they may cause damage.

High-heels are popular with many women because they accentuate the female form and add height. But try to wear them occasionally – worn all the time, they can cause serious long-term damage to the feet, knees, hips and back, and may lead to the development of joint disorders and varicose veins. There is no reason why flatter, more practical shoes should be boring or unflattering. Slightly chunky shoes or boots are hard-wearing and can be very stylish.

SHIVER ME ARMPITS!
T-shirts were invented in the last century, it is believed, when the British Royal Navy ordered sailors to sew sleeves onto their undershirts to screen their hairy armpits from royal view.

7 ways to **improve body shape**

**Staying active is the best way to retain your youth and vitality.
Follow this plan to keep your body looking great
and feeling flexible and young.**

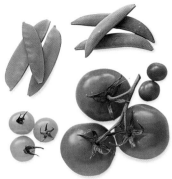

ENCOURAGE SMOOTHER SKIN

Dry skin brushing or massaging with a rough mitt are techniques that improve skin texture and tone by removing dead skin cells and other debris that block the pores and lead to dull, dry and blemished skin. They also help the body detoxify itself by promoting lymphatic drainage and increasing blood flow to the skin. Skin brushing can also target areas prone to cellulite (see page 75), such as the buttocks and thighs. Afterwards, massage in your favourite rich moisturising cream – you should feel fabulous.

1 Brush your skin with long, sweeping strokes using a dry natural-fibre bath brush. Begin gently – once your skin tone improves you can gradually brush more vigorously. Move up the limbs from fingers to shoulders and toes to hips. Brush up over the buttocks from thighs to waist. Cover as much of the body as you can reach, always brushing in long strokes towards the heart.

2 After brushing, have a warm bath or shower and cleanse your skin thoroughly. Dry your skin by patting it gently with a soft towel and then moisturise thoroughly.

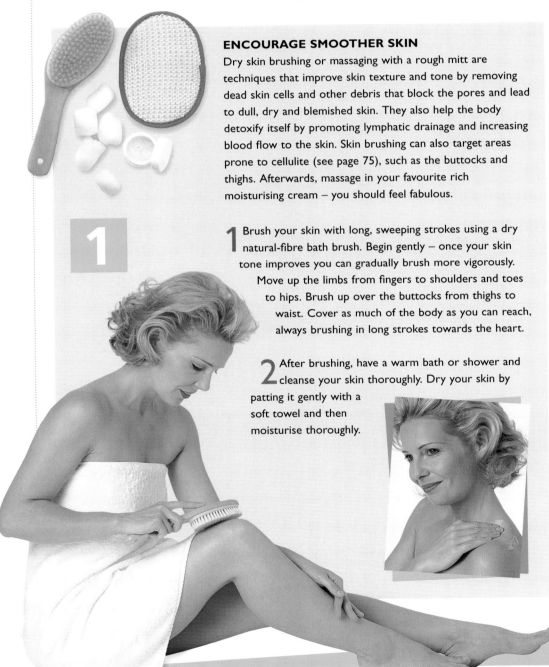

Eat more fibre

Fibre is not digested in the stomach and therefore passes through your entire system in its raw form, cleansing it and clearing out other undigested foods. Include plenty of fibre in your diet to keep your system running smoothly and prevent constipation.

Fibre is also an excellent component in any weight-loss programme, filling you up, but with few kilojoules (calories). So eat plenty of fruit, vegetables and whole-grain cereals to keep your body functioning smoothly and healthily.

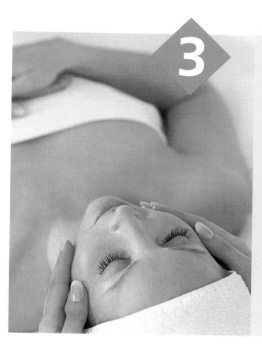

3

INDULGE IN A BEAUTY TREATMENT

Many beauty salons and spas offer wraps and mud treatments to improve skin tone and alleviate water retention. For example, thalassotherapy involves applying mineral-rich sea water, sea mud, seaweed, algae and sea salt to the skin, usually in the form of baths, compresses and poultices. The absorption of sea minerals is said to improve skin condition and restore the body's natural mineral balance. By encouraging sweating, thalassotherapy also helps remove impurities from the body. However, probably the most beneficial aspect of a beauty treatment is the way it makes you feel afterwards – relaxed, fresh and scrubbed clean all over.

TRY MARTIAL ARTS

4

The active martial arts, such as judo, karate, kung fu, kick boxing and ju jitsu, are all very good for flexibility, muscle toning and all-round aerobic exercise. Join a local class and enjoy meeting new friends while learning a new skill. Self-defence sports can also help to boost your confidence, putting you on a new, positive course for the future.

Keep your weight constant

5

Your body is living evidence of your experiences, and if you have been overweight, your skin will have stretched and will need extra-special care and treatment to recover its former elasticity. Stretch marks and cellulite are a particular problem for those who suddenly lose or gain weight. Finding your optimum weight and keeping it constant can help you to improve and maintain your body shape.

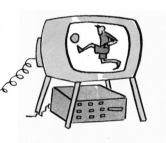

SHAPE UP AND STRETCH

The following yoga exercise helps to firm up the hips and abdominal muscles. Lie flat on your back with your arms straight out to the sides, palms down. Raise your knees, keeping them together and put your feet flat on the floor. Keeping your shoulders on the ground, twist your knees to the left and lower them to the floor; look to your right. Hold for 10 seconds and then do the same on the other side. Repeat the exercise 5 times on each side.

6

WORK YOUR JOINTS

7

Starting with your neck and working down, slowly move all of your joints one by one through their whole range of motion. For example, start with a head roll, carefully rolling your head all the way around, and then turning your head from one side to the other to loosen your neck. Then move on to the shoulders, thinking of every conceivable movement that they can make, without straining. Follow with your arms and hands, waist, hips, legs and feet, making each movement a few times. Do not attempt to move joints that are arthritic, and if you feel particularly stiff, you should see your doctor. You can do this exercise in bed or while watching television. It helps you retain flexibility by keeping the joints supple.

Hair care

When it comes to appearance, your hair is one of your most important features. A regular hair-care routine and a good diet can keep your hair shiny and healthy, so that it forms a pleasing frame for your face.

Choosing a style that suits your face is the first step towards good-looking hair. Once you have a cut that works for you, a healthy diet and getting into good hair-care habits will keep your hair in great condition. With all the products on the market today, there is a solution for nearly every hair-care problem.

Hair is a barometer of health and well-being and often shows the first sign of ill-health or stress.

Your hair is mostly made up of the protein keratin. To keep it healthy, aim to incorporate a range of proteins, such as lean meat, soya, tofu and eggs, into your diet. Variety rather than quantity is the key. Like the skin, the hair visibly benefits from specific nutrients in food (see page 47), particularly zinc, magnesium, potassium and iron (see page 48 for food sources).

LOOKING AFTER YOUR HAIR

The condition of your hair is mainly determined by its moisture content. An oily secretion called sebum protects the outer coating of each hair and helps to keep it hydrated. Triggered by hormonal changes, the production of sebum is prolific during puberty, but reduces over the years. Older people, therefore, often find that their hair becomes dry and lacklustre and increasingly requires the help of hair-care products to bring out shine and bounce.

Hair is a dead structure so it cannot heal itself, although some hair-care products can repair minor problems. It is easily damaged by excessive brushing, blow-drying, styling, perming and by overuse of chemical treatments, such as colourants, that cause breakage and split ends. Sun, wind, air pollution and chlorinated water can also dry out your hair and increase the risk of damage.

CLOSE-UP ON HAIR

Deep inside the skin's lower layers are hair follicles, each fed by its own blood vessel and producing a single hair. Hair is made up of an outer layer of scaly cells, a middle layer that gives the hair its colour and bulk, and a central core made from transparent cells and air spaces. Hair cells grow from the root and all that is visible is made from dead keratin proteins. Each hair has a life cycle of about three to five years, after which it is pushed out of the follicle by new hair growth. Hair grows at different rates throughout the year – faster in summer and slower in winter – and it may even have a moulting season in spring or autumn.

The average person has about 120,000 hairs on his or her head, and loses 20–100 hairs every day.

The action of shampooing cleanses and stimulates scalp circulation, resulting in healthier and faster hair growth. There is some debate on how often you should wash your hair, but the best approach is to wash it as often as it needs – more frequently if it is greasy and less if it is dry. If your hair looks good, don't change your routine.

Always rinse your hair thoroughly in clean water – inadequate rinsing is one of the commonest causes of dull, lifeless hair.

Body-building shampoo is protein-based to increase hair growth and add volume to fine or thin hair. Moisturising shampoos should be used by those with dry or treated hair – it may be too rich for those with normal hair and might lead to greasiness. Colour-protective shampoos help retain the tones of coloured hair by keeping cuticles smooth and the cortex moistened. Medicated shampoos can effectively treat dandruff and some other scalp problems.

Conditioners are basically anti-aging creams for the hair, smoothing the cuticles, preventing tangles, improving the shine and replacing lost moisture. They are also important for buffering against moisture loss and other damage. Deep-moisturising formulas are essential for those with dry, permed or coloured hair. Keep the conditioner on for a few minutes before rinsing, to get the best results. A leave-in solution may improve the health of curly or coarse hair, which often needs more thorough conditioning. Fine or wispy hair needs a lightly moisturising formula as heavy conditioners may pull it down, making it look thin and lank.

After shampooing and conditioning, blot hair with a towel – hair is at its weakest when wet, so take care not to rub or pull it. Choose

Magic ingredients?

Although many shampoos and conditioners promise new and special ways to make your hair better, the reality is that many hair-care products contain the same ingredients and offer no superior treatments to rival brands. Choose the right type for greasy, normal or dry hair and find the product that your hair likes best. Special ingredients to watch out for include:

AHAs (alpha-hydroxy acids) These speed cell renewal and regulate the oils in the hair. Shampoos with AHAs are also considered to be good alternatives to antidandruff shampoos.

Vitamin E This natural ingredient lubricates and protects the outer layers of the hair and provides nourishment.

Protein-based shampoos Proteins, especially keratin, are added to thin hair to give it body, although a good diet is also beneficial.

Colour-protective protein shampoos Helping to prevent colour-fade in dyed hair, these products offer added moisture and conditioning for chemically treated hair.

Leave-in conditioners These are good for very dry hair as they keep the hair moisturised between washes and protect against external drying and polluting elements. They may, however, build up in the hair, causing matting.

Natural ingredients Egg yolk, aloe vera and coconut oils are particularly good for moisturising and nourishing hair.

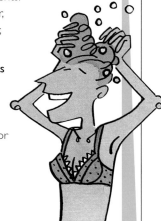

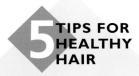

5 TIPS FOR HEALTHY HAIR

1. Keep your hair covered in bright sunshine.
2. Rinse your hair after swimming.
3. Avoid using chemicals on your hair.
4. Do not use medicated shampoos for long periods.
5. Eat a balanced and healthy diet.

the moderate setting on your dryer and hold it about 20 cm (8 inches) from the hair, aiming the nozzle down the hairshaft away from the roots. Damage from hairdryers usually occurs when the hair is nearly dry, so stop blow-drying while the hair is slightly damp.

Thoroughly brushing and combing your hair improves circulation and removes loose hairs, dust and excess hair products.

However, don't overdo it – you may be working your scalp more than it needs and end up removing too much hair. Use a good-quality brush that is gentle on your scalp. A comb should be wide-toothed and smooth – seams and roughness can split and damage the hair.

With countless new styling aids marketed every year, choosing the right product to enhance your hair can be a real headache.

SCALP MASSAGE

For healthier, shinier hair, a scalp massage works wonders. Try it for yourself. It will relax you, relieve stress and enhance blood circulation to the scalp to feed and revitalise the hair follicles.

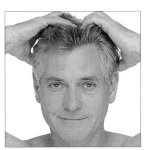

1 Rub a little coconut oil or a deep conditioner on to your fingertips and apply to the scalp with a firm motion as if shampooing.

2 Massage the scalp with the fingertips and thumbs, working from the forehead to the base of the skull in straight lines. Use a rotating motion to cover the whole area.

Use this quick run-down of hair-care products to choose one that best suits your hair type and style.

▶ *Mousses* One of the easiest ways to bring body and control to any hairstyle, mousses are simple to apply and are widely available.
▶ *Gels* Although gels can be useful for some styles, they can be quite heavy, leaving the hair stiff and difficult to restyle. They may also leave a white residue behind when dry.
▶ *Thickening solutions* These contain keratin, which coats each strand to make it thicker. Spray it onto your hair, blow-dry to bond the liquid and your hair will appear thicker until the next wash.
▶ *Serums* Revolutionising styling for dry, frizzy and coarse hair, serums provide suppleness and deep moisture without stiffness or greasiness. A single drop can cover a whole head of hair, although you may want to focus on the ends if they are damaged or split.

▶ *Waxes* Popular with many men, wax creates a sheen reminiscent of the 1960s. A little blended evenly can give weight to dry or flyaway hair without stiffness or grease.
▶ *Putties and styling creams* For a more specialised market, putties and creams can stiffen hair into peaks or ruffles for a sophisticated and structured look.
▶ *Finishing sprays* These are very useful for setting many styles, but they can also leave the hair stiff and solid if used in excess.

HAIRSTYLES

Good hair days start with a good cut. The best styles make the most of the natural qualities of your own hair by, for example, enhancing curl or giving thin hair extra body. If you have thick, straight hair, a jaw-length bob is often more light and bouncy than longer styles, which can look very heavy and unflattering. Avoid jagged-edged styles, unless you plan to live up to it with plenty of dramatic clothes and make-up. If your hair is naturally curly, have it cut to help it curl rather than frizz. Your hairdresser may want to cut your hair when it is dry to style with the natural direction of the curls. If you have a delicate face, it may be necessary to layer or wisp your fringe so that your hair doesn't overpower your face. For fine hair, try a perm or a demi-wave, which lifts the hair at the roots to add body without touching the drier, more vulnerable tips of the hair.

Before choosing a hairstyle, study the shape of your face and head. The shape is defined by your hairline, the width and length of your face and its proportions.

In general, faces come in five different shapes – oval, round, long, square and heart-shaped, although you may find that your own face is a combination.

▶ *Oval* This is a good shape for most hair styles, but avoid styles where the hair is cut very close to the face.

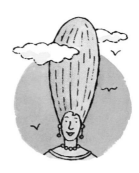

► **Round** The hair should be feathered onto the cheeks to narrow them, or pulled back at the sides to emphasise the bone structure.

► **Long** Reduce the length of your face with a fringe and avoid long hair, particularly styles that cover the sides of the face.

► **Square** Opt for curves that hide or soften the jaw. Avoid symmetrical styles, which accentuate the square shape.

► **Heart-shaped** A flip (jaw-length hair that curls up at the ends) is ideal for this shape because it gives volume around the bottom of the face.

STYLES FOR THE OLDER WOMAN

There are no hard and fast rules about the best styles for an older woman; the main idea is to wear your hair the way you feel most comfortable. Long hair can look good on an older woman, but avoid the 'curtain' look by layering the hair to create body.

Short styles are often preferred by women over 50 because they are more practical and often more stylish.

Sharp, short cuts can look clean and fresh. Styles that are very short at the nape of the neck and longer on top can be easily dressed up for a glamorous evening look.

Keep styles bouncy, lifting off and away from the face to add vitality and draw attention away from aging skin. A fringe can be good for covering wrinkles on the forehead – a wispy or parted fringe can be used if a thick fringe does not suit you.

Avoid very young looks, such as a swingy bob or a pony tail, that draw attention to your age. Keep your hair well-groomed and regularly styled – it will make a real difference to your overall appearance.

TURNING GREY

Hair turns grey when the pigment-forming cells at the root of the hair become inactive. The first signs of greying occur when the hairs growing from the first deactivated follicles are long enough to be seen. Around

HAIR-RAISING STYLES

Wigs and toupees were popular in the 17th and 18th centuries. The wigs were large and ornate to denote class and wealth, but they looked unnatural and were impractical.

Types of colouring

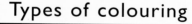

COLOURING	SUITABLE FOR	UNSUITABLE FOR
Colour-enhancing shampoos/ conditioners	Adding temporary colour. Particularly suitable for fair, auburn or medium brown hair and for maintaining the colour of previously dyed hair. Can achieve a subtle effect; good for creating warm or red tones, and the colour is semi-permanent.	Bleached hair, which can turn orange, or for a dramatic colour change, or for concealing a lot of grey hair.
Temporary colours	Creating a subtle colour change and safe for permed or chemically treated hair. Easy to use, they contain a higher percentage of pigment than colour shampoos, so they can last for up to three washes.	Grey hair or for dramatic colour changes.
Semi-permanents	Boosting natural colour and adding shine. Simple to use, they are good for hiding some grey hair, and can be used on chemically treated hair. In addition, if you decide you don't like the colour you can wash it out without any regrowth problems. Choose a colour that is within two shades of your own and always use the gloves supplied.	Permanent colour. These are wash-in formulations that glue colour polymers to the hair cuticle without penetrating the hair. They fade after six to eight washes.
Demi-permanents	Adding depth and tone. They provide more colour options than semi-permanents. They do not contain damaging ammonia, so do not affect the condition of your hair. They can cover up to 70 per cent of grey hair and go deeper into the hair shaft so are longer-lasting – around 15 washes. Follow instructions carefully.	Lightening your natural shade or on highlights, bleached, chemically treated or permed hair, or hair that is very dry or damaged.
Permanent colour	Replacing the natural pigment. These penetrate each hair shaft, allowing you to choose any shade you like. The further you go away from your natural hair colour, however, the more obvious the regrowth will be.	Temporary effects.

COLOUR YOUR PERSONALITY

The colour of your hair plays an extraordinary role in your appearance and, to a degree, defines your personality. Look at the model in the pictures below: it is actually the same photograph but the colour of her hair has been altered graphically. Her appearance is startlingly different according to the change in hair colour. Does your own hair colour, whether you have experimented with dyes or not, match your natural complexion? It may help if you ask your friends or family to advise how a hair colour change may alter or improve your whole image.

Blonde hair can be uplifting, or make your complexion appear pale.

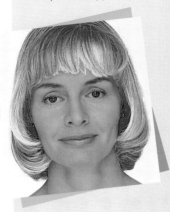

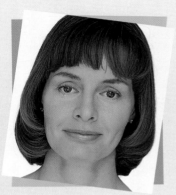

Dark hair can be subtle and natural, although it can be drab and mousy.

Combination or streaked hair offers a natural-looking variation.

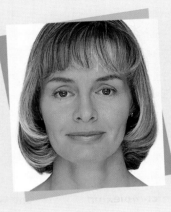

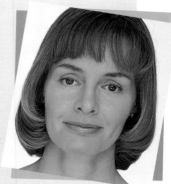

Auburn is warm and full of character, but only if you have the right skin colouring.

4 TIPS FOR HAIR STYLING

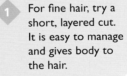
1 For fine hair, try a short, layered cut. It is easy to manage and gives body to the hair.

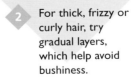
2 For thick, frizzy or curly hair, try gradual layers, which help avoid bushiness.

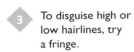
3 To disguise high or low hairlines, try a fringe.

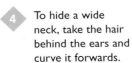
4 To hide a wide neck, take the hair behind the ears and curve it forwards.

50 per cent of the population has predominantly grey hair by the age of 50, but for some people, greying occurs much earlier or later for a variety of reasons. How soon and how much hair turns grey is usually determined by heredity. If your parents went grey early on, it is likely that you will too.

Grey hair can look wonderful – it is now considered chic, particularly in the fashion industry – and special products can enhance the silver in grey hair.

Because fair hair contains less pigment than dark hair, it tends to go grey earlier. Grey hair can seem coarse in comparison with other hair. This is because it usually appears at a time when the sebum-secreting glands in the scalp have become less productive, producing drier hair.

Premature greying can be attributed to stress and other factors, such as nutrition deficiencies caused by excessive dieting. Research suggests that more women are turning grey prematurely, partly as a result of taking hormones such as the contraceptive pill and hormone replacement therapy (HRT, see pages 137–139). A lack of calcium, phosphorus, potassium, magnesium or the B vitamins are other possible causes. Stress exacerbates this problem by depleting the levels of B vitamins in the body.

If you prefer to disguise grey hair, you can colour it, either professionally or at home with a home rinse, natural or ammonia-based dye. Do not try to recreate your natural, youthful hair colour – hair changes with age and the deep, lustrous colour of your teens or 20s may be too much with an older complexion. Use a colour that is close to your natural colour but warmer in tone, such as a soft brown or chestnut. Highlights, lowlights and streaks are an alternative to a complete change of colour and can look more natural than bold all-over dyes. You can also add subtle highlights and lowlights to coloured hair to produce a softer, more natural look.

COLOURING YOUR HAIR

Dying your own hair is an easy and inexpensive way to change your appearance. Read the instructions carefully beforehand and carry out a sensitivity and a strand test to judge the colour – choose a strand next to your face so that you can see how it looks with your skin colouring. Do not use tints on hair that is already coloured or treated with henna or colour-restoring lotions. If you need to dye the roots of your hair as they grow through, carefully cover the roots with dye first and only coat the rest of your hair a few minutes before rinsing. Since hair grows at different rates, you alone need to decide how often you should dye your roots, although between six and ten weeks is considered normal by most professionals.

Choosing the right shade is crucial; try to match your own complexion and natural hair colouring.

▶ **Black** This colour is suitable for dark, olive or clear ivory skin types, and those whose natural hair colour is medium to dark brown. Black makes a dramatic, confident statement – it's not for the faint-hearted. Since black hair tends to drain colour from your face, it best suits those with strong skin tones or bold make-up. It looks modern and makes the hair look glossier. However, black is prone to fading.

▶ **Brunette** This is best for those with light to very dark brown hair and should be avoided if your hair is light blonde (natural, highlights or tint) as it can turn green. Rich brown is great – it can be as bold or as subtle as you like – especially if you want to enhance your natural colour but do not want anything too dramatic. Brunette can vary from mahogany to plum, and the deeper the tone, the richer the shine.

▶ **Red** This is suitable for those with pale skin, green or blue eyes and medium to brown hair. It should be avoided if you have

Technology battles on to find the definitive hair-loss prevention treatment. Regaine is the 'cure' currently available in the West, but others are fast being developed to compete in the lucrative hair-loss market.

Baldness busters

Regaine is a topical solution containing the active ingredient Minoxidil. It works by dilating the blood vessels in the scalp – increasing blood flow and nourishing the hair follicles. The success of the product has been limited to those with minimal baldness and without a receding hairline. The treatment must be taken for life to have a permanent effect – which could be very expensive.

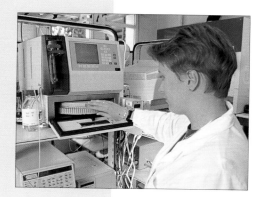

PRODUCTS IN THE PIPELINE

Propecia, already available in the U.S., contains Finasteride. It is taken in pill form and has worked for some men, but is not considered safe for women. It shares the drawbacks of Regaine in its limitations and expense. Other new products in development are Tricomin – which is said to stimulate and sustain hair follicle growth – and Diazoxide, which, like Regaine, dilates the blood vessels in the scalp.

Scientists have discovered that balding men are deficient in an enzyme called aromatase, and a new product is being refined that supposedly boosts levels of this enzyme and prevents baldness.

The most effective medication to date stimulates blood vessels, increasing the flow of blood to each hair follicle.

olive skin or a rosy complexion. Red hair is vibrant and striking which, on the right person, can make the complexion glow. It is a difficult colour to maintain, however, since it has a tendency to fade rather quickly.

▶ *Golden blonde* This is suitable for those with a light tan or slightly sallow skin, and hazel, green or blue eyes. Avoid it if you have a rosy complexion. Golden blonde will give you a healthy, vibrant, sun-kissed look.

▶ *Platinum or ash blonde* This is best for those with pale, rosy, freckly skin whose hair is in good condition. It is best avoided if you have dark brown eyes, or a sallow, olive complexion. White–blonde creates a glamorous look and, because it is a neutral colour, it allows you to have fun with make-up and clothes. Nevertheless, bear in mind that the lighter the shade you choose, the greater the risk of damaging your hair, so if you have blonde hair keep it well conditioned.

HAIR LOSS

From your mid-20s onwards, the rate of hair growth slows down and your hair becomes thinner. This often occurs earlier in men, because the female hormone oestrogen protects women from hair loss until later in life.

Around 50 per cent of men experience serious hair loss before the age of 30, whereas 30 per cent of women will notice major hair thinning by the age of 50.

Serious hair loss – or alopecia – has two main causes. The most common form is male pattern baldness, or alopecia androgenetica, which is an inherited condition. It is thought to be related to the effect on the hair follicles of a substance called dihydrotestosterone (DHT), which is a by-product of the male sex hormone testosterone.

Solutions to male pattern baldness

Hair transplants Hair from the back of the head, which seldom goes bald, is transplanted to the hairless areas either as a series of individual 'plugs' or in strips, depending on the technique.

Hair implants Strips of synthetic hair are implanted into the hairless area. The synthetic hairs are easily damaged by heat so a hairdryer must not be used.

Electrotherapy Using a TENS machine, electrotherapy has restored growth in some cases, although results are usually better in those who have not been balding for more than five years.

Hair weaving This is a non-surgical procedure in which strands of new hair are braided onto existing hair in order to cover bald patches.

Hairpiece The right toupee or wig can be quite natural-looking, giving you confidence and making you appear younger. Seek professional advice.

Other treatments Depending on the cause of baldness, oestrogen or vitamin D lotions have been successful, and in some cases treatment with UV light.

The other main cause of hair loss is illness. Alopecia areata is the usual culprit, resulting in small patches of baldness. A more severe but rarer form of the disorder – alopecia universalis – causes total hair loss, from the body and head.

In women, severe hair loss is usually caused by stress, illness or hormonal changes – one half of all cases is stress-related, especially following a severe shock, operation or childbirth (over 50 per cent of women suffer hair loss up to seven months after giving birth). Women can usually expect 30–40 per cent regrowth once the underlying cause has been tackled.

Other causes include cancer treatment, antibiotics, anaemia, endocrine (hormone gland) disorders, psoriasis, eating disorders, zinc deficiency, pollution and an excess of vitamin A in the diet. Overuse of chemical hair treatments can also lead to hair loss.

To combat hair thinning, regularly apply hair-thickening products, such as body-building shampoos and protein conditioners. A perm can give body to fine or thinning hair. Scalp massage may also help by improving the blood circulation to the follicles.

Looking after your teeth

Good oral hygiene and regular dental check-ups are the basis for healthy teeth. Many further treatments now exist to straighten or whiten teeth and correct other dental problems.

A warm smile is a sterling asset and it's well worth spending several minutes each day taking care of your teeth to keep them looking healthy. It is also necessary to visit a dentist every six months or so to make sure that any teeth or gum disorders are caught early and treated properly.

In childhood and early adulthood, the most common dental disorder is tooth decay (dental caries). After early adulthood, the enemy becomes periodontal disease, also known as gum disease or pyorrhea.

More teeth are lost through periodontal disease than cavities, according to a 1997 Canadian study.

As collagen levels in the gums decline with age, the gums shrink, exposing more of the tooth – hence the expression 'long in the tooth'. Periodontal disease, which affects up to 95 per cent of adults, adds to this problem, weakening the support for the tooth, often leading to tooth loss. Your best defence is to brush with a fluoride toothpaste, morning and night, and floss once a day to reach the areas that the toothbrush cannot clean.

Choose a soft- or medium-bristled brush and apply modest pressure to the teeth and gums. The key to effective brushing is the motion used rather than the force. Dentists recommend a gentle back and forwards movement over teeth and gums for the most effective cleaning. Make sure you replace

CLOSE-UP ON TEETH

The core of every tooth is a living pulp, containing blood vessels and nerves, which is surrounded by a protective layer of a hard substance called dentine. Above the gum line, each tooth is coated with enamel, and below the gum line, the root of the tooth is connected to the jaw by a layer of cementum.

Teeth erode over time – the main culprit is bacteria from the sugar content in food. Tooth decay resulting from erosion is known as dental caries. Common locations for tooth decay are in the grooved grinding surfaces of the back teeth, the lateral edges of adjacent teeth and just above the gum line. If decay occurs below the gum line, gingivitis can develop, making the gums swell and eventually become chronically infected.

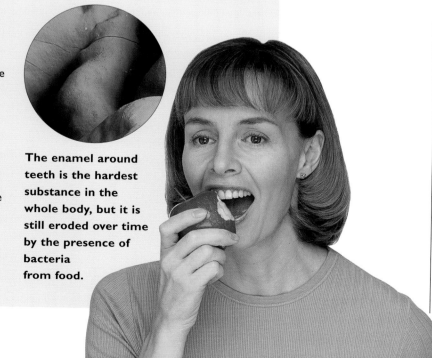

The enamel around teeth is the hardest substance in the whole body, but it is still eroded over time by the presence of bacteria from food.

Years of eating, drinking and smoking discolour and wear down your teeth. Get the best out of your toothpaste by choosing the one that suits your own personal dental requirements.

Toothpaste plus

Extra-special toothpastes are being developed all the time, but comprehensive research to test their success and side effects often lags behind, so don't believe everything you read on the label.

EXTRA-SPECIAL TOOTHPASTES

Stain-removing toothpaste The active ingredient in this is sodium fluoride, a natural chemical that helps to remove stubborn stains. Although no abrasives, bleaches or acids are used, some studies have revealed that long-term use results in the thinning of tooth enamel.

Micrograin cleansing formula Micrograins gently abrade the teeth to help cleaning. Overuse can cause gum damage or too much enamel abrasion.

Tooth whitener This usually contains an abrasive protein-dissolving agent, such as papain. Some brands also use hydrogen peroxide and a micrograin cleansing formula.

Sensitive-teeth toothpaste This contains potassium nitrate, strontium acetate or chloride which have a numbing effect on exposed areas of nerve tissue. This can be effective, but only temporarily. Consult your dentist if your teeth are extremely sensitive.

Specialty toothpastes can be expensive and ineffective. Before you buy, check first with your dentist.

your brush every three months – beyond this it is no longer doing its job properly.

The arch enemy of teeth and gums is plaque, a sticky coating made up of millions of bacteria, that forms on the teeth. The bacteria feed on sugar residues left in the mouth after eating and drinking and produce acids that attack the tooth enamel. Plaque acids also attack the gums, leading to inflammation and bleeding – known as gingivitis.

The acid level rises for up to 30 minutes after you eat certain foods, eroding the teeth and inflaming the gums, until your saliva slowly neutralises it.

Sometimes, holes develop inside a tooth that can't be cleaned. Known as dental pocketing, this condition is one of the leading causes of bad breath in those over 40. The only treatment available is surgery.

In addition to brushing and flossing, you can take the following steps to limit the damage that plaque causes. Reduce your intake of sugar, particularly in coffee, tea and colas, as plaque quickly converts it into acid. Whenever possible, brush your teeth after eating to remove plaque deposits. Chew sugar-free gum, which encourages saliva flow to neutralise acid levels. Even swilling your mouth out with water following a meal will help to remove a great amount of plaque. Alternatively, eat a small piece of hard cheese at the end of the meal. This is high in calcium which counteracts the acidity from the plaque deposits and also strengthens the teeth. Areas of tooth that have been lost through erosion are gradually replaced – in a process called remineralisation – by calcium and other minerals in saliva. For example, minerals from fresh, green leafy vegetables and dairy products aid this process, provided that sugar is not eaten too often.

If you suffer from periodontal disease, you may require frequent removal of tartar, a deposit that forms on the teeth and leads to discolouration. Root problems and underlying gum disorders can be detected in X-ray.

If you have lost any teeth, it is important to have a bridge, denture or implant fitted to fill the space. Otherwise, remaining teeth will spread across to fill the gap, leading to further gaps and weakening their connection with the jaw. Brush dentures regularly with a suitable cleansing solution, particularly the top surfaces and the gaps between the teeth. As your gums recede, dentures fit less well, so have them checked every five years and altered, if necessary. There is no reason why dentures should be uncomfortable or prevent you from enjoying certain foods. They should fit snugly and look natural. Seek dental advice if you encounter any difficulties with denture wear.

TOOTH CLEANSING AGENTS

In addition to fluoride, other chemical agents can be added to toothpaste to improve the cleaning function. For example, anti-plaque agents combat bacterial build-up and prevent plaque formation. Some of these should not be used long-term, because they may stain your teeth and affect your sense of taste. Anti-tartar agents prevent the build-up of tartar, or calculus – plaque that has hardened from calcium in the saliva – and is difficult to remove.

Some mouthwashes and rinses contain alcohol or other caustic chemicals that accelerate tooth wear. A fresh breath mouthwash that is too strong, might feel refreshing initially, but it may be killing off the good bacteria in saliva as well as the harmful variety. This is disastrous for your teeth, whose natural defences against decay are broken down. If you use a mouthwash, ask your dentist to recommend a suitable brand for optimum benefit. Persistent bad breath can be a sign of gum disease. If a mouthwash does not appear to counteract this problem, it may be that there is a more deep-seated cause.

TOOTH WHITENERS

Whiteners can be applied by your dentist or can be bought over-the-counter in the form of whitening toothpaste.

Those administered by the dentist contain high quantities of hydrogen peroxide or carbamide peroxide which, up until very recently, were banned in cosmetic dentistry in Europe because of safety concerns. The ban has now been lifted, but there is still a question mark over the effectiveness of tooth-whitening products.

There is no evidence that whitening-formula toothpastes, which contain a small amount of hydrogen peroxide, will produce successful results for everyone. Moreover, some people have found that they cause permanent damage to their teeth, leaving them feeling rough and uneven.

Toothbrush technology

The array of toothbrushes on the market can be overwhelming. Below are some of the more popular types.

Angled-head toothbrush The head is positioned to reach the corners of the mouth more easily than a regular brush. Some people may find them awkward to use, however, and the benefits are often minimal.

Electric toothbrush Electric toothbrushes not only clean your teeth well, but also massage your gums. A rotating action is considered better than a vibrating action.

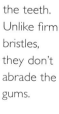

Ridged-bristle toothbrush The central bristles are slightly longer than the others to reach between the teeth and help clean and clear the gums.

Round-head toothbrush If the head is large and round, your gums may be taking a beating. A slimmer, smaller head, which is gentler on the gums, is better.

Soft- versus firm-bristle toothbrushes Dental experts recommend that you use a brush with soft bristles, which are flexible and reach between the teeth. Unlike firm bristles, they don't abrade the gums.

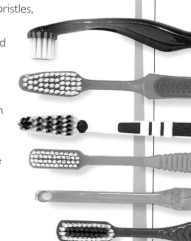

COSMETIC
dentistry

No matter how diligent you are in your daily oral hygiene, your teeth may still become chipped, worn or stained over time. This can add years to your looks, but help is at hand since teeth can be corrected by cosmetic dentistry.

Before you visit the cosmetic dentist, give some thought to the look you want to achieve. If you want to repair wear or damage, ask your dentist's advice on what can be done. You may dream of recapturing the way you looked when you were younger – bring along some old photographs to show the dentist the effect you wish to create. If you want to totally change your teeth's appearance, show the dentist a picture of someone with the look you're after.

Many cosmetic dentists now use computer-imaging techniques so that you can see and alter on the screen how you would look after undergoing various forms of dental procedure. This will help you decide the best course of action.

In some cases, however, damage to existing teeth may be too far gone and your dentist may advise replacing the teeth with a bridge or dentures. There is no reason to find this alarming – your gums will benefit from getting rid of unhealthy teeth and your whole mouth may start to feel cleaner and more comfortable. Many older people wear dentures but these are often so natural-looking that only they themselves know. Your dentist will advise you about tooth replacement.

Cosmetic procedures

Bleaching Using oxidising or bleaching agents, the dentist lightens or removes discoloration caused, for example, by tea or coffee.

Cosmetic contouring Teeth that are worn or slightly uneven can be reshaped by contouring. It is a relatively inexpensive and quick procedure – around one hour – and may be combined with composite resin bonding and laminating.

Composite resin bonding This involves etching the tooth to make it slightly porous and then applying a plastic material onto the surface, to make it smooth and healthy-looking.

Laminating A thin veneer of porcelain, preformed plastic or composite resin is bonded to the front of the teeth to effectively cover up any damage, wear and staining.

Crowning This involves fixing a crown, or cap, to replace part of a tooth. Crowns are available in a wide range of materials including porcelain, acrylic, steel, aluminium, gold or combinations of these materials.

Bridge This is an appliance that replaces one or more missing teeth. It is usually attached to the adjacent teeth by means of cement or wires on the roof of the mouth which are hidden from view.

Orthodontics Clear plastic plates and lingual braces are worn to reposition misaligned teeth. Braces can be used to straighten crooked teeth or to correct a bad bite that is causing uneven wear. Orthodontal treatment can be time-consuming, often taking up to 18 months to be completely effective.

BEFORE

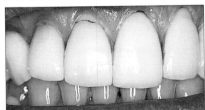

AFTER

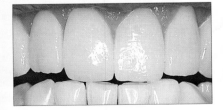

Healthy, attractive teeth can keep you younger for longer. These teeth have had a range of dental treatments, including bleaching, contouring and laminating.

Chapter 4

Health matters

Physical health

By keeping your body in good working order, you greatly increase your chances of living a long life. Examine your body for physical changes that may require medical attention and get regular medical check-ups.

Your body is a living miracle that, with care and attention, you can maintain in great shape throughout your life. Yet it is easy to neglect your physical health in today's busy world. Many people look after their cars better than they do their own bodies – taking them for an annual service and keeping them running smoothly while expecting their bodies to function without proper maintenance. Prevention is the key to good health, so schedule regular check-ups.

One of the best ways to care for your body is to get to know it: how it feels, how it looks and how it works. Understanding your body, both inside and out, can help you monitor your general health and spot potential problems. Many disorders can be treated and cured more effectively if diagnosed early. Regularly examining yourself may also help you become more confident about your body and your physical health.

HEREDITY

Some conditions have a strong genetic link, meaning that the disease or a predisposition towards the disease is passed on from generation to generation. They include diabetes, heart disease, high blood cholesterol levels (hypercholesterolemia) and cancers of the colon, breast, cervix, uterus, ovaries and prostate. To discover whether you are at risk, find out about the medical history of close

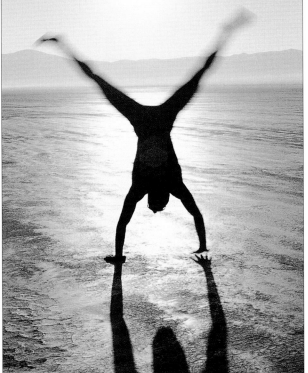

Know yourself, inside and out, to monitor your health and vitality.

relatives – grandparents, parents, aunts, uncles and siblings – to see if a pattern emerges. Even if there appears to be a genetic link, it does not mean that you will automatically be affected. You may not have inherited the gene or there may have been other factors, such as smoking or obesity, involved that don't apply to you.

Many disease genes have been identified and located on a particular chromosome, and you can be tested to see if you carry the offending gene. If you know a particular disease runs in your family, you are more likely to be alert to symptoms, if they appear. You may also adopt preventive measures, such as stopping smoking if there is evidence of heart disease in your family. Your doctor may also recommend regular screening for signs of the disease. Prostate screening, for instance, is recommended only for those with a family history of prostate cancer.

CHECK-UPS AND SCREENINGS

Your doctor may have already recommended routine screening, that is tests designed to pick up diseases before symptoms appear. Although your doctor should recall you at appropriate intervals, it's a good idea to keep track of when you last had a test and when you are due for your next (see pages 116–117). As you age, expect to be tested for certain cancers, such as colon and breast cancer, especially if members of your family have had the disease.

You should visit your doctor for routine check-ups throughout your life, but with increasing frequency as you grow older. Don't feel that you have to wait for a check-up to talk to your doctor about anything that is worrying you. Make an appointment and be frank and honest about your concerns.

SELF-EXAMINATION

To begin the process, take time out each month to stand in front of a full-length mirror and take a good look at your hair, face and body. It may help to use a hand-held mirror to see all parts of your body.

If you have never studied your body before, it may take a while to take in your marks, scars, moles and blemishes – those you were born with and those you have accumulated over the years.

Make a note of these marks, taking into account their colour, shape and size to create a map of your body that you can refer to. This map will help you spot new developments or changes in existing marks. Work methodically down your body; remember to note the positive and beautiful aspects, too!

Be alert to any changes in your general health. Your weight should remain fairly constant, unless you are dieting or exercising strenuously. Any dramatic, unexplained weight loss warrants investigation by your doctor. Similarly, any change in bowel habit, such as persistent diarrhoea or constipation, should be brought to your doctor's attention. Also, be aware of how often you urinate, if you've experienced severe shortness of breath or unusual or inexplicable fatigue.

Most of the signs you discover during your self-examination will be minor and harmless. They will simply alert you to the fact that you may need to fine-tune your diet and lifestyle. But there is always the possibility of a more serious underlying cause, so watch your body

and listen to what it tells you. This will help catch a disorder as early as possible and give your doctor the best chance of treating you.

THE SKIN AND HAIR

Your skin is a barometer of your health, so keep a close watch on any changes in its colour or texture. If it looks dull and grey, it may mean that you're not eating a healthy diet, or that you're simply a little under the weather. Vitamin deficiencies can cause rashes, as can food allergies and medications, particularly antibiotics and sulfonamides. Some viral infections, such as chickenpox, cold sores and shingles, affect the skin, but these look different from other skin rashes – each has a characteristic pattern – and are often experienced with a fever.

Rashes and/or eczema can be caused by a variety of factors, from a simple and easily controlled allergy to a severe stress disorder. If you are prone to these types of skin complaints, try to control them through changes in diet and lifestyle or simple home remedies. Make a note of when your condition tends to appear, monitor it and try to assess what exacerbates it and/or what appears to clear it up. This information may help you tackle the problem yourself, and if the irritation persists or worsens, it will also be useful to your doctor.

Look for raised bumps, lumps or newly pigmented areas. Most moles never grow bigger than the blunt end of a pencil, so look out for ones that grow larger, have an irregular outline, bleed, itch or change colour.

Cases of skin cancer are increasing dramatically each year, all over the world, but if caught early cure rates are high.

However, the most deadly of the skin cancers, malignant melanoma, often starts in or near a mole – so it's vital to monitor any changes in a mole. Check, too, for wounds or ulcers that do not heal, and for spots or warts that change shape, size or colour.

BLOOD CHOLESTEROL LEVELS

A simple home kit will give you an indication of your total blood cholesterol level. Scores below refer to millimols per litre.

Score 6.2 and over (6.5 and over in ANZ)
Risk High
Action See your doctor for further tests and keep to a low-fat diet. You may need cholesterol-lowering drugs.

Score 5.1–6.1 (5.5–6.5 in ANZ)
Risk Increased
Action Visit your doctor for a confirmatory test. Keep to a low-fat diet.

Score 5.0 or less (under 5.5 in ANZ)
Risk Low
Action Carry on as you are, although an annual check is advisable to register any changes.

Professional tests also provide triglyceride, LDL and HDL levels. (The National Heart Foundation of Australia doesn't recommend home testing.)

GENETIC LINKS

There are a number of conditions you can inherit from your parents, including some that neither parent appears to have. A gene can pass through generations via 'carriers', who are not affected by the gene but can pass it on to their offspring. A good example of this is colour-blindness, which affects only male members of a family. Although women aren't affected, they can pass the gene on to their children. This diagram illustrates how colour-blindness is inherited. It is a sex-linked gene, which is found on the X chromosome. A dominant gene means children need receive only one copy (from either parent) to be affected. A recessive gene, on the other hand, requires both parents to have the gene in order to pass it on.

▲ X chromosome
△ Affected X chromosome
● Y chromosome

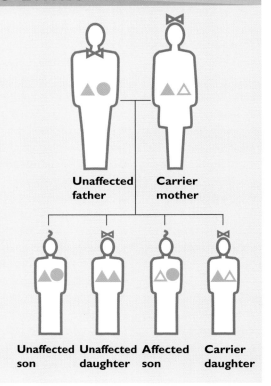

Unaffected father   **Carrier mother**

Unaffected son   **Unaffected daughter**   **Affected son**   **Carrier daughter**

Your hands and feet are also good indicators of some health problems – discolorations or rough surfaces on the nails can indicate poor nutrition. Clubbing, or broadening of the tips, of fingers and toes may indicate a chronic lung disease or a heart abnormality.

If you find a lump or other unusual sign on the skin, don't panic; it may be perfectly harmless. Nothing is gained, however, by putting off a visit to your doctor if you think there may be a problem. Many tumours, for example, are either benign (that is, non-cancerous) or respond well to treatment. The sooner a condition is diagnosed, the greater the likelihood of successful treatment.

THE HEART AND LUNGS

Each day your heart beats over 100,000 times – that's over three billion beats in an average lifetime. This unique muscle works incredibly hard throughout your life and the best way to keep it in tiptop condition is to exercise regularly. As you grow older, you may notice occasional signs, such as chest

pain, that mean you need to change some aspect of your lifestyle or visit your doctor for a cardiovascular check-up. This could include an assessment of your heart's activity via an ECG (resting and during exercise), heart function using echocardiography, heart size and shape as revealed by a chest X-ray, and how the muscles are working and blood is flowing using various imaging techniques.

After the age of 50, heart problems become more common, but if you have kept your heart fit and healthy you will fare well. A common symptom of angina – a lack of oxygen in the heart due to a narrowing of the heart arteries – is pain in the chest or arm. If you often feel pain in your left arm or shoulder (it's referred pain from your heart), you should bring this to your doctor's attention.

You can take preventive measures to reduce your risk of angina and other problems associated with heart disease, such as atherosclerosis. If your risk factors for heart disease are high (overweight, high cholesterol level and/or a high-fat diet), you should make some simple lifestyle changes; your doctor may also recommend drug treatment. Start with a healthy eating plan (see pages 42–51), paying particular attention to reducing your intake of cholesterol-rich foods and saturated fats. As well as adjusting your diet, you may need to lose some weight (see pages 59–65). Drinking large quantities of alcohol is ill advised, and smoking should be cut out completely. Get regular exercise – aim to raise your heart rate for over 20 minutes three times a week (see pages 14–19).

Many studies have confirmed that stress and high blood pressure contribute greatly to angina and heart disease. Taking time off to relax and reducing the stressful factors in your life can help to improve your cardiovascular health.

As you grow older, your lungs lose some of their former elasticity and you may find that you can become short of breath more easily. Again, exercise works your lungs hard, which helps them remain more elastic. Smoking greatly increases your chances of developing diseases such as emphysema and lung cancer, life-threatening conditions for which treatments are limited and often ineffective. The mechanisms that protect your lungs from infections, such as the action of cilia (tiny hairs) and mucus, become less effective as you age, so you are more liable to infections, such as flu and bronchitis. These can be uncomfortable and draining, requiring rest and, if appropriate, a course of antibiotics. Asthma, which affects up to a fifth of the population in some Western countries, is increasingly common. It is mostly caused by pollen (see box), house dust mites and/or animal fur. Most asthma sufferers can manage their asthma themselves, using inhalers (or puffers) to deliver a dose of bronchodilator drug directly to their lungs when they feel they need it.

HIGH BLOOD PRESSURE

Your blood pressure varies throughout the day (see page 118). Normally, blood pressure increases when you are under stress or are involved in physical activity. In these

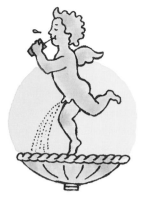

FLUSH OUT GERMS
Cranberry juice is highly effective at treating cystitis. The juice contains an unidentified substance that stops the offending bacteria from attaching to the bladder lining. Drinking plenty of fluids can also help flush the infection away.

circumstances, your heart responds to your body's activities and needs by increasing the resistance to the force of blood through the arteries – this puts extra stress on your arteries and major body organs. People who suffer from abnormally high blood pressure (hypertension) have, therefore, an almost constant stress on their bodies, which puts them at higher risk of certain diseases.

High blood pressure makes you 12 times more likely to have a stroke and 6 times more likely to suffer a heart attack.

It is estimated that hypertension affects 15–30 per cent of the adult population of most Western countries – usually people over 55 years old. Although it's often thought of as a 'man's disease', it afflicts just as many women after menopause as men. Many of the sufferers of hypertension are unaware of their condition because there are no noticeable symptoms. Most people find out only when their doctor carries out a simple blood pressure test – a part of most routine check-ups.

continued on page 118

Hay fever
Some people don't look forward to late spring and early summer because of the havoc pollen wreaks on their respiratory system. Hay fever is an allergy to air-borne pollen from trees, grasses and moulds, which irritates the bronchioli (tiny air passages) in the lungs, causing breathlessness and wheezing. Subsequent inflammation of the bronchioli can also lead to excess phlegm production and sufferers often acquire a chesty cough as they try to remove mucus. Treatments include the use of inhalers and/or antihistamine drugs. Although the best policy is to stay away from the triggers, this can prove difficult when the sun is shining and you want to get outside.

What's happening inside your body? Advances in the screening techniques available enable doctors to pinpoint early warning signs of a range of conditions, so that preventive forms of treatments can be enacted.

CHECK-UPS FOR
men and women

Screening techniques allow your doctor to check your body for hidden and potential problems so that they can be treated before they become well established. For example, a physical exam might turn up precancerous cell changes in the cervix or high blood cholesterol levels – both could lead to a serious disorder, but if caught early can be treated successfully. Take control of your health by making changes in your lifestyle to live a healthier, longer life. Help your doctor, too, by being self-aware and looking out for any changes from the norm.

SCREENING TEST	HOW OFTEN YOU NEED A CHECK
BLOOD PRESSURE MEASUREMENT	
Your blood pressure is checked during a routine physical examination. Your doctor records your diastolic and systolic pressures (see pages 118–119).	Once you reach 50, you are advised to have an annual blood pressure reading. You should have check-ups twice a year if you suffer from heart disease, high blood pressure or if anyone in your family has high or low blood pressure.
CHOLESTEROL BLOOD TEST	
A cholesterol test involves taking a pin prick of blood to test for blood cholesterol. High levels of cholesterol and other fats (triglycerides) in the blood indicate an increased risk of heart disease. (You can also buy home-testing kits at a pharmacy.)	After 40 years of age, you should have a blood cholesterol test every five years. If you smoke, have high blood pressure or if a close family member suffers from diabetes or heart disease, you should have one more frequently.
ELECTROCARDIOGRAM (ECG)	
Your doctor should listen to your heart with a stethoscope, monitor its activity via an ECG and/or check chemical levels in a blood sample. Other tests include MRI scanning of damaged heart muscle and coronary angiography to check artery health.	If you have a family history of heart disease, are overweight, smoke and rarely exercise, you should have an annual heart check-up over the age of 35.
BONE DENSITOMETRY	
The standard technique is to use a low-level radiation scan of the wrists, hips and spine. Other techniques include the use of ultrasound and blood tests. Bone densitometry can indicate whether you are at risk of osteoporotic fractures.	You should have an annual check-up if you are a post-menopausal woman who is not taking HRT. Regular testing is particularly important if there is a history of osteoporosis in your family or you keep breaking bones.
FAECAL OCCULT BLOOD AND COLONOSCOPY	
Colorectal screening involves a faecal occult blood test to detect the presence of hidden blood in the stool. The colon may be examined with a viewing device – a sigmoidoscope or colonoscope – to detect polyps or precancerous growths.	Colorectal cancer is a common killer of people over 50. An annual screening for men and women over 50 is advised, especially if there is a family history of ulcerative colitis or colonic polyps.

SCREENING TEST	HOW OFTEN YOU NEED A CHECK
DENTAL EXAM	
During a dental check-up, your dentist can spot the signs of gum disease, fill cavities and look out for structural problems. Your gums can be good indicators of a more general disease and your dentist may be able to spot early warning signs.	See your dentist every six months or, if you notice a problem, at the first opportunity. Extra check-ups may be needed during pregnancy when the teeth are particularly prone to difficulties.
VISION CHECKS	
An eye exam should include routine testing for glaucoma, cataracts and macular degeneration. Tell your optometrist or ophthalmologist if any family member has suffered from glaucoma or other eye conditions.	Have your eyesight tested every two to five years from the age of 35 onwards.
AUDIOMETRY TESTS	
If anything simple is found to be impairing your hearing, such as a build-up of wax, this is easily treated. If you are experiencing hearing loss, you may be advised to use a hearing aid to amplify sounds and reduce stress on your inner ear.	If you have noticed a decline in your hearing or your doctor has some cause for concern, you will be referred for audiometry tests. Hearing loss is not an inevitable part of aging – but it is quite common as age progresses.
HORMONE LEVEL TESTS	
As well as detecting whether or not you are in menopause, these tests can show up conditions such as hypothyroidism (an underactive thyroid), which is more common in postmenopausal women.	If you have the following symptoms without reason, you may benefit from a hormone level test: fatigue, depression, weight loss or gain, and thinning hair. A thyroid function test should be carried out every year after the age of 55.
BLOOD-SUGAR TEST	
Type II diabetes mellitus is more common from the 40s onwards in men and women and occurs when the body cannot produce sufficient insulin, or is resistant to its effects. Blood-sugar and urine tests are required to confirm diabetes.	Get a test if you have the following symptoms; fatigue, excessive thirst and urination, frequent urinary or vaginal infections, weakness and blurred vision. The test should be carried out every three years, or more if you have symptoms.

SCREENING FOR WOMEN

Some experts recommend yearly mammograms for all women over the age of 50 as the incidence of breast cancer rises significantly after menopause. Below this age an X-ray is less useful because the breast tissue is usually too dense to show up a tumour, and so an ultrasound scan may be preferred. To confirm or disprove the presence of cancer, a biopsy is performed. This involves taking a small tissue sample for laboratory examination.

A smear test can detect the precancerous changes that could lead to cervical cancer. Checks are recommended every one to three years. (Ask your doctor how often you should have one.) The test should be combined with a pelvic examination. Life-threatening conditions such as ovarian cancer are often detected during these check-ups.

SCREENING FOR MEN

Doctors may recommend prostate screening every year for men over 50 (and over 40 if there is a family history of prostate cancer). Routine screening includes a rectal examination, in which the physician uses a finger to detect whether the outer core of the prostate is enlarged. With age it is common for the inner core of the prostate to enlarge, causing symptoms such as awakening at night with the need to urinate, reduced urine flow, urgency and a dribble at the end of passing urine. This is usually due to a common and treatable change called benign prostatic hypertrophy. A more serious indicator is a chemical called prostate specific antigen, which rises slightly with age but more significantly with cancer. To confirm the presence of cancer, a biopsy is taken so that tissue samples can be analysed in a laboratory.

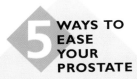

5 WAYS TO EASE YOUR PROSTATE

1 Drink lots of water.

2 Urinate as often as you feel the need.

3 Ejaculate regularly to unclog your prostatic ducts.

4 Avoid fats and cholesterol, and eat more vegetables.

5 Don't just sit there – get some exercise to relieve the pressure on your prostate.

The exact causes of hypertension vary from person to person. Blood pressure rises with age, usually because of changes in hormone levels, weight gain and physical inactivity. Your family history is important and if any members of your family suffer from high blood pressure, you may be at risk.

Being overweight certainly does not help – 60 per cent of people with hypertension are overweight. Women taking the contraceptive pill increase their risk of high blood pressure, particularly if they are smokers. The more recently developed low-dose contraceptive pills have less of an effect on blood pressure.

Stress and other psychological factors have been found to have a significant effect on blood pressure. Students in Vancouver were found to have higher blood pressure if they had little social support from friends and family, and many studies have linked high-stress jobs with high blood pressure.

Sodium is the other main contributor to high blood pressure. Commonly eaten as table salt, it makes your body retain water. The more water, the more blood in circulation, and the more your heart has to work to pump the blood around. Cutting down on salt can significantly improve your blood pressure.

A British research team found that reducing salt intake to 3 grams per day – about a teaspoon – could prevent 26 per cent of all strokes and 15 per cent of heart attacks caused by blood clots.

Further studies, carried out at the Johns Hopkins University in Baltimore, have found that the combination of a high-sodium diet with a high-stress lifestyle makes a person ten times more likely to develop high blood pressure than either of these factors on its own.

HEALTHY BLOOD PRESSURE

Your blood pressure rises and falls throughout the day, according to your activities. As you sleep, your blood pressure is relatively low, and on waking, it starts to rise, usually reaching its normal pressure within the first few hours after getting out of bed. Vigorous exercise raises blood pressure greatly, more so if you are unfit. Other highs in the day may be caused by stress, smoking or drinking alcohol. You will not recover quickly from a period of high blood pressure if you are overweight, inactive or a smoker. Blood pressure can be lowered with rest and relaxation techniques (see pages 198–199).

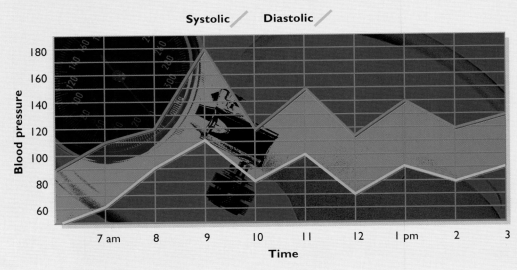

The lesson is clear – try to manage stress, reduce your salt intake, keep your weight down and exercise. Read food labels to find out how much sodium is in each product, and use low-sodium alternatives.

A balanced diet can also help keep sodium down and blood pressure normal. Studies have shown that potassium, magnesium, calcium and fibre supplements may help to regulate blood pressure (see pages 47–49). Smoking is especially bad for people with high blood pressure; make the decision to stop now!

THE HEAD AND BRAIN

Headaches are probably the most common physical complaint in adults. They can be caused by food allergies, food additives, cold or flu, sinusitis, stress, anxiety, hypertension, hangover, fever, migraine or environmental factors, such as bright lights or loud noises. The best way to deal with headaches is to avoid the things that cause them. Treatments usually involve relaxation, possibly with the addition of a mild painkiller.

Migraines are very severe headaches that persist for long periods, ranging from a few hours to a number of days. They are often sparked by certain foods, particularly red wine, chocolate, dairy products, citrus fruits and certain drugs and additives. They can also be caused by stress, anxiety or depression. Avoidance of known triggers is the best policy, and treatments include painkillers, stress management (see pages 192–197) and complete rest in a darkened room.

A more serious condition, and one that becomes more likely as you age, is stroke – damage caused by interruption of the blood supply and consequent starvation of oxygen to the brain. Recent studies have found that a healthy lifestyle reduces the chance of stroke to a great extent. Taking a quarter of an adult's dose of aspirin daily from age 60,

Blood pressure monitoring

Have a blood pressure test at least once every two years if you are over 40, more frequently if you suffer from health problems. You can use a home monitoring machine to check your own blood pressure, although this should not take the place of professional monitoring. Blood pressure is recorded as two sets of numbers – the higher figure (systolic pressure) represents the pressure during the heart's contraction phase, and the lower figure (diastolic pressure) is the relaxation phase. Normal blood pressure for an adult is below 140/90. Persistently high blood pressure readings – over 150/90 – put you at serious risk of heart disease, stroke and kidney failure. You can lower your blood pressure significantly by getting more exercise and making sure your diet is healthy. It's especially important to reduce your salt intake.

with your doctor's agreement, can reduce the risk of stroke. A balanced diet rich in potassium and beta-carotene (see pages 47–49) and low in cholesterol and saturated fats (see pages 43–44), makes for a great insurance policy against stroke. Research at Duke University in North Carolina has indicated that you should also stop smoking and moderate your alcohol consumption. Regular exercise and stress reduction are also strongly advised.

THE DIGESTIVE SYSTEM

Starting at your mouth, this system continues through your stomach and intestines to your anus. Particular problems can affect different parts of the digestive system, so be aware of what to look for. Look inside your mouth and throat for inflammation, ulcers, white patches and lumps. Some of these signs might indicate common problems such as infection, vitamin deficiencies or stress. If you smoke a pipe, be extra vigilant for potentially cancerous mouth and throat lumps.

PHYSICAL THERAPIES

Don't suffer any joint or muscle pain unnecessarily – get some hands-on therapy.

Physiotherapy is the oldest established form of conventional manipulative therapy. Many people are referred by their doctor for a course of physiotherapy to restore mobility, strength coordination and motor skills following stroke, injury, disease or surgery. Others benefit from physiotherapy to ease the pain and stiffness caused by years of bad posture, occupational disorders and osteoarthritis. Practitioners may use a combination of massage and joint manipulation, and sometimes heat treatment, ultrasound and other sophisticated techniques.

Chiropractic and osteopathy are often used for chronic back pain or injuries. These therapies involve hands-on manipulation of the spine, joints, muscles and surrounding tissues. The manual targeting of bone and soft tissue can

not only help restore bone and joint health but also re-establish proper functioning of the nerve pathways.

There are certain differences between the two approaches. Osteopathy aims to improve the function of your skeletal frame, using gentle manipulation of your joints to stretch and loosen muscles and ligaments, and so restore their normal range of movement and alleviate pain. Chiropractic concentrates on the realignment of the vertebrae in your spine, and so, although a chiropractor uses similar movements to an osteopath, they are often combined with sharp, rapid thrusts of the affected joints.

Both methods can alleviate pain in a single session, but it may take several visits before long-term relief is obtained.

One of the most common digestive problems is nausea, mostly a harmless response to consuming something that disagrees with the system. Pain in your stomach could be caused by excess acid attacking your oesophagus, indigestion, infection or gastritis (irritation of the stomach lining), and the body usually quickly deals with these problems. If nausea, vomiting or stomach pains persist, you should visit your doctor.

Intestinal pains can occur for the same reasons as stomach disorders. Bouts of flatulence, diarrhoea and constipation can cause discomfort and necessitate a change in your diet if you find such episodes are frequent. Irritable bowel syndrome causes abdominal pain and distention, and changeable bowel function. It is thought to be caused predominantly by anxiety, and sufferers are advised to adjust their diet, manage stress and, sometimes, take medication to control symptoms.

As you get older, you may experience a change in your bowel functioning, often resulting in constipation. To eliminate the problem, add plenty of fruit and fibre to your

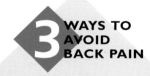

3 WAYS TO AVOID BACK PAIN

1 Adopt a well-balanced sitting and standing posture.

2 Avoid twisting and bending at the same time.

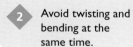

3 Keep your back in good shape with stretching exercises.

diet and increase your fluid intake. If you still have trouble after adjusting your diet, visit your doctor – constipation can aggravate other problems, including haemorrhoids (swollen veins in the anal canal).

Bleeding from the anus or blood in the stool may be a sign of irritable bowel syndrome, although haemorrhoids are the more usual cause. In most cases, haemorrhoids can be treated by adopting a high-fibre diet or, failing that, they can be removed surgically.

THE MUSCLES

There are more than 300 pairs of muscles in the human body, all working together to give us the energy, strength, flexibility and mobility to carry out our everyday tasks. Muscles provide freedom of movement and play a major part in determining your body shape and strength. Without muscles, your body would stop functioning altogether – your heart is a vital muscle itself – yet muscles are rarely looked after as well as they should be.

We place great physical demands on our muscles and all too often ignore the warning signs that can lead to damage. Unless they are regularly exercised and looked after, muscles can become weak and stiff and they may even atrophy (start wasting away). Simple, regular exercise – not necessarily strenuous – will tone the muscles. For advice on managing your muscles see pages 28–33.

BACK PROBLEMS

Sooner or later, most people experience backache of some kind. It could be a slight nagging annoyance to one side of your lower spine, or a massive explosion of pain that renders you bed-ridden for a few weeks.

By far the greatest cause of back pain is muscle strain. If you don't exercise regularly, the muscles that support your spine weaken from lack of use. So when you try to do something a little more strenuous than usual, such as lifting a heavy box, your muscles are unprepared and strain as a result.

As soon as you get a back strain, you should apply ice to reduce the pain and swelling. Wrap ice in a towel and apply it to the affected area for 10 minutes every hour until the initial ache subsides. Never apply ice directly to the skin. After the swelling has reduced, apply heat to the injured area by placing a warm cloth on it for 10 minutes every hour, or take a warm shower or bath.

Usually, the best home treatment for back pain is gentle exercise, especially walking and swimming, combined with stretching, such as the yoga positions shown on pages 122–123. Ask your doctor for advice – there are some more serious back conditions for which exercise is inappropriate. Painkillers, especially those with an anti-inflammatory action, such as ibuprofen, can reduce pain and swelling, but keep to the recommended dosage.

Although most back problems subside within a week or two, you should see your doctor if pain persists or worsens, or if you experience numbness or tingling in your legs or abdomen. You may want to visit a chiropractor or physiotherapist, who can also help if the condition is not complicated.

With a little thought and effort you can help prevent back pain. The best preventive

LIFTING TECHNIQUE

A large percentage of back problems result from improper lifting. When attempting to pick up something heavy, let your leg muscles – not your back – take the strain.

▶ Keep your spine as vertical as possible and bend your knees, not your back.

▶ Place your feet comfortably apart, on either side of the object, if possible.

▶ Tense your abdominal muscles to provide support.

▶ Hold the object as close to your body as possible.

▶ Lift slowly and avoid twisting your body as you stand.

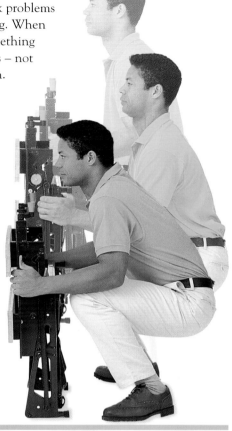

action is to exercise. Walking, swimming, cycling and other aerobic exercises help to condition your whole body without placing too much strain on your bones. Stretching is also important – your back is more likely to strain if the muscles are unaccustomed to use. Stretching exercises, found on pages 36–37, should be performed regularly, and always to warm up your joints before undertaking any arduous physical task (see pages 20–21).

Good posture will also help your back. Spend a little time considering your usual standing and walking postures and then adjust them to balance weight and take excess strain from your back. You can help support your back by strengthening your abdominal muscles – your back and abdominals work together. Don't wear high-heeled shoes or tight-fitting clothes that restrict movement and ruin your posture.

Make sure that your bed mattress is firm and does not sag. If you have discomfort while sitting, buy a small foam roll (lumbar support) which you can position in the small of your back when you sit down to give extra support to your lower back. These are available from pharmacies and other shops.

When tackling a heavy object, think twice. First, do you really need to move it? Can someone else help you? Is there an easy lifting technique that can lessen the load? Test the load to make sure that it isn't going to cause serious damage. Second, if you need to move it, follow the correct lifting technique described on page 121.

Back problems can result from a disease, such as osteoporosis or osteoarthritis. Sufferers are often prescribed specific back and lower-abdominal strengthening exercises to help prevent associated back pain. Some people with arthritis find that practising t'ai chi helps enormously.

THE BONES AND JOINTS

One of the most strenuously used parts of the body, the skeletal system can be desperately painful when damaged. The individual bones need to be strengthened with a diet that includes a regular, moderate intake of calcium, plus adequate amounts of phosphorus, fluoride and vitamin D. This must be combined with regular weight-bearing exercise, such as walking or jogging, to ensure these minerals are deposited into the bones and not allowed to pass out of the body.

The skeleton is constantly accumulating and losing minerals, such as calcium. These minerals are released from the bones by cells known as osteoclasts in order to meet the needs of other parts of the body. The minerals are regularly replaced by other cells in the bones called osteoblasts, which build up the bones and maintain bone density. By putting steady moderate pressure on the bones, through regular weight-bearing exercise, you

YOGA FOR BACKS

Yoga can be very helpful for maintaining a healthy back. The following postures (asanas) are especially recommended.

THE SPINAL TWIST

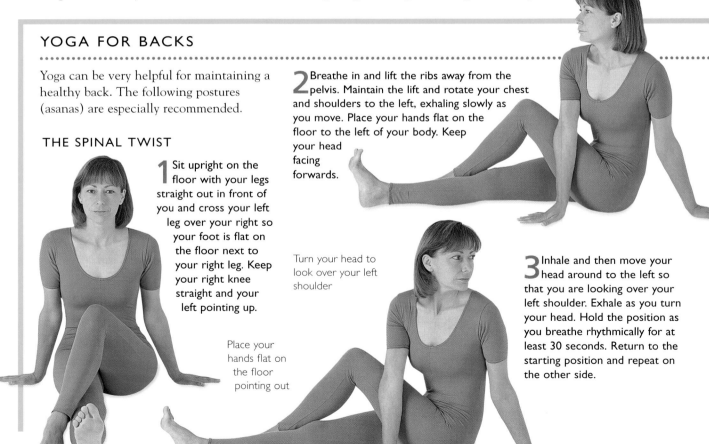

1 Sit upright on the floor with your legs straight out in front of you and cross your left leg over your right so your foot is flat on the floor next to your right leg. Keep your right knee straight and your left pointing up.

Place your hands flat on the floor pointing out

2 Breathe in and lift the ribs away from the pelvis. Maintain the lift and rotate your chest and shoulders to the left, exhaling slowly as you move. Place your hands flat on the floor to the left of your body. Keep your head facing forwards.

Turn your head to look over your left shoulder

3 Inhale and then move your head around to the left so that you are looking over your left shoulder. Exhale as you turn your head. Hold the position as you breathe rhythmically for at least 30 seconds. Return to the starting position and repeat on the other side.

can slow down the rate of bone loss and increase the rate of build-up. Inactivity leads to rapid bone loss, which is hard to reverse.

As you grow older, your risk of developing the bone-thinning disease osteoporosis increases. Osteoporosis mainly affects your vertebrae, wrists and hips.

Osteoporotic bone is much less dense and so is more liable to fracture. Unfortunately, there are no treatments for this disease, but experts advise that building up bone mass before the age of 35 can do more to prevent or delay its onset than any other measure. They recommend increasing your daily calcium intake to 700–800 mg and some suggest 1000–1500 mg over the age of 50 (see end of book). The following are risk factors: a sedentary lifestyle; the menopause; a family history of the disease; excessive alcohol

consumption; and a calcium-deficient diet. If one or more of these factors apply to you, you should take some preventive action (see page 124).

Remember that staying in the same position for long periods of time places extra stress on your bones and joints. If you spend a great deal of time sitting down during the day, make an effort to get up and move around and stretch briefly every half an hour.

ARTHRITIS

The single leading cause of disability in people of all ages is arthritis, affecting millions of people around the world. Although there are a number of different types of arthritis, they all result in stiffness of the joints and an inability to move normally. The two most common types, rheumatoid arthritis and osteoarthritis, occur about three times more often in women than in men, and become more common with age.

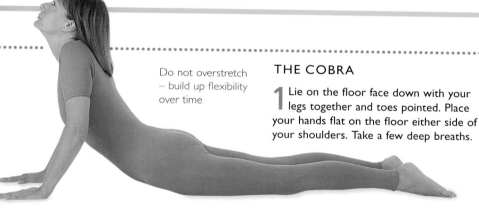

Do not overstretch – build up flexibility over time

THE COBRA

1 Lie on the floor face down with your legs together and toes pointed. Place your hands flat on the floor either side of your shoulders. Take a few deep breaths.

2 Push yourself up into the cobra position by straightening your arms. Keep your legs and hips on the floor, look up and feel your back flexing. Do not overstretch your back; as you practise you will find your back becoming more flexible. Practise regularly and work towards straightening your arms.

THE CAT

1 Get on to all fours with your knees under your hips and hands under your shoulders. As you breathe in, allow your belly to drop towards the floor and lift your head to look straight in front.

2 Exhale and arch your back towards the ceiling, like a cat stretching. At the same time, allow your head to drop towards the floor. Hold this position and your breath for as long as is comfortable. Repeat the sequence, breathing rhythmically, 10–20 times.

Keep your arms and legs at right angles to your back

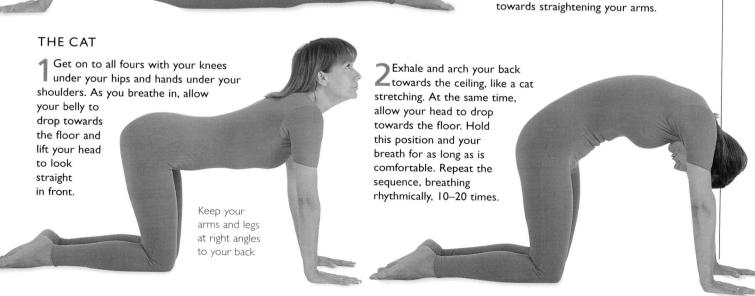

Rheumatoid arthritis affects 0.8–1 per cent of any population and occurs when the immune system inappropriately attacks the body's own tissues – but what triggers this response is not yet fully understood. It is thought to be linked to hormones and the childbearing process, but women who have not had children can still be affected. As a result of the unknown triggers, it is hard to identify risk groups or prescribe methods of prevention.

Osteoarthritis, the most common type of arthritis, occurs when the cartilage in joints deteriorates due to repetitive stress injury, poor nutrition and general wear and tear. It is estimated that almost everyone over the age of 60 has osteoarthritis to some degree, though the symptoms may not be noticeable.

You can't stop osteoarthritis once it occurs, but you can help prevent it, or reduce its effects, by eating and exercising properly. Excess body weight exacerbates the condition so, if you are overweight, try to shed some weight. If you are underweight, you can also be hit hard by osteoarthritis because your body lacks sufficient calcium to keep bones healthy. A calcium supplement will help keep your joints strong for longer. If you are a woman undergoing or past menopause, consider hormone replacement therapy (see pages 134–139), which reduces the risk of osteoarthritis by 60 per cent.

Exercise is another way to stop your joints from becoming stiff. Improve muscle strength and flexibility (see pages 32–33 and 36–37) to ease pressure on the joints. Strengthen the muscles in your abdomen to support your back and in the thighs to protect your knees.

Avoid injuring your joints as much as possible; an injured joint will almost certainly contribute to osteoarthritis later in life.

Choose low-impact activities that do not strain your joints – try swimming and avoid running on hard roads. Footwear is particularly important for protecting bones and joints – poor shoes can damage the toes, feet, ankles, shins, knees, thighs and pelvic bones.

PREVENT OSTEOPOROSIS

Up to around the age of 35, bones tend to gain more minerals than they lose, thus remaining strong. After 35, this process often reverses, leading to decreased density, or bone mass, making the bones more porous and liable to fracture. Known as osteoporosis, this condition affects both sexes, although women are at higher risk, particularly after menopause. There is no cure, but you can take steps to reduce the effects. These include hormone replacement therapy (HRT) if you are undergoing or past menopause, exercises to strengthen the back and limbs, and daily calcium supplements – around 1000 mg for those on HRT and 1500 mg for others (see end of book). You may also be prescribed bisphosphonates to inhibit calcium loss and increase bone density.

Arthritic pain can be eased with heat or ice. Place a hot-water bottle or ice pack on the painful area for 10–15 minutes several times a day. Avoid exercise or any other strenuous activities if you are in pain – it will not only aggravate the pain, but can also cause further damage. A balanced diet can help ease the symptoms of arthritis, according to a number of studies. Reduce your intake of saturated fats and increase the amount of fruit and vegetables, fish with omega-3 fish oils (see page 44), and fibre. People with arthritis may have a reaction to certain foods, similar to a food allergy. In these cases, the offending foods should first be identified and then eliminated from the diet.

THE HORMONAL SYSTEM

Some hormone levels decline with age, such as growth hormone and DHEA, while others remain constant through life, such as cortisone and thyroid hormones. Any changes in your inner chemicals or fluctuations in hormones, nutrients and subtle chemical functions can have a surprisingly big impact on your health. You will need to have some tests to discover a specific problem, but common symptoms of imbalances include fatigue, constant thirst, propensity for infections and illnesses, blurred vision, hearing loss and muscle tiredness.

One of the most common hormonal disorders is diabetes mellitus, which affects 2–5 per cent of the Western population.

Untreated, diabetes is a life-threatening condition and its management and associated complications should be monitored closely by your doctor. It tends to run in families, so look into your family history.

Diabetes occurs when a lack of insulin prevents sugar from being absorbed into the cells that need it for energy. As the body can't get its energy from sugar, it turns to fat supplies, but the chemical breakdown process is often faulty and produces dangerous substances called ketones, which can cause coma and even death. Common symptoms of undiagnosed diabetes, resulting from high levels of blood sugar, include an excessive thirst and need to urinate. High sugar levels in blood and urine impair your body's fight against infections such as cystitis and candidiasis, which are common in women.

There are two principal types of diabetes mellitus – insulin-dependent and non-insulin-dependent. Insulin-dependent, also known as type I, diabetes typically develops in younger people (usually appearing before the age of 16) and demands regular injections of insulin, because the pancreas cannot produce enough, or any, itself.

The other type, type II or non-insulin-dependent diabetes, develops gradually, mainly in people who are over the age of 40 and overweight. It is more common than type I diabetes, affecting 90 per cent of the diabetic population. It may produce no symptoms and be discovered only during a routine check-up. In this type of diabetes, insulin is produced but the body appears to have a resistance to its effects. Instead of using insulin injections, this type of diabetes can usually be treated, and sometimes reversed, through dietary control and weight loss.

Other hormonal problems include thyroid and adrenal gland disorders (affecting metabolism), anaemia (lack of iron in the blood),

Foot ailments

Many common problems affecting the feet are easily avoided.

Bunions and blisters Often a direct result of badly fitting shoes, these are particularly aggravated by wearing high heels over extended periods of time. They may also be due to arthritis or heredity, so watch out if you fall into these categories.

Corns and calluses These are lumps of hardened dead skin that form on bony areas due to friction. They usually don't need treatment if they do not cause pain, but avoid tight shoes and moisturise the area properly. Many of the over-the-counter remedies sold in chemists contain salicylic acid and should be applied only to the hard skin.

Foot infections Athlete's foot and other infections are due to perspiration and a lack of aeration. Use an antifungal cream if you have the initial itchiness and blistering of the skin. Avoid the problem by wearing ventilated shoes, cotton socks and exposing your feet to fresh air.

Verrucas Also called plantar warts, verrucas are caused by a virus and are often acquired in swimming pools or communal showers. Prevent them by wearing flip-flops. Treatments include pharmaceutical preparations, laser surgery and cryosurgery.

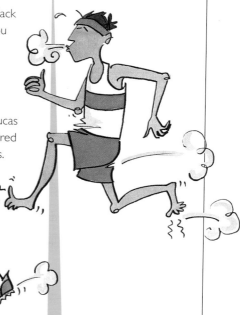

EXAMINING YOUR BREASTS

Check your breasts a day or two after your period or, if you are no longer menstruating, on the same day each month. Feel for lumps or areas of dense tissue. If you notice anything in one breast, check the corresponding area of the other breast. If both feel the same, it is likely to be your natural shape.

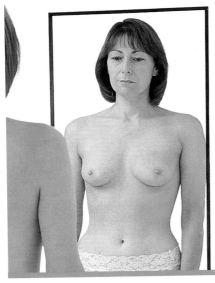

1 Stand naked in front of a large mirror and study your breasts for any abnormalities, such as dimpling, changes in shape or skin texture, or nipple changes. Put your hands on your waist, lean forwards and check again. Be aware of any discomfort.

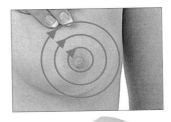

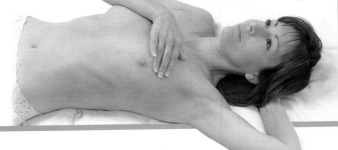

2 Lie on your back, placing your left hand under your head. Feel your left breast with the flat of your right fingers. You may feel soft, normal glandular lumps, but if you feel anything unusual you should visit your doctor. Squeeze the nipples gently to check for discharge.

hypoglycemia (low blood-sugar), and a range of nutritional deficiencies. If you have been experiencing tiredness or feeling ill for over a month, you should discuss the above possibilities with your doctor. Simple tests to measure hormone levels in the body can confirm or rule out a problem. Treatments, including HRT, are available if a disorder is identified.

THE FEMALE REPRODUCTIVE SYSTEM

Monitor your reproductive health with regular self-examinations. Make a note of any changes to your lower abdominal area and in your menstrual cycle. Abdominal discomfort, painful intercourse, irregular or abnormally heavy menstrual bleeding, or lower back pain at the end of a period may indicate endometriosis – a condition in which some of the uterine lining (the endometrium) becomes displaced and attaches to other organs within the pelvis.

Benign fibroid tumours occur in about 20 per cent of women over 30, and in many cases present no symptoms at all. But, they sometimes cause heavy or prolonged periods, frequent urination, constipation, or sharp lower abdominal pain. They often shrink in size after menopause.

Examine your breasts every month to feel for irregular lumps, and see your doctor if you find anything unusual. Although nearly 90 per cent of the lumps women find are non-cancerous, the importance of regular self-checks cannot be overemphasised. Have a smear test every one to three years (check with your doctor) and an annual mammogram if you are over 50, or more often if you are at high risk.

THE MALE REPRODUCTIVE SYSTEM

Men should check their testes for lumps at least once a month and discuss any abnormalities with their doctor. Problems with the prostate gland are harder to diagnose than those with the testes, but symptoms include difficulty in starting to urinate, poor flow of urine and increased urination. An enlarged prostate (also known as benign prostatic hypertrophy) is common in men over 50. If the symptoms are severe, then surgical removal of the prostate gland (prostatectomy) is necessary. Your doctor may recommend an annual prostate-specific antigen test if you are over 50 (and over 40 if there is a family history of prostate cancer). However, the test can be inaccurate: a high proportion of positive results turn out to be false alarms, while 20 per cent of tumours go undetected by the test. More accurate tests are in development, such as one using insulin-like growth factor as an indicator.

CANCER

According to the World Health Report, cancer claimed the lives of over six million people worldwide in 1997 – lung cancer and stomach cancer were the biggest killers.

The likelihood of cancer developing in a 20-year-old is very low, but it doubles every ten years. By age 90, there is a strong chance that a cancer has developed, even if there are no symptoms.

So, although cancer appears to be more common now than in the past, this is actually because people live longer and thus increase their risk of cancer. However, by being alert to any bodily changes and avoiding known cancer-causing agents (carcinogens), you can help to reduce your risk of cancer.

The main carcinogens, accounting for over a third of cancers, are found in food and drink. Reducing fats, particularly saturated fats, in your diet has been found to lower the risk of cancer considerably. Keep your diet high in fibre and the nutrients found in fresh fruit and vegetables, which can help prevent cancer in the digestive system as well as at a number of other sites. If your diet is inadequate, take a broad-spectrum supplement with vitamins A, C and E. These are antioxidants that will help to eliminate cancer-causing free radicals (see pages 47–48). Limit your consumption of pickled, cured, smoked and charred food – if you like barbecues, avoid inhaling the smoke and eating the blackened pieces of food. Also, keeping your weight down and exercising regularly could cut your risk by half.

Smoking is a major cause of lung cancer and you should stop now; research shows that you gain benefits within days of giving up (see pages 144–146). You should also try to avoid pollution, particularly chemical pollutants, as much as possible. Alcohol increases the risk of cancers in the digestive system and some studies suggest a limit of one unit a day.

Women who regularly use a feminine deodorant, regardless of the liquid used, increase their risk of cervical cancer fourfold. Practise safe sex, especially if you have different partners, as a sexually transmitted disease also increases the chance of cervical cancer.

Trace your family tree to see if any of your relatives have suffered from cancer. Although less than 10 per cent of cancers are directly inherited, the risk increases if you have a genetic susceptibility. Ask your doctor to evaluate your risks so that you can take extra measures to prevent it or detect it early.

TESTICULAR EXAMINATION

Get into the habit of examining your testicles every month to check for any lumps or abnormalities. If they are caught early, problems can be treated more effectively.

1 After a shower or bath, palpate each testicle, with the middle and index fingers below the testicle and the thumb on top. Gently roll the testicle between fingers and thumb. Look out for lumps, areas of pain or discomfort, swelling or ulceration of the scrotal skin.

2 Feel all round the testicle. Cancerous lumps usually feel firm to the touch and are not tender when pressed.

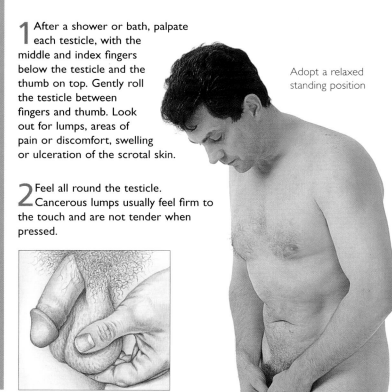

Adopt a relaxed standing position

9 health-giving **supplements**

Therapeutic plant and animal substances are available in a host of supplements. Some have been used medicinally since ancient times, while others were only discovered this century.

SELENIUM THE CELL PROTECTOR

1 Some researchers believe that selenium, found in meat, seafood and whole-grains, can slow the aging process. Moreover, research at the Arizona Cancer Center showed that subjects who took 200 micrograms of selenium daily for five years had 46 per cent less lung cancer, 58 per cent less colorectal cancer and a 39 per cent overall drop in cancer deaths. Selenium is thought to work with an antioxidant enzyme to protect against cancer, and to prevent age-related cell mutations and preserve the skin's elasticity. The recommended daily amount for women is 55–70 micrograms, and 70–85 micrograms for men (see end of book), although you may need 100–400 micrograms for optimal nutrition – ask your pharmacist or doctor about a supplement.

CALCIUM FOR YOUR BONES

2 Calcium is the main constituent of your bones and is essential for keeping them healthy. However, if your body needs calcium for other reasons, and there is none in the system, it will simply take it from the bones, reducing bone density over time. Calcium also helps stablise your blood pressure and protects against stroke and cancer. The recommended daily dose is 700–800 mg (see end of book), so consider taking a supplement. Choose one containing zinc, magnesium, boron and silica so that the calcium is metabolised for bone formation and does not gather elsewhere, causing other health problems.

Co-enzyme Q-10 for energy

3 **Co-enzyme Q-10 is made in the body, yet up to half of the population may be deficient in the nutrients required to produce it. Proponents of Q-10 supplements say that it improves heart function, fitness and general wellbeing; it may also protect against gum disease, heart disease, cancer and aging. Daily dosages range from 50 to 100 mg and some experts recommend up to 300 mg for optimum benefit.**

GINKGO BILOBA, A MEDICINE FROM PREHISTORY

4 The ginkgo biloba tree dates back to the Jurassic age, and was first described in a Chinese medical book in 2800BC. In the West, studies have shown that ginkgo biloba dilates blood vessels and so increases blood flow to the brain, thus enhancing memory and mental alertness. It also promotes cardiovascular health, and being an antioxidant, combats cancer-causing free radicals. A daily supplement of 120 mg (split into two or three doses) is often recommended.

GINSENG, THE ANCIENT TONIC

5

Used throughout the ages as a tonic to help maintain the body's balance, ginseng has oestrogenic properties said to reduce menopausal hot flushes. Some people believe that it may also help other menstrual irregularities, boost libido, alleviate depression and overcome fatigue. Ginseng is said to counteract problems with sexual desire and impotence in men. It should only be used as recommended on the packet. There are side effects if it is taken in excess.

St John's wort to lift your mood

6

Clinical tests have shown that St John's wort (hypericum) may be helpful in the treatment of mild to moderate depression – it's often prescribed in Germany as a substitute for Prozac – and may alleviate insomnia and high blood pressure. In one study on a group of depressed patients, almost 67 per cent of those taking the herb showed significant improvement in their symptoms compared with only 27 per cent of the placebo group. There were no side effects reported.

HEALTHFUL BEE PRODUCTS

7

Two substances produced in bee hives – propolis and royal jelly – are claimed to have health-giving properties. Propolis, an antibacterial agent used by bees to insulate the hive, contains essential oils and concentrated bioflavonoids, which may help to protect against cancer, heart disease and premature aging. Royal jelly is fed to the queen bee by worker bees to help her grow. It is claimed to enhance the immune system, increase stamina and boost energy levels. Some believe that royal jelly helps protect the body against the side effects of chemotherapy and radiotherapy.

FLOWER OILS FOR BALANCED HORMONES

8

The seeds of the evening primrose contain large amounts of the essential fatty acid omega-6 (gamma linolenic acid or GLA), which your body can convert into prostaglandins. These are used to regulate several body functions, including hormone balance, blood pressure and inflammation; as a result they can alleviate premenstrual and menopausal symptoms. To supplement the linolenic acid in their diet, some people take evening primrose oil, which also counteracts the effects of stress, alcohol, smoking, illness, aging and vitamin deficiency on prostaglandin production.

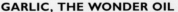

GARLIC, THE WONDER OIL

9

Known for its medicinal properties since 3000BC, garlic was used by ancient Egyptians, Vikings, Greeks and Chinese. It is best known for promoting a healthy heart. It is said to contain over a dozen antioxidants, which contribute to its effects of lowering cholesterol levels and blood pressure and helping to thin the blood to prevent harmful clots. It is also believed to help guard against infection and some cancers, and is a rich source of selenium. Research suggests that supplements equivalent to between one and three garlic cloves a day offer maximum benefits.

Hormonal changes

Over time, hormone levels in the body alter and this can cause physiological changes that vary in intensity and effect. Metabolism, energy levels and emotions may all be affected.

If you've been feeling out of sorts recently or you've noticed your body's behaviour becoming erratic, your hormones may be to blame. They affect a huge range of bodily functions, from energy levels to emotions and mood. Hormones, released from specialised glands in your body, travel in your bloodstream to their target organs. For example, a hormone produced in the pituitary gland in your brain may act on your thyroid to control metabolic reactions that regulate energy. Unusual fluctuations in hormone levels can cause both physical and emotional symptoms. Fluctuations can occur throughout life, but women around the age of 50 experience a complex change, called menopause, that can greatly alter the way their bodies function.

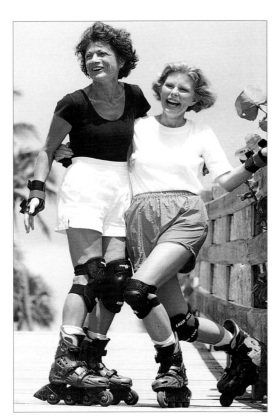

Time to take charge: many women find their own feet during middle age and menopause.

MENOPAUSE

The type and severity of the symptoms experienced as a result of menopause will vary from one woman to another, so there is no single answer that works for everyone. However, there are a number of things that you can do yourself to manage your menopausal symptoms, and your doctor can provide further advice and medical treatment, if necessary.

Menopause literally means your last menstrual period. It is the time when your ovaries cease functioning and menstrual periods stop, marking the end of the reproductive years. Menopause is a culmination of a gradual process that begins about three to five years before your final menstrual period. A woman is past menopause when she has stopped having a period for 12 consecutive months. It is impossible to know the exact moment when your menopause begins, because the start of menopause can only be worked out retrospectively.

On average, menopause occurs around the age of 51, but it can start much earlier or later. Around 1 per cent of women experience menopause before age 40 and, in rare cases, it may begin before 30.

You may hear your doctor refer to this time of your life as the climacteric, which can be divided into different stages: premenopause (the time when you menstruate regularly); perimenopause (the transitional stage leading up to menopause, which lasts about three to five years) and postmenopause (the years after menopause). Because of uncertainty about your final ovulation, it would be sensible to continue with contraception for at least a year after your last period if you don't want to conceive.

The timing of menopause is determined from birth, because it is the potential limit of ovulation. A baby girl is born with a set

HORMONE LEVELS

Until menopause, oestrogen and progesterone are produced and released in an approximately 28-day cycle. As the supply of eggs runs out in midlife, hormone production becomes erratic. With progression towards menopause, levels of progesterone and then oestrogen diminish.

Oestrogen peaks in the first half of the cycle and then falls off after ovulation, which is when progesterone levels start to rise. Both levels decline, which starts the bleeding period.

Oestrogen is produced in the ovaries. Progesterone is secreted (by the corpus luteum) after ovulation, which may be sporadic in perimenopause. There may not be bleeding every cycle.

Oestrogen is present in small amounts; it's now mainly produced by fat cells, which convert the male hormone androstenedione.

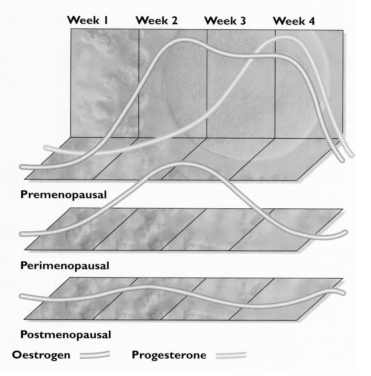

Week 1   Week 2   Week 3   Week 4

Premenopausal

Perimenopausal

Postmenopausal

Oestrogen   **Progesterone**

number of immature eggs in her ovaries. Each month an egg is released, so that by about age 45 few eggs remain and some of those that do may be defective. As the number of available eggs diminishes (and hormone levels also decline), there is irregular ovulation and periods become sporadic. This phase, the perimenopause, lasts until periods have stopped for 12 months. Levels of oestrogen fluctuate throughout each menstrual cycle; gradually the ovaries slow down and eventually stop producing oestrogen, as it is no longer needed for reproduction (see above).

Certain factors hasten the onset of menopause – smoking, for instance, can bring menopause forward by as much as three years, as can undernourishment. Women who have their ovaries removed during a hysterectomy are immediately thrown into menopause and are often given hormone replacement therapy (HRT, see pages 137–139). HRT aims to smooth out the dramatic changes and decline in hormone levels, by restoring the level of oestrogen and/or progesterone, thus alleviating many menopausal symptoms.

THE EFFECTS OF MENOPAUSE

Virtually every important body tissue contains oestrogen receptors, proof that oestrogen plays a vital role in the body's functioning. So, when levels begin to fluctuate, the effects can be felt throughout the body.

In addition, there are disruptive effects due to fluctuating levels of other hormones. Amplifying reactions in the brain can lead to larger amounts of two important sex hormones – follicle-stimulating hormone and luteinising hormone – being secreted. High levels of these hormones can seriously disturb

Effects of fluctuating hormone levels

PART OF BODY	POSSIBLE PROBLEMS
Head	Migraines and other forms of headache
Brain	Mood changes, irritability, depression, anxiety, binge-eating
Lungs	Asthma
Breasts	Lumpiness and tenderness
Digestive system	Lowered intestinal motility, leading to constipation and bloating
Muscles	Tiredness, backache, loss of muscular coordination and strength
Joints	Loss of mobility, stiffness
Body fluids	Fluid retention leading to weight gain, increased blood pressure, swollen ankles, swollen face, tendency to cystitis
Skin	Increased sensitivity to heat, blushing, hot flushes, acne and pimples
Uterine system	Pelvic pain, erratic periods

many aspects of a woman's metabolism, including blood-sugar levels, fat metabolism, bone integrity and mood. It may also depress thyroid function.

PHYSICAL SYMPTOMS
Because of the wide-ranging nature of menopausal symptoms, many women find a holistic (whole body) approach works best.

Not all women experience physical problems during menopause, but most experience some of the following symptoms:

▶ *Hot flushes* A widespread complaint, hot flushes affect 75–85 per cent of menopausal women. They range from a glowing sensation to a burning heat, usually with some sweating, which may be particularly bad at night. Hot flushes can be aggravated by stimulants and certain drugs. Avoid caffeine, alcohol and smoking, and ask your doctor about any interactions with your current medication.

▶ *Vaginal problems* Thinning of the vaginal walls, leading to dryness or soreness, can make sex uncomfortable, even painful, and reduces a woman's desire for lovemaking. The walls also become less acidic, which encourages infections to develop.

▶ *Headaches* Tension-type headaches (tightness at the back or top of the head) and migraine-like headaches (with nausea, a preceding light-headedness and lights in front of the eyes) are common complaints.

▶ *Fluid retention* Abdominal bloating and weight gain may occur due to increased fluid retention.

▶ *Aging skin* Thinning and loss of elasticity in the skin may be caused by low oestrogen levels. This may be compounded by years of sun and wind exposure, smoking and drinking alcohol. A good skin care regimen and regular moisturising are very important at this time – in particular, you should ensure that your skin is always properly protected from the sun's damaging UV rays (see pages 73–75).

▶ *Incontinence* You might experience stress incontinence, in which you leak a small amount of urine when you sneeze, cough or lift a heavy object. It can often be alleviated by Kegel exercises to strengthen the pelvic floor muscles and so improve bladder control.

In addition to the physical signs of menopause, you are at increased risk of certain conditions, including osteoporosis (see pages 122–124) and heart disease (see pages 114–115). Your doctor will monitor your individual risk for these conditions.

PSYCHOLOGICAL EFFECTS
Most women experience some emotional swings during menopause. Hormonal imbalances are probably partly responsible, but these ups and downs can be exacerbated by difficulties in adjusting to changes – perceived or real – in a woman's sexual and social roles at this point in her life. However, emotional fluctuations are not necessarily a bad thing. Some doctors say facing up to and working through the past is an essential part of any transformation.

Some women, however, suffer severe and wide-ranging psychological effects. These may include exaggerated mood swings, irritability, loss of self-esteem, memory lapses, difficulty in concentrating, tearfulness, anxiety and reduced libido. Some of these symptoms may be the direct result of falling oestrogen levels on the hormone receptors in the brain; studies have linked reduced oestrogen levels with memory loss. Others may be caused indirectly by the physical symptoms – night sweats may bring on sleeping problems.

You should bring any concerns that you have to the attention of your doctor, even if only to rule out another cause. Your doctor will also be able to recommend various methods of treatment and relief, such as HRT or possibly counselling.

SELF-HELP TREATMENTS

Some women effectively manage menopause by making a few simple but well-chosen changes to their lifestyle and diet. Regular physical exercise has been shown to relieve menopausal symptoms greatly, and it can also help compensate for the reduction in muscle mass caused by declining hormone levels.

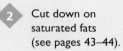

4 WAYS TO EASE SORE BREASTS

1. Wear a good, comfortable and supportive bra.

2. Cut down on saturated fats (see pages 43–44).

3. Take an evening primrose oil supplement, which has been found to reduce breast pain in 70 per cent of women.

4. For particularly sore breasts, consult your doctor, who can recommend a suitable therapy.

Blood circulation, heart and lung function, and psychological health can all be improved with exercise. Try to exercise for 20 minutes three times a week (see pages 14–19).

Smoking increases the risk of osteoporosis and can exaggerate other symptoms of menopause. Women who stop smoking at the onset of menopause may reduce their risk of hip fracture by up to 40 per cent and the risk of spinal compression fractures even more.

Migraines can be caused by foods or by environmental factors. If you are prone to migraines, try to identify and avoid any trigger factors, such as alcohol, dairy products, coffee, fatigue and stress. Yoga, meditation, visualisation and other stress-reducing practices may also be effective in limiting migraines (see pages 152–153).

DIET AND DIETARY SUPPLEMENTS

A balanced diet is the basis for good health and a strong body (see pages 42–51) and can have a huge beneficial effect on menopausal symptoms. Keeping your fat (especially saturated fat) intake down and fibre intake up are the first steps to a healthy diet.

continued on page 136

Stay cool

Hot flushes are at best an inconvenience, at worst uncomfortable – or even embarrassing. Luckily, other people probably won't notice, so try to just keep calm and take deep breaths until they pass. Keep an account of when they tend to occur: you may need to adjust your lifestyle slightly if you are prone to flushes at a particular time of day.

Choose your clothes carefully Avoid synthetic fabrics, such as polyester, and clothes with high collars and long sleeves. Keep your clothes loose and well aerated, and dress in layers; that way you can peel them off as necessary.

Exercise regularly Studies have found that if you take regular aerobic exercise you reduce the frequency and intensity of hot flushes.

Drop your temperature Take a refreshing shower if you're at home or spritz your face with cold water if you're out and about. A small thermos of iced water in your bag is a good standby – or you might like to try a small, handheld, battery-operated fan.

Stop smoking Smoking intensifies hot flushes because it affects your circulation.

Avoid flash triggers Many women find that certain foods, such as chillies or chocolate, trigger hot flushes. Try to identify any such triggers and cut them out of your diet for a while. You might reintroduce them at a later date.

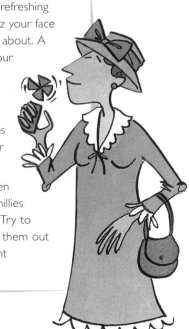

HRT METHODS
pros and cons

Hormone replacement therapy is available in various forms and dosages. Many women gain immediate benefit from HRT, but others discontinue treatment because it is less effective than they hoped or because of unacceptable side effects. In many cases, problems can be avoided by keeping your doctor informed about your body's response. The dosage may need to be increased if your symptoms are still severe, or reduced if you experience unpleasant side effects.

If the oestrogen dose is too high, for example, you might experience nausea, weight gain, tender breasts or leg cramps. Progesterone opposes the oestrogen reactions but, in excess, it may lead to digestive disorders, acne, 'pre-menstrual' mood changes and loss of sex drive.

Which type of HRT is best for you?

Some side effects might be only temporary, while your body adjusts to HRT, so unless they are very unpleasant, persevere for a few months before requesting a change.

Some forms of HRT aim to mimic the hormone levels that regulate the menstrual cycle so, while HRT will not restore a woman's fertility, it may cause premenstrual symptoms.

TYPE	PROS	CONS
Pills, Cyclical sequential therapy: oestrogen is taken from day 1 to day 21 of the menstrual cycle and progestogen from day 9 to day 21. There are seven days without medication.	Effective at relieving physical symptoms; you are in control of your medication and can stop taking it when you choose.	Withdrawal bleeding occurs on the medication-free days; side effects may include breast tenderness and nausea. May be unsuitable for those with a history of high blood pressure, blood clotting or liver trouble.
Pills, Continuous therapy: oestrogen is taken throughout the cycle and progestogens from day 14 to day 25. For convenience, progestogens can be taken only one cycle in three to reduce frequency of withdrawal bleeding.	Effective at combating physical symptoms; you are in control of your medication and can stop taking it when you choose.	Withdrawal bleeding occurs within two days of progestogen being stopped; side effects may include breast tenderness and nausea. Unsuitable for those with high blood pressure, blood clotting or liver disorders.
Pills, Combined continuous therapy: oestrogen and progestogen are taken together throughout the cycle. This may avoid withdrawal bleeding, although this can take up to a year to do so and does not work in every case.	No withdrawal bleeding for some women; effective at combating symptoms; you are in control of your medication and can stop taking it when you choose.	Side effects may include breast tenderness and nausea. Irregular bleeding may occur in the first year of treatment, before the body has adapted; unsuitable for those with a history of high blood pressure, blood clotting or liver disorders.

During a woman's fertile years, oestrogen levels rise each month until ovulation (egg release), which occurs around day 14 in a 28-day cycle. If the egg is not fertilised it develops into a structure called the corpus luteum, which produces progesterone. Falling hormone levels signal the menstrual bleeding. To mimic the natural cycle, oestrogen replacement may be given for part of the monthly cycle, with progestogen given later on. Some days are progestogen-free and it is then that women may experience menstrual symptoms and withdrawal bleeding. Fifty per cent of women taking HRT find that these effects subside after four months.

Taking continuous combined oestrogen/progestogen formulations may help avoid these side effects.

TYPE	PROS	CONS
Implants: Up to six months' supply of oestrogen is given through an implant inserted into the fatty tissue in the abdomen. The oestrogen dose is lower than with pills, but progestogen is still needed.	Highly effective at relieving both physical and emotional symptoms. As the hormone is absorbed directly into the bloodstream, bypassing the liver, it may be suitable for those with liver disorders.	Requires minor surgery; dose can't be varied once implant is inserted and removal is difficult; increased dosage may be needed to limit menopausal symptoms (for reasons that are not clear) so risk of overdose is higher than with other methods.
Skin patches: A patch containing oestrogen is placed on the lower trunk and changed every three or four days. Progestogen is taken from day 14 to 25, as a pill or as a combined oestrogen/progestogen patch. In some types the oestrogen is in alcohol in a small 'bubble' held against the skin. Less bulky is a matrix patch, in which oestrogen is impregnated in a spongy material lying flat against the skin.	Effective at relieving physical and emotional symptoms; low-dosage so few side effects; you can remove the patch when you choose.	The skin may become red, itchy or sore following the use of some types, especially in hot weather.
Cream or pessaries: These contain oestrogen and are inserted into the vagina with an applicator twice a week. Progesterone-only creams are applied to the skin (see page 139).	Effective at treating vaginal symptoms (a dry, sore, itchy vagina) and slight incontinence. Easy to apply.	Only limited absorption of oestrogen occurs, so it is unsuitable for treating other menopausal symptoms. Must not be used just prior to intercourse or partner may absorb some of the hormone.
Gel: This provides an alternative to the patch. It is applied to the lower trunk and rubbed in daily. Progestogen is taken from day 14 to 25 as a pill.	Effective at relieving physical and emotional symptoms; low-dosage so few side effects; unlike patch it does not cause skin reaction.	Only a limited amount of oestrogen absorption occurs, and in inconsistent amounts.

Nutrients for menopausal complaints

NUTRIENT	SOURCES	COMPLAINT
Vitamin A	Carrots, spinach, turnips, apricots, liver, melon, sweet potatoes	Excessive menstrual bleeding, breast problems, skin conditions
Folic acid (folate)	Leafy green vegetables, nuts, beans, liver, kidney	Cervical abnormalities, osteoporosis
Niacin	Meat and poultry, fish, pulses, whole-grains	Hyperlipidemia (high blood lipid levels), hypoglycemia
Vitamin B6	Meat and poultry, fish, bananas, whole-grains, dairy products	Deficiency as a result of HRT, cervical abnormalities and cancer, diabetes mellitus
Vitamin B12	Fish, poultry, eggs and milk, B12-enriched soya products	Anxiety, depression, mood swings, fatigue
Vitamin C	Citrus fruit, strawberries, broccoli, peppers (capsicums)	Excessive menstrual bleeding, cervical abnormalities
Vitamin D	Sunlight, oily fish, fortified products	Poor calcium absorption, osteoporosis
Vitamin E	Vegetable oils, leafy green vegetables, whole-grains, beans	Hot flushes, vaginal problems, skin conditions, osteoarthritis, fibrocystic disease of the breast
Calcium	Milk and dairy products, green leafy vegetables, citrus fruits, peas and beans	Osteoporosis, hyperlipidemia, high blood pressure
Magnesium	Green leafy vegetables, nuts, soya products, whole-grains	Osteoporosis, fatigue, coronary artery disease, anxiety, depression
Potassium	Orange juice, bananas, dried fruit, peanut butter, meat	Fatigue, heart disease, high blood pressure, anxiety, depression
Zinc	Seafood, meat, liver, eggs, poultry	Osteoporosis
Iron	Nuts, liver, red meat, egg yolk, green leafy vegetables	Excessive menstrual bleeding
Iodine	Seafood, seaweed	Hypothyroidism, fibrocystic disease of the breast
Chromium	Meat, cheese, whole-grains	Hypoglycemia
Selenium	Seafood, meat, whole-grains	Fibrocystic disease of the breast and breast cancer
Bioflavonoids	Citrus fruit, especially the pulp and pith	Hot flushes, excessive menstrual bleeding, vaginal problems, anxiety, irritability

Eat at least five portions of fruit and vegetables every day and vary your meals during the week, trying to include at least one portion of oily fish, such as salmon or tuna, and an organ meat, such as liver. Avoid high-sugar, high-salt and highly processed foods as humans are not adapted to deal with them.

Foods such as soya increase the amount of oestrogen in your body. Reports of menopausal complaints are less common in the East, where the diet is relatively low in fat, high in fibre and rich in soya products. Such a diet may increase levels of chemicals with an oestrogen-like effect, thereby reducing the need for, or at least the dosage of, any hormone replacement therapy (see right).

Be aware of how much water your drink each day – you may need to drink extra to replace that lost in hot flushes or night sweats. If your urine becomes a dark orange rather than a light straw colour, then it's probably a sign you're dehydrated, which can cause headaches and fatigue.

For the body to rebalance itself naturally, it needs an ample supply of vitamins and minerals. Vitamin E has been one focus of

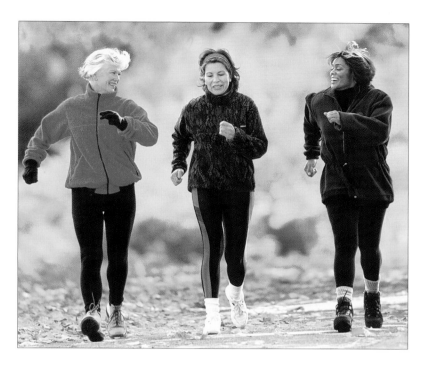

fat cells after menopause. Recent studies have suggested that taking a supplement of the mineral boron helps to increase calcium absorption from the digestive system. Factors that impede calcium absorption include alcohol, smoking, drugs, stress and caffeine.

HORMONE REPLACEMENT THERAPY

A major breakthrough in managing menopause, HRT eliminates many of the problems associated with this time of life. HRT involves taking supplements of oestrogen and /or progesterone. By rebalancing your hormone levels, you reduce your risk of symptoms and associated conditions.

Because of ongoing research, the frequent changes in the field of HRT can be confusing. The immediate benefits are the reduction in menopausal symptoms, especially hot flushes, night sweats, mood swings and poor concentration. It has also been found to relieve anxiety, depression and irritability, improve sex drive, vaginal problems, skin and hair condition, and help control weight.

The long-term oestrogen boost from HRT reduces the risk of osteoporosis by as much as 60 per cent, and the risk of heart disease or stroke by 35–50 per cent.

Recent research has found that HRT helps to lower blood cholesterol levels in women. HRT may also delay Alzheimer's disease and reduce the risk of cancer of the colon.

Although some studies have suggested a link between HRT and breast cancer in postmenopausal women, others have shown little or no relationship. Conflicting press reports mean that many women choose not to take HRT because of their fear of developing breast cancer. The fact is, the average Western woman is far more likely to die of heart disease or stroke and many times more likely to develop osteoporosis than breast cancer.

Your family history and your individual susceptibility to certain conditions play a large role in whether you could benefit from

attention in the last decade, with some research confirming it relieves symptoms of menopause, heart disease and Alzheimer's disease. Other nutrients are also thought to relieve menopausal complaints (see left).

Many women take a multinutrient supplement to ensure that they get all that their body needs. However, taking a megadose has no proven benefits and may be detrimental to your health. Unless your doctor or nutritionist has specifically prescribed megadoses, you should stick to the standard dosage.

Menopausal and postmenopausal women are now encouraged to take a calcium supplement to help prevent osteoporosis. Ask your doctor to recommend a calcium supplement suitable for you. Calcium comes in different forms and reacts in various ways with your body. Calcium carbonate and calcium glutonate are the easiest to absorb, although the former may cause constipation. Calcium citrate is better tolerated by those with the low stomach acid common in menopausal women. A calcium–magnesium combination supplement is ideal because the two nutrients function together. To absorb calcium effectively, you need small amounts of vitamin D and oestrogen, which is provided mostly from

Discuss your menopause problems with your friends and the women in your family; you may discover some helpful tips.

BENEFITS AND RISKS OF HRT

You may benefit from HRT if you have:

▶ **Symptoms of menopause such as hot flushes, night sweats or vaginal dryness**

▶ **Osteoporosis or a family history of the disease**

▶ **A high cholesterol level or low HDL ('good' cholesterol) level**

▶ **A family history of heart disease**

▶ **Gone through menopause or have had a hysterectomy that involved the removal of the ovaries**

▶ **A family history of colon cancer**

You may not be a good candidate for HRT if you have:

▶ **Had breast cancer**

▶ **Had a blood clot in the vein of your legs, lungs or eyes during pregnancy or while taking birth-control pills**

▶ **Active liver disease or severely impaired liver function**

HRT. Investigate your family medical history and discuss it with your doctor, who may run some tests, including bone densitometry, to help decide whether HRT is suited to you.

The immediate benefits of HRT – the reduction of symptoms and the maintenance of energy and libido – are well known. Many millions of women in the Western world are now prescribed HRT as a matter of course. So, it's surprising to discover that current studies indicate only 15–25 per cent of women eligible for HRT use the treatment. Furthermore, another 20–30 per cent receive a prescription but never fill it. As the benefits of HRT are publicised and increasing numbers of women take it, it seems likely that HRT will be perceived as the standard way of helping women through menopause.

CHOOSING A FORM OF HRT

A variety of HRT treatments is available and you should discuss with your doctor which ones you might try. You may need to experiment with different types or vary the dosages before you find one that suits you. Usually, women with an intact uterus take oestrogen and progesterone in combination. Taking

oestrogen alone increases the risk of cancer of the endometrium (uterus lining), so taking synthetic progesterone (progestogen or progestin) is recommended to reduce that risk. Your doctor will be able to explain in detail which type of HRT will best suit your lifestyle – but a summary is given on pages 134–135.

HRT can be taken in one of various forms – pill, patch, implant, cream or gel.

The oestrogen pill is taken every day of the month or for the first 25 days of the month, depending on the pill. The progestogen is usually taken for 10 to 14 days of the oestrogen pill cycle. After this time some women may experience withdrawal bleeding, which is usually lighter than a menstrual period and does not cause cramps. Some pills give a continuous daily dose of both oestrogen and progesterone, which may cause irregular bleeding through the first few months of use, but no bleeding from then on.

Skin patches are usually about 5–8 cm (2–3 inches) wide and are impregnated with oestrogen, which is absorbed gradually through the day. The patch is placed on your abdomen or buttocks and replaced every three to seven days. Again, doctors advise an additional progesterone patch for 10–14 days of the month to reduce the risk of endometrial cancer. Patches are better than pills if you are at risk of gallstones, but you may experience bleeding at the end of the month.

Oestrogen creams and gels are applied directly to the vagina to alleviate dryness. They have a lower, more erratic dosage and so do not provide all the benefits offered by the other forms of HRT.

CHANGING FORMS OF HRT

It is essential to have an annual check-up if you are taking HRT; see your doctor more frequently if you have any concerns. Your doctor will examine your breasts and perform a pelvic examination to look for any abnormalities. Your blood pressure will also be checked, as it could fluctuate with HRT.

Your dose may be changed as you get older and should be reduced gradually if you decide to stop treatment. You should, however, view HRT as a long-term treatment, especially if you are at risk of osteoporosis or high blood cholesterol levels. It's important to realise that some health benefits gained from HRT may be lost when you stop treatment.

The choice and combination of hormones available for HRT, and their methods of application, have increased hugely over the years, but treatments can be broadly categorised as traditional and non-traditional. Traditional HRT has been available since the late 1930s and involves the use of the female sex hormones oestrogen and progesterone (or synthetic forms of these hormones) to treat and alleviate symptoms of menopause. Non-traditional HRT involves therapy with oestrogen, progesterone, testosterone, de-hydroepiandrosterone (DHEA), growth hormone and pregnenolone, all of which are discussed on pages 140–141.

MALE MENOPAUSE

The male equivalent of menopause – the andropause – is not as clearly defined as the female version (see page 130). In fact, levels of testosterone often stay at near normal levels until late in life. In older men, however, a sex-hormone-binding protein may lock onto the hormone and reduce the level of free testosterone available in the blood. Body tissues may also become more resistant to testosterone over time. The resulting testosterone deficiency is now referred to as the male menopause or andropause.

Testosterone replacement therapy may be recommended when there are symptoms of testosterone deficiency, such as hot flushes, fatigue and reduced sex drive, or demonstrably low levels of free testosterone. Factors affecting testosterone production include damage to the testes or infections such as mumps. Symptoms of low testosterone levels include joint pain, loss of stamina and strength, reduced sexual fantasies and reduced or absent spontaneous erections during the night.

'Natural' hormone treatments are growing in popularity. The hormones usually come from plants, although some modifications are often needed to allow them to be used by a woman's body.

'natural' HRT

Natural progesterone is at the forefront of the natural hormone developments. The Mexican yam plant (*Diascorea villosa*) contains a substance called diosgenin that needs to undergo only one change to become a form of progesterone identical to that found in women. It is usually applied as a cream, but you can take it as a pill or pessary.

Critics of natural progesterone claim that for this form to be effective it must still be synthesized. However, tests have shown that as well as relieving menopausal symptoms, natural progesterone strengthens bone and reduces the risk of fractures.

Whereas natural progesterone may be preferred to progestogens and progestins, which are considered alien to the body, oestrogens (as oestradiol, oestrone and oestriol) are prescribed in the proportions naturally present in premenopausal women. Natural oestrogen can be given in pill or cream form, and its effectiveness has to be monitored regularly.

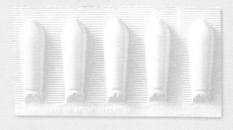

Many of the new 'natural' hormones are still only available in creams and pessaries.

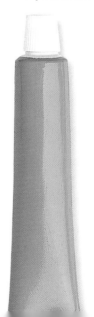

TESTOSTERONE AND AGING

Andropause is the term describing a decline in free testosterone in aging men. This often occurs in combination with an increase in a sex-hormone-binding globulin, which binds testosterone and makes it less available.

Although male menopause is more gradual than the female, some men suffer both physiological and psychological changes after the age of 40 as a result of decreasing testosterone levels.

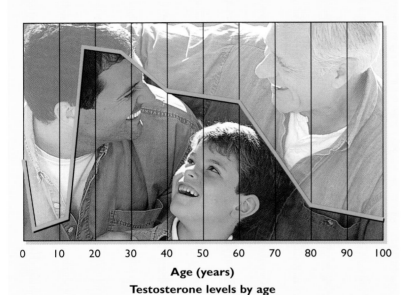

Age (years)
Testosterone levels by age

Researchers refer to the loss of libido that occurs in some older males (60 plus) as a result of reduced testosterone as the 'involutional syndrome'. Such men are likely to seek treatment because their sexual self-image is important to them.

Testosterone is administered by mouth, skin patch, cream or injection. Slow-release testosterone implants are occasionally used. Treatment leads to extra energy, improved wellbeing, increased sexual fantasies and spontaneous erections. When therapy is combined with an exercise programme, increased muscle power, bulk and physical endurance result. If higher than normal doses are given, the individual may seem 'hyped-up' and irritable to others, while feeling agreeably energetic to himself.

The main potential risk of testosterone is that, in being taken up by receptors in the prostate gland, it can aggravate pre-existing prostate cancer or benign enlargement of the prostate. Some doctors believe it may cause cancer. New research implies that oestradiol, which is metabolised from testosterone, is the causative agent of cancer both in men and in women. If you have a family history of prostate cancer, your doctor will monitor the condition of your prostate closely. If levels of prostate specific antigen rise – an indicator of possible prostate cancer – treatment will be stopped. In those with pre-existing liver disease, testosterone may be given by patch or injection to bypass the liver.

OTHER HORMONE REPLACEMENTS

Following the success of HRT in treating menopause, medical research has started investigating other hormone replacements to combat the symptoms of aging. Hormonal deficiencies, whether or not they are related to menopause in men and women, can be relieved and remedied by hormone replacement. The preliminary findings of these treatments are described below, but research into the long-term effects is still ongoing.

TESTOSTERONE

Often thought of as exclusive to men, testosterone plays a crucial role in women's health, too, maintaining sexual desire. Replacement therapy can take the form of a pill or cream and restores optimal levels and sexual function. However, too high a dose may lead to hirsutism (excess hair).

DEHYDROEPIANDROSTERONE (DHEA)

This chemical is produced by the adrenal glands and, in small amounts, by the testes and ovaries. It attaches to receptor sites throughout the body, including the brain. DHEA production declines significantly with age, unlike other steroid hormones produced by the adrenal gland. DHEA levels also seem to be associated with longevity.

The clinical benefits of DHEA replacement were highlighted in a study in 1994. In this study, in which 13 men and 17 women aged 40–70 were given DHEA sulphate

(DHEAS) for six months, 84 per cent of the women and 67 per cent of the men showed marked improvements in energy, mood and the ability to deal with stress; resistance to infection also improved. Other studies have shown links between high DHEA levels and reduced risk of high blood pressure, obesity, heart disease and improved memory.

DHEA is available without prescription in most Western countries, but it is regulated in others – you should ask your doctor's advice. The effects of long-term use are unknown at this time. DHEA should be taken only under medical supervision and requires regular monitoring.

GROWTH HORMONE

Growth hormone is secreted by the pituitary gland, a peanut-sized organ situated under the brain, and is needed during childhood and adolescence for the growth of bones, muscles and other tissues in the body. Age brings with it a reduction in muscle bulk and bone strength, and an increase in fatty tissue, and this is matched by a corresponding decrease in the amount of growth hormone secreted. In our 70s, the hormone level is only 20 per cent of that when young.

Some evidence suggests that frail older people whose growth hormone levels are very low may benefit from replacement therapy using synthetic forms of growth hormone. Possible benefits include increased energy, improved wellbeing and greater bone density, reducing the risk of bone fractures. Growth hormone improves the muscle to fat ratio, particularly around the abdomen. In studies of those taking hormone supplements, middle-age spreads 'melted away', thereby reducing the risk of heart disease. Short-term side effects of too much growth hormone include fluid retention, joint pain and increased tendency to develop diabetes.

PREGNENOLONE

Pregnenolone is manufactured by the adrenal glands, which also produce DHEA, other sex hormones and cortisol. It reportedly fights the effects of stress.

5 WAYS TO A BETTER LIFE AFTER MENOPAUSE

1. Be self-aware and focus on you.

2. Treat yourself to a pampering weekend.

3. Assert your independence and join a new club.

4. Keep doing stress-reducing and relaxation exercises.

5. Continue to watch your diet and keep up a regular exercise programme.

Pregnenolone is also said to relieve osteoarthritis by stimulating the production of natural corticosteroids, which alleviate inflammation. As it is derived from cholesterol, it is sold legally as a food supplement in some countries, but is classed as a controlled drug in Australia and the U.K., where it is regulated. It is too early for studies to substantiate claims made about this drug.

LIFE AFTER MENOPAUSE

The years after menopause, especially once any bothersome symptoms have disappeared, are often a time for reassessment. Perhaps there are changes you'd like to make in your life which you've put off because of the needs of others. Seize the opportunity now to reach your full potential. You may decide to give up work, or take up work; or you may want to run the local marathon next year – go for it!

Continue to eat healthily, keep active and have fun – it'll help you live longer and have a happier life. Maximise your time so that you have more for yourself, and for friends and family. Plus, you don't have to worry about contraception any more. How many more reasons do you need to get going?

Researching future possibilities

Following the success of HRT in treating menopause, research is focusing on other hormone therapies. Here are some preliminary findings. To learn more, contact your doctor.

DHEA This chemical is thought to boost energy levels and improve the immune system.

Growth hormone Stronger bones and increased muscle mass may be gained from this therapy.

Pregnenolone This may help to combat mood swings, fatigue, memory loss and depression.

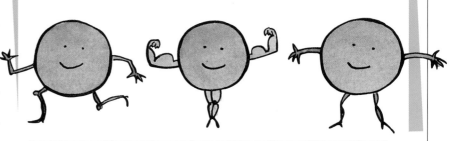

Healthy lifestyle

Wellbeing depends not only on keeping fit and eating well, but also on living in a supportive environment. It's also important to get enough sleep and to avoid drinking to excess, smoking and pollution.

The environment in which you live can have an enormous impact on you and your health – often without you being aware of its effects. To live a long and healthy life, therefore, you need to be vigilant, taking care to avoid external pollutants, such as dirty air, and internal pollution, such as smoking and excessive drinking, and be sure to get the quantity and quality of sleep you need.

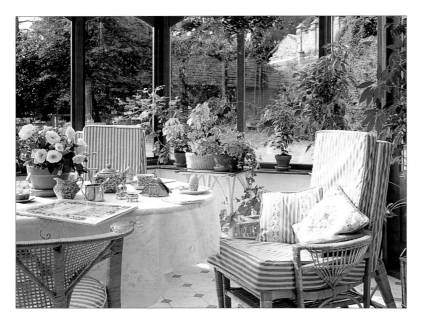

A calm, supportive environment with plenty of fresh, green plants can help boost your health and vitality.

ENVIRONMENTAL POLLUTANTS
Pollution – be it in the air that you breathe, as a noise you can hear, or in the food that you eat – exerts pressure on your body that increases the risk of many illnesses, besides putting a strain on your wellbeing. Be conscious of your environment; you can avoid many pollutants if you are aware of them.

The main causes of air pollution are industry and transport vehicles. Fortunately, most industrial areas are located away from the places where people live and work; unfortunately, busy roads are not. If you live on a main road, open the back windows instead of those at the front of the building. Avoid walking along motorways; try to find a quieter route. Always wind up your windows before entering a tunnel or parking garage.

Air can be polluted at home by gas leaks, chemical fumes from cleaning or do-it-yourself products, or from an open fire. To create a healthy home environment, get all gas and electrical appliances serviced on a regular basis, choose eco-friendly household products wherever possible, and make sure that you keep all your rooms well ventilated. Extremes of heat or cold can also be bad for you; try to keep the temperature at a happy medium. Improve the air quality in your home with lots of green plants: they absorb carbon dioxide and produce oxygen, as well as adding colour to a room.

> *Noise pollution contributes significantly to stress because you simply can't switch your ears off.*

Make sure that you are not exposed to unnecessary noise by taking measures to reduce the amount of background noise in your home or at work.

Radioactive pollution can also affect your health. Radon is a naturally occurring radioactive gas which is released from certain types of rock. If you live in an area with high radon levels, make sure the foundation or basement of your home is well-ventilated at all times, to prevent a build-up of radon gas. TV and radio masts and overhead power lines generate a considerable amount of electromagnetic radiation, and concerns have been voiced about their safety. If you are worried about radioactive pollution where you live, contact your local environmental protection organisation.

FOOD AND DRINK

Colouring, preservatives and other chemicals are added to many foods. Some of these are natural and have been used safely for centuries, but others can be harmful – indeed, some have been withdrawn from use following evidence of possible links with health problems. For optimum health, choose fresh, organic foods; check the ingredients of processed foods, which often contain additives.

Caffeine is a chemical found in coffee, tea, cola and chocolate products. Smaller but substantial quantities may also be found in a number of medicinal preparations, such as painkillers and some cold and flu remedies. Caffeine is both a central nervous system stimulant and a diuretic (it promotes urine production). Its stimulant· effect occurs because it encourages the production or release of the hormones adrenaline and noradrenaline into the bloodstream. These hormones accelerate the flow of blood around the whole body, including the brain, increasing alertness and motivation.

Caffeine has been used for many centuries as a minor stimulant, but the ease with which it can now be purchased and prepared has led to overuse. The consumption of caffeine in the Western world is increasing considerably, despite the health risks that are associated with excess caffeine. You're probably familiar with the 'wired' feeling of one cappuccino too many, but consistent excesses can lead to serious side effects and dependence.

Some of the adverse effects resulting from constantly overindulging in caffeine-containing drinks include:

▶ *Psychiatric symptoms* Anxiety, depression and insomnia, and any pre-existing psychiatric conditions, such as paranoia, can be aggravated by caffeine overload.
▶ *Withdrawal symptoms* The typical features of caffeine withdrawal include headaches and irritability.
▶ *Urinary symptoms* Excessive urination results from caffeine's diuretic effect.

THE CAFFEINE HIGH

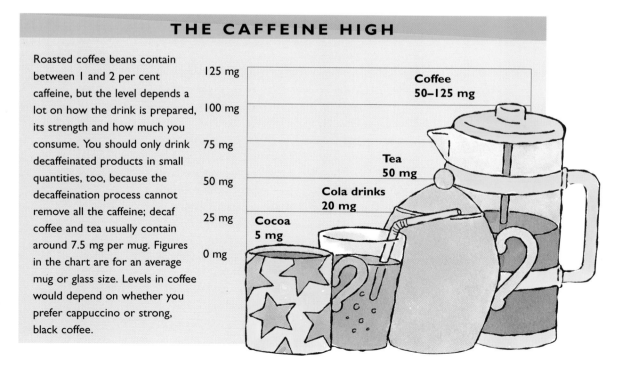

Roasted coffee beans contain between 1 and 2 per cent caffeine, but the level depends a lot on how the drink is prepared, its strength and how much you consume. You should only drink decaffeinated products in small quantities, too, because the decaffeination process cannot remove all the caffeine; decaf coffee and tea usually contain around 7.5 mg per mug. Figures in the chart are for an average mug or glass size. Levels in coffee would depend on whether you prefer cappuccino or strong, black coffee.

Coffee 50–125 mg
Tea 50 mg
Cola drinks 20 mg
Cocoa 5 mg

125 mg
100 mg
75 mg
50 mg
25 mg
0 mg

▶ **Digestive symptoms**
Excess caffeine is associated with diarrhoea, gas, increased stomach acidity and a greater risk of digestive disorders, such as ulcers and dyspepsia.

▶ **Cardiovascular problems** Caffeine can cause abnormal heart rhythms, rapid heartbeat, high blood pressure and an increased risk of heart disease. It also raises blood cholesterol levels.

▶ **Sleeping difficulties**
Restlessness, poor-quality sleep, insomnia and restless leg syndrome are all exacerbated by caffeine.

▶ **Premenstrual syndrome** Caffeine is known to aggravate PMS.

Nevertheless, caffeine also has some potential health benefits. It is chemically similar to theophylline, for example, a potent medicine used to help open the airways in asthma sufferers, so caffeine can have a positive bronchodilatory effect on people with asthma. It also appears to improve the effectiveness of some painkillers, which is why certain brands contain caffeine.

SMOKING

Smoking is responsible for 3 million deaths a year worldwide. So, one of the single most positive actions you can take to safeguard your health is to stop smoking.

It is now accepted that smoking can shorten your life by as much as 24 years. Up to 40 per cent of deaths due to coronary artery disease each year are smoking-related.

> **If you are a heavy smoker, you have 15 times the risk of dying from a heart attack before age 45 than a non-smoker.**

One-third of all smokers die of a smoking-related disease, such as lung cancer, heart attack or stroke – half of these before the age

TOBACCO – THE HIDDEN DANGERS

Nicotine is not the most dangerous ingredient of tobacco. There are over 4000 components in tobacco smoke, including minuscule amounts of poisons such as arsenic, formaldehyde and DDT. Collectively, these can cause lung disorders such as chronic bronchitis, emphysema and lung cancer; an increased risk of cancers of the mouth, throat, oesophagus, kidney, bladder and pancreas, and a four-fold increase in heart attacks. Smokers also inhale high levels of carbon monoxide, which reduces the amount of oxygen available for the brain and other organs. Tobacco smoke damages the tiny hairs (cilia) that help protect the lungs from infection, so smokers are much more likely to suffer from coughs, colds and flu than non-smokers. Smoking increases the risk of osteoporosis, leads to premature menopause and accelerates aging of the skin.

of 70! If these facts alone aren't enough to make you stop, bear in mind that you're probably not the only person who will suffer – passive smoking, inhaling another person's cigarette fumes, increases the risk of lung cancer in non-smokers by 30 per cent.

Smoking triggers the release of the stress hormone adrenaline, which speeds up the heart rate and raises blood pressure with consequent long-term effects on health (see pages 114–115). It is also the most potent promoter of free radicals known; not only does it encourage the body to create free radicals, but also cigarette smoke itself is rich in free radicals.

There is no evidence that low-tar brands of cigarettes are less damaging to the lungs; they are just as harmful to the heart. While pipe and cigar smoking are generally considered slightly safer than cigarettes, because less tobacco smoke is inhaled, they still carry major health risks. Cigar and pipe smokers run a much higher risk of developing mouth and throat cancer than cigarette smokers. Marijuana smoke can be especially harmful to the lungs because it is usually inhaled unfiltered. It may also contain more cancer-causing agents than tobacco smoke.

Studies show that nicotine is one of the world's most addictive substances, right up there with cocaine and heroin. If you have smoked for a long time, stopping may be the

6 ways to **stop smoking**

You'll find it easier to give up smoking if you focus on the danger times and avoid situations that trigger your desire to light a cigarette.

STICK ON A PATCH

1

Wear a nicotine patch to help break the smoking habit. They won't help you get over the craving instantly, as you've become addicted to the nicotine in tobacco. But, when used as directed, you will receive ever-lower amounts of nicotine, making withdrawal easier.

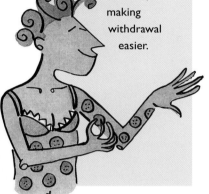

SHUN STIMULANTS

2

Avoid stimulants such as coffee, tea, alcohol and chocolate during the early weeks of your stop-smoking campaign as they can increase your desire for a cigarette. Instead, drink plenty of fruit juices, caffeine-free herbal drinks and water.

SEEK HELP

3

Consult a therapist who practises hypnosis or acupuncture to help people stop smoking. These methods are not effective for everyone, but many ex-smokers have found that, when combined with other measures, they can help to reduce the desire for cigarettes. Contact a local support group, which can provide advice and encouragement as you need it.

EAT HEALTHILY

4

Giving up smoking can make you want to snack more, so instead of sweets and high-fat junk food, fill yourself up on fresh fruit and vegetables. Buy healthy snacks you can nibble on during the day. Chewing gum can also help you resist the urge for unhealthy nibbles, but choose sugar-free types or you risk tooth decay.

Don't be tempted

5

Avoid having even a few puffs of a cigarette: it may weaken your resolve. Don't despair if you do give in to temptation, however. Simply tell yourself that you had a momentary lapse. If you fail on the first attempt, keep trying until you succeed. Take heart from the fact that, while many ex-smokers were successful the first time, many more managed to stop on the second or third attempt.

KEEP BUSY

6

Don't sit around, bored and wanting a cigarette. Take up walking, jogging, swimming or cycling. Research shows that ex-smokers who exercise regularly are less likely to smoke or to want to smoke and have a healthier attitude towards life.

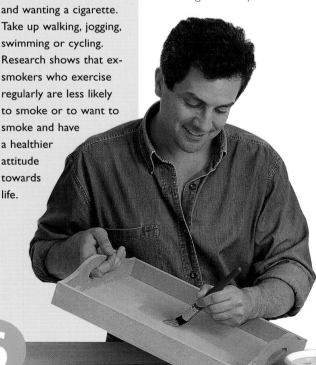

4 WAYS TO DRINK SENSIBLY

1. Identify problem times and situations and focus on cutting alcohol intake at these times.

2. Have three alcohol-free days each week to get yourself out of the habit of drinking daily.

3. Try non-alcoholic cocktails – they are tastier than you think.

4. Give up habitual alcoholic drinks after work or at home – you'll soon find that you feel better without them.

hardest thing you will ever do. Nicotine is a powerful and highly addictive stimulant that reaches the brain within seconds of inhaling tobacco smoke. But when you do manage to kick the habit, you'll start enjoying the health benefits immediately. The level of oxygen-depleting carbon monoxide in the blood will decline right away so you'll very quickly have much more energy and stamina.

Studies show that only five years after giving up cigarettes, the risk of stroke among ex-smokers equals that of people who have never smoked. This applies regardless of the age at which the individual stops smoking or of the length of time they have smoked.

ALCOHOL

Alcohol depresses the nervous system and decreases the activity of the brain and spinal cord; it therefore reduces anxiety, tension and inhibitions. In addition, studies show that a glass or two of wine or beer a day can actually improve your health. In small quantities, alcohol stimulates the appetite and aids digestion by encouraging the flow of gastric juices. It may also help to boost levels of high-density lipoproteins (HDLs or 'good cholesterol'), thereby reducing the risk of

heart attack and stroke. Red wine, in particular, is considered beneficial in moderation because it contains phytochemicals, which are strongly antioxidant and so protect against heart disease and cancer.

According to studies in Europe, teetotallers are at greater risk of death from cancer, heart attack and stroke than those who drink alcohol in moderation.

In larger quantities, however, alcohol can impair physical and mental functioning. Chronic drinkers are at increased risk of heart attack, stroke, liver disease, ulcers and cancer. Alcohol can also adversely affect mental faculties, such as memory, judgement and concentration, affecting work performance and driving skills.

Alcohol dependence is a major problem worldwide, affecting the health and emotional wellbeing of alcoholics and those around them. Alcoholism is also a major cause of violence and marital breakdown.

Most health organisations suggest safe limits of alcohol consumption. These vary from country to country, but they are usually

KNOW YOUR ALCOHOL LIMITS

On average, it takes around one hour for one unit of alcohol to be eliminated from your body. (It varies, depending on your weight.) However, alcohol has a cumulative effect, which means that if you have a couple of drinks at lunch and then two more early in the evening, your blood alcohol level could be over the drink-driving limit. Watch out if you are driving early in the morning after drinking heavily the night before – you may still be over the limit!

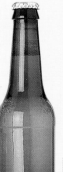

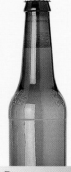

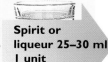

Non-alcoholic cocktail 375 ml 0 units

Low-alcohol beer 375–425 ml 1 unit

Beer 275–285 ml 1 unit

Wine 100–125 ml 1 unit

Spirit 25–30 ml and mixer 1 unit

Spirit or liqueur 25–30 ml 1 unit

three to four drinks per day for men (one an hour) and one to two drinks a day for women. A drink is generally defined as 275–285 ml of beer, 100–125 ml of wine or 25–30 ml of distilled spirits. A small amount daily is healthier than binging at the weekends.

Excess alcohol can lead to serious dehydration. It acts as a diuretic, so you urinate more, and also dilates the blood vessels under the skin so that you feel warmer and have to perspire more to cool down. To minimise the risks of dehydration, try to have the same number of glasses of water as you have had of alcohol.

Drinks vary widely in their alcohol content and their effect on the body. Drinking with a meal slows the rate at which alcohol is absorbed into the body, while gassy drinks, such as beer, or drinks with carbonated mixers, such as whisky and soda, speed up absorption.

DRUGS AND YOUR HEALTH

Prescription and over-the-counter drugs have a number of medicinal uses – many prevent or treat life-threatening conditions.

There are drug side effects that may harm your health. Some well-known drugs that have effects to be aware of include:

▶ *Aspirin and ibuprofen* Taken over a long period of time or with alcohol, they can cause bleeding of the stomach wall. People with particularly sensitive stomachs should use an alternative, such as paracetamol.

▶ *Paracetamol* A common painkiller, paracetamol can be tolerated in small doses by

the liver and kidneys. It can be easy to take too much, however – there is no antidote for an overdose and the resulting liver damage cannot be reversed; monitor the amount of paracetamol in your medicines.

▶ *Viagra* The new anti-impotence pill increases the risk of heart attack, so if you have a heart condition you should discuss it with your doctor (see page 219).

▶ *HRT* Hormone replacement therapy can reduce your risk of osteoporosis but can increase the risk of breast cancer (see pages 137–139). Your doctor may advise you to stay off HRT if breast cancer runs in your family.

▶ *Contraceptive pill* This increases the risk of heart disease, high blood pressure and thrombosis. The progesterone-only pill can lead to ovarian cysts. All women are cautioned not to smoke while taking it.

Be aware that some drugs can be addictive if taken over long periods of time. Most famously, withdrawal from Valium has proven problematic for many people; as a result, doctors are much more careful about the length of time for which it is prescribed.

Before taking any over-the-counter drugs, always read the side effect and warning information. Your doctor and pharmacist should note the side effects of any prescription drugs that you are given, and they can also advise you about the risks of over-the-counter drugs, if you are concerned.

SLEEP AND YOUR HEALTH

While you sleep, certain systems in your body are highly active – replenishing and replacing cells, building tissues, releasing growth hormone, producing antibodies to fight

What happens during sleep?

During the night you go through different levels of sleep. There are two types of sleep: rapid eye movement (REM) sleep, when you dream, which makes up about one-third of sleep, and non-REM sleep, which accounts for the rest.

REM sleep The dream period of sleep occurs about once every 90 minutes throughout the night, lasting for longer periods as the night goes on. It is identified by rapid, jerky movements of the eyes under the lids – from which it gets its name – an increase in brain-wave activity and fluctuating blood pressure. REM sleep is thought to be a time of processing information from the day and integrating it into the memory, and therefore has a big impact on mental and emotional health.

Non-REM sleep The non-dream sleep has four stages: stage 1 is the lightest, stage 4 is the deepest. Deep sleep occurs mostly in the first three hours of sleep, after which sleep becomes progressively lighter. It is thought that bodily repair and growth occur during non-REM sleep.

infection and relax muscles. In effect, sleep rebuilds you. The restorative powers also work on the mind so that you wake from a good night's sleep feeling refreshed and energised. Some research indicates that much of the information gained during the day is sorted and processed during the night.

Sleep is a fundamental human need. If you have trouble getting to sleep – perhaps personal problems are making you too tense – your emotional health suffers and you wake up feeling drained. Poor-quality sleep also affects the way you look, producing dark circles under the eyes, often accompanied by puffiness and poor skin tone. Usually, an early night is all it takes to restore mind and body. But if the cycle of sleep disturbance continues, it affects not only your appearance, your energy levels and peace of mind but also your concentration.

Research suggest that most of us are getting far less sleep than we did at the end of the last century.

This is mostly because sleep is now viewed as a luxury rather than a necessity – if you need to fit more activities into your life, the chances are you will do this by cutting down on your sleep. Too much stress can result in the inability to get adequate sleep; sleeping problems are linked to stress and anxiety more than any other cause.

Excess caffeine or other stimulants can prevent you from sleeping properly. The general rise in caffeine intake during the last few decades has been reflected in a general trend towards reduced sleep and in reports of sleeping problems becoming increasingly widespread.

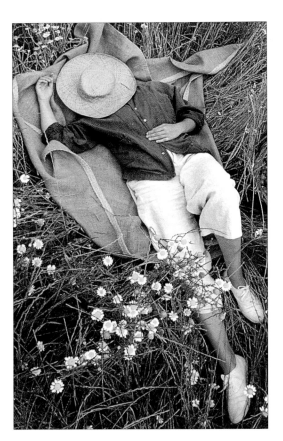

The siesta is a way of life in southern Europe, where people sleep through the hottest and least productive part of the day.

CIRCADIAN RHYTHM

The body has its own internal clock, called the circadian rhythm, which governs cycles of sleep and wakefulness, fluctuations in body temperature, intellectual performance, digestion, and cell growth and renewal throughout a roughly 24-hour period.

It is thought that the circadian rhythm is controlled by melatonin, a hormone produced by the pineal gland in the brain. Enzymes in the pineal gland are activated by darkness and release melatonin every night. If you are exposed to daylight when you would normally be asleep, the body becomes confused and melatonin is not produced in sufficient quantities at the proper time. This most commonly happens when you travel through different time zones, causing jet lag; some people find that taking extra melatonin in pill form helps combat jet lag. Blind people and shift workers can also suffer from reduced melatonin, resulting in the body becoming out of step with its natural clock.

Excess melatonin can result in seasonal affective disorder, or SAD, in which people suffer repeated episodes of depression due to decreasing light levels in certain seasons of the year.

The darker months enhance melatonin production and consequently some people feel lethargic and depressed.

Rhythms can also be disturbed by stress or poor nutrition, which reduces the availability of tryptophan, an amino acid needed for melatonin production. You can boost the body's production of melatonin by including tryptophan-rich foods in your diet, such as low-fat dairy products, tuna and poultry.

If your body does not produce enough melatonin during the evening, you will still feel wakeful at bedtime and have difficulty sleeping. If secretion continues to be depressed, you may wake up early. If your pineal gland secretes too much melatonin the next day, you will feel sleepy and have trouble waking or staying awake during the day.

Naps during the day are usually seen as a benefit to health – especially if we don't get the sleep we need at night. Some people try to exist on cat naps alone, but it is preferable to sleep for a long stretch at least once during any 24-hour period so that you reach deep sleep. Keep napping to around 20 minutes; any longer and you may jeopardise your night-time sleep pattern, and you will also wake feeling unrefreshed. The art of napping during the day enables you to keep your concentration high, boost your energy and stop you from feeling tired.

ENCOURAGING SLEEP

Can't sleep? Never stay in bed fretting about it, it just makes the situation worse. Instead, get out of bed, drink a cup of warm milk and read a book until you feel tired. You could use the time to catch up on paperwork, write letters or do a little light housework. Mundane, undemanding tasks will probably make you sleepy so you can return to bed.

Make sure your bedroom is quiet, well-ventilated and at a comfortable temperature. Adjust the lighting so that it is relaxing – if necessary, fit heavier curtains to block out disruptive light.

Harvard University researchers have found that low lighting has a sedative effect on your body.

Low light levels stimulate the pineal gland to secrete more melatonin, which makes you sleepy. Keeping lighting at the level of candlelight for several hours before bedtime can help you fall asleep.

Your bed needs to be comfortable, but not too soft, as this often encourages a bad sleeping posture that can lead to back trouble. If

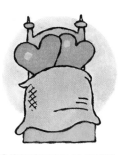

SOPORIFIC SEX
Sex is good for overcoming insomnia. According to experts, orgasm triggers a release of endorphins in your brain. These chemical agents promote slumber-inducing alpha brain waves, helping you into the relaxed state of early sleep.

your mattress is more than ten years old it may need to be replaced. Your body may have changed over a decade and need more support or firmer springing. Replace pillows when they begin to harden with age.

The average person moves 60 or 70 times a night, so a restless partner may disturb your sleep. If this is a problem for you, consider getting a bigger bed. If you sleep better alone, explain this need to your partner in a loving way. Times when you do snuggle up together will then have their own special quality.

A recent study by the Henry Ford Sleep Disorders Center in Detroit concluded that married couples sleep better than those who are single or in unmarried relationships. The report emphasised the role of behavioural patterns. Married people have a more stable and regular sleeping pattern, whereas singles are more likely to stay out late and tend to drink alcohol and coffee more often.

SLEEP NEEDS

Sleep requirements are highly individual – some people may need as much as ten hours, others can get by on five hours. Take a note of how long you sleep and how you feel the next day to work out your optimum sleeping time. The majority of people find that they function best on a sleep time of around seven or eight hours.

As you grow older, the amount of sleep you require changes, so you may find that you sleep less during the night than you did a decade ago. This reduction in night time sleep may be due to the age-related decline in melatonin production. You may find, however, that you take more naps during the day.

Sleep needs (hours)

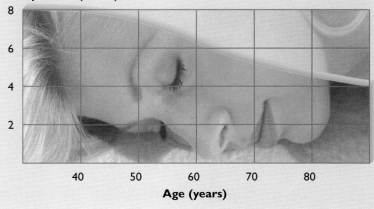

Age (years)

RELAXING BEFORE SLEEPING

Record the following message on a tape. 'Feel your toes relax, release the tension and rest. Feel your feet relax, release the tension and rest...' And continue all the way up your body to your head.

Play the tape softly when you get into bed at night, relaxing each body part as directed. If you need to relax further, you may then want to follow with some meditation and deep-breathing exercises (see page 153).

Getting yourself in the mood for sleep is one of the crucial factors in combating sleep problems. One tried-and-tested method is to induce the slower alpha brain waves associated with early sleep. This can be achieved through meditation and visualisation (see pages 152–153) or through making and playing a relaxation tape like the one above.

If you have sleeping problems, you may want to examine your lifestyle. Try out some of the following tips:

▶ *Feeling sleepy?* Don't go to bed until you feel tired.

▶ *Avoid smoking* The nicotine in tobacco is a stimulant that can keep you awake for up to two hours after smoking.

▶ *Watch what you drink* Limit alcohol intake and don't drink any caffeinated drinks for six hours before bedtime.

▶ *Stick to a sleep pattern* Find a sleep routine you are happy with and don't vary it.

▶ *Acclimatise your room* Adjust the temperature and level of ventilation (open the window slightly); make the room as dark and quiet as possible – use earplugs if necessary.

▶ *Avoid eating big meals* Filling up on food before you go to bed can keep you awake.

▶ *Wear yourself out* Get regular aerobic exercise but make sure it is at least three hours before bedtime. Stretch your muscles to relieve tension before climbing into bed.

▶ *Relax, relax* Have a warm, relaxing bath before bedtime to ease the joints and muscles and promote sleep. You could add a few drops of an essential oil, such as lavender.

▶ *Listen to soft, relaxing music* Try some soothing music or a guided meditation tape to ease you into peaceful slumbers.

▶ *Drink a calming herbal tea* For an overactive mind, try camomile or lemon balm – both are caffeine-free. For a stronger sedative effect, try limeflower or passiflora.

▶ *Try a herbal remedy* Studies have shown that valerian can relieve sleep problems and help improve the quality of sleep.

▶ *Read something light* Easy reading often distracts an overactive mind; don't read anything too stimulating or work-related.

If you've tried every self-help measure going and you are still not getting a good night's sleep, consult your doctor. He or she will ultimately want to find out what's causing your insomnia, but in the meantime may prescribe a short course of sleeping pills. Although these will make you sleepy, they don't provide the same quality of sleep as you would naturally experience, so you may wake feeling slightly unrefreshed. Discuss any concerns you have about sleeping pills with your doctor.

CAUSES OF SLEEP PROBLEMS

Most people go through short bouts of sleeping problems, but more serious, long-term disorders are relatively uncommon. Anxiety and depression are the most common causes, responsible for 85–90 per cent of sleep problems. Stress is another culprit since it can cause anxiety and depression.

During the day, your body steadily pumps out adrenaline and cortisone—hormones that keep you alert and functioning. Towards the end of the evening, their levels reduce while melatonin production rises, making you feel pleasantly sleepy and ready for bed. However, if adrenaline and cortisone are still being released because of stress or elation, sleep will not occur – and neither will the replenishing and restoring melatonin. Anxiety stimulates excess adrenaline production, which blocks the activity of growth hormone, the chemical that helps the body to repair and renew its cells during the day and, to a greater extent, when you are asleep.

Sleep is essential for restoring the body. Research on people who were hospitalised for illness or surgery found that if their sleep was interrupted they didn't recover as quickly as those who had a good night's sleep.

Failure to develop a regular sleeping routine also causes problems. For sound, restful sleep you should go to bed at the same time each night and, more importantly, get up at the same time each day. Changing your sleep pattern can confuse your circadian rhythm.

A common mistake is to change your sleep routine at the weekend, staying up later and then making up the time by staying in bed longer in the morning. This is one of the main causes of the 'Monday morning feeling' experienced when people return to their weekday routine. Stick to your routine as much as possible. If you do go to bed late, keep your alarm set at your usual time; you may feel tired at first but you'll soon adjust.

Shift work can cause long-term sleeping problems because the body's clock is programmed to sleep at night. The best way to deal with shift work is to try not to alter your sleeping pattern too often – reverting to a 'normal' sleep pattern over the weekend will disrupt your routine. Shift work can cause stress so you may want to limit the amount you do, if possible. Use relaxation techniques and exercise to reduce stress and help you regulate your sleep regimen.

Sleep apnoea is a common cause of sleeping problems. It is widespread among overweight people, especially middle-aged men who snore heavily, and becomes more common in women after menopause. Sleep apnoea causes the sleeper to stop breathing for a minute or more at frequent intervals throughout the night. The brain then restarts the breathing response, usually with a gasp that partially wakens the sleeper, thus disturbing sleep. This pattern causes tiredness during the day and a loss of concentration. Sleep apnoea is potentially serious because oxygen levels drop very low and carbon dioxide levels rise extremely high during the non-breathing stages. This increases the risk of high blood pressure, stroke and heart disease.

Heavy snoring is the main cause of sleep apnoea. Thirty per cent of men and 14 per cent of women snore, and this problem often gets worse with age. Snoring occurs when the muscles of the soft palate in the throat become over-relaxed and sag into the airway, vibrating as you breathe. Sleep apnoea occurs when the soft palate blocks the air passage.

If you snore, you can reduce the risk of apnoea by losing weight, limiting your alcohol intake and avoiding sleeping pills, all of which are linked to a flabby soft palate. There are devices available that improve air flow by expanding the nasal passages, restraining the tongue or altering the position of the jaws. In extreme cases, doctors may recommend a breathing mask at night or minor surgery.

Tips to reduce snoring

Correct your sleeping position Sleep on your side to keep the air passages open. Some people attach a small ball to the back of their nightwear to prevent them from turning over in their sleep. If you sleep with someone who snores, simply turning him or her over often stops it.

Avoid high pillows Keeping your head higher than your body with several pillows or a very soft bed only encourages snoring.

Clear your passages To help prevent snoring when you have a cold, inhale steam from a herbal infusion to remove excess phlegm. You can also use a room infuser or dab a little menthol and eucalyptus oil on your bedclothes.

Try an anti-snoring device An adhesive strip that pulls the nasal passages open is the easiest to use. More specialised equipment is available through a doctor.

MEDITATION
and visualisation

By tapping into the power of your mind, you can take control; anxiety, depression and negative thinking will be things of the past. Meditation and visualisation techniques help calm your mind and totally transform your outlook.

Benefits of meditation

► Reduces stress
► Improves mental alertness
► Calms an overactive mind
► Improves memory
► Boosts regenerative processes
► Slows biological aging

Meditation is an ancient practice originating from the spiritual traditions of Asia, where it is used to reach a higher state of being – often known as Nirvana. It is thought to work by relieving the mind of day-to-day worries and transferring attention to the greater wonders of living and simply being.

The health benefits of meditation come about because it calms and refreshes the mind, freeing it of disturbing thoughts and worries. Studies of brainwave patterns during meditation show a relaxed mental state similar to that of sleep. Indeed, many meditation exercises are designed to be performed as a prelude to sleep.

Visualisation can also be used to calm the mind and encourage sleep. The important factors in visualisation are to focus on the image in your mind and not be distracted or feel forced to achieve a particular state of mind.

Meditation and visualisation should be pleasant experiences, so you'll want to include them in your life on a regular basis.

MEDITATION POSITIONS

Don't be put off meditation by visions of trying to squeeze yourself into the classic lotus position: you can meditate in almost any position. The most important considerations are to choose a position that is comfortable and that does not put pressure on any part of your body.

First of all, pick a quiet spot where you won't be disturbed. Next, choose your position. If you are using meditation to help you sleep, you could practise lying down, but an upright position is generally more effective because you will be able to concentrate better. The most commonly used position is to sit cross-legged, which keeps the back upright and balanced, yet tension-free. Meditation takes some practice: at first you may find it difficult to keep focused, but you will soon learn to maintain the relaxed alertness of the meditative state for 15 minutes or more.

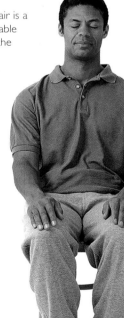

Sitting on a chair is a more comfortable alternative to the cross-legged position. Keep your feet flat on the floor and your back straight. You may lean on the back of the chair, but take care not to let your shoulders slump.

Lying on your back is the best position if you are using meditation to help you drift off to sleep. Lie with your arms by your side and your hands flat on the bed. Do not cushion your neck and head with a high pillow.

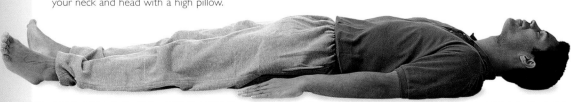

MEDITATION EXERCISE

If you are experiencing difficulty in sleeping or are waking up often in the night, perhaps due to a menopausal night sweat, carry out the following exercise for as long as you can.

1 Begin by clearing your mind of all thoughts. Now try to focus on your breathing and relax so that you feel each breath reach deep within your abdomen. Watch your abdomen rise and fall as you breathe in and out. Concentrate on this movement and notice how, as you relax, it develops an even, rhythmic pattern.

2 Once your breathing has become regular, each time the abdomen rises mentally acknowledge the action. Each time the abdomen falls you should do the same. Do this calmly and don't try to force the rising and falling.

3 If you begin to feel sleepy, acknowledge and give in to this feeling rather than fight it. But if you are still wide awake, keep doing the exercise for as long as possible. You could try to add a visualisation (see below) if sleep continues to evade you.

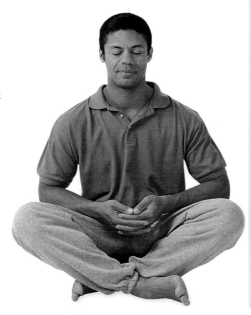

Affirmations

Similar to mantras, affirmations are words or phrases that can be repeated during a meditation to encourage positive thinking. You can devise your own affirmation or use one of the following examples:

▶ Relax
▶ Peace
▶ Love
▶ I will succeed
▶ I have unlimited potential
▶ I am calm
▶ I am in control
▶ I am attractive
▶ I enjoy life
▶ I am willing to change and grow
▶ I am complete

VISUALISATION

Visualisation is a technique for directing your mind using your imagination and positive thinking. By freeing your mind from stress and the pressures of life, you can let your imagination take you to calm and restful places.

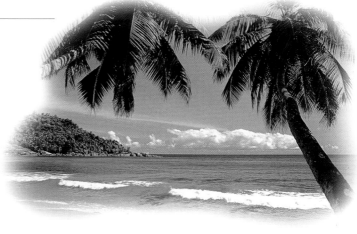

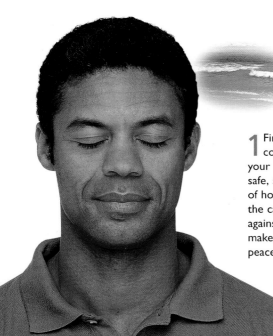

1 First decide on the image you want to conjure up. It may be a past event in your life or a place that made you feel safe, secure and calm. Popular images are of holidays: lying on a beach listening to the calming sounds of the waves lapping against the shore. Whatever your image, make sure it is a happy, relaxed and peaceful one.

2 Still your breathing by performing the breathing exercise above for a few moments and try to empty your mind completely.

3 Once your mind is clear, introduce your image. Explore it in great detail; try to visualise the smells, tastes, textures and colours of your experience as if it were real. Allow the warmth of that image to bathe and nurture you. Experience the serenity of the moment. Keep your breathing steady and calm.

GETTING INSIDE
your dreams

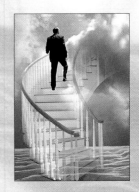

We dream during a particular type of sleep – rapid eye movement (REM) sleep (see page 147). There are several theories as to why we dream, but none has been proven completely. What we do know, however, is that most people dream, even those who can't remember their dreams. REM is fundamental to psychological health; if you are deprived of sleep for a long period, your body will try to catch up on dream time when you next fall asleep. Long-term sleep deprivation may lead you to dream while you are awake.

During REM sleep, the only inactive parts of the brain are the frontal lobes, which organise your thoughts and create order and meaning. The most active part of the dreaming brain is the limbic system, which is responsible for emotions. During REM sleep you leave the rational world behind and enter a world governed by emotions.

It was Freud who reaffirmed the concept that dreams are both meaningful and significant. He saw them as coming from the irrational part of the unconscious or psyche. He deduced that one of dreaming's functions is to defuse a sense of inner frustration by allowing the satisfaction of desires.

According to sleep expert Professor Rosalind Cartwright, of the Rush Presbyterian Hospital, Chicago, the mind uses dreams to resolve emotional problems and, in effect, keep you sane. In the first period of REM sleep, the brain acts out negative emotions in the form of a dream. This dream is the most disturbing of the night. In the second REM period, the brain taps into its memory network looking for similar experiences in the past to find a solution to the problem. From then on through the night, the dreams become progressively less disturbing as, by showing your fears in a different light, they help you to come to terms with them.

What do your dreams mean?

Although symbolism in dreams is largely personal and idiosyncratic, there are certain events and images that therapists associate with particular latent thoughts.

Flying Soaring through the air can be an expression of sexual desire or, more generally, a desire for freedom.

Swimming Often viewed as an emotional and spiritual communion between your inner self and the world around you, swimming and water dreams tend to be calming. Drowning, though, may indicate difficulties in facing your emotions.

Being chased Although this may mean many things, it is often interpreted as escape from a difficulty.

Falling Many people experience dreams of falling; it may suggest a tumble from a precarious or stressful position in real life.

Driving Symbolic of progression, the car that you are driving is important. If you are carefully driving a large, unwieldy vehicle, it may indicate that your life is slowed down by caution and unnecessary baggage. A speeding sports car may suggest that your life is careering out of control.

Nudity Associated with social fear, nudity is often interpreted as anxiety about being seen as one really is.

Other people Apart from close friends and family, most people in your dreams characterise parts of yourself. A mean old scrooge, for example, may be telling you to watch your money.

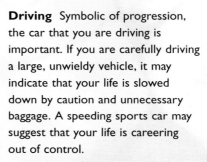

Animals Similarly to other people, animals often represent parts of you that need more attention. A dog, for example, may symbolise the loyal, friendly side of you.

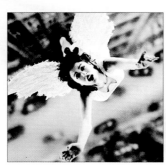

Chapter 5

Mind and senses

Staying sharp

Get your mind working to the best of its ability with practice and exercise. Take up mental and intellectual challenges and stay up to date with the world around you to boost your brain power.

The mind develops rapidly from birth and continues to grow through childhood and adolescence and into adulthood. It is often said, however, that from midlife onwards there is an inevitable decline in mental faculties. Recent research shows that much of the supposed decline is greatly overstated or is related to a specific illness, such as Alzheimer's disease, which causes the steady degeneration of the brain. This is not an inevitable part of aging.

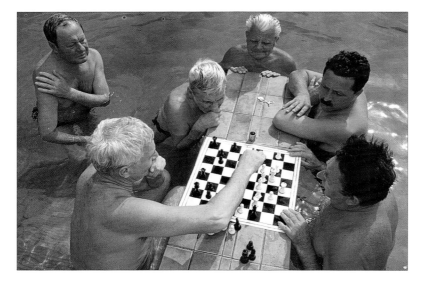

Challenging games help to stimulate and maintain brain activity, promoting mental health and longevity.

A 1995 study of the mental capabilities of 65,000 older men and women, carried out at Manchester University in the U.K., showed that IQ declines by, at most, 5 per cent between the ages of 50 and 80. This is a negligible amount in people of all levels of intelligence, but especially in those whose IQs are already relatively high to start with. In fact, other research suggests that the average decline is only 5–15 per cent over an entire lifetime, from a peak at around the age of 25. If you find your brain function reducing as you age, it may be from lack of use.

Take charge and don't let your mental capacity slow down as you get older. One of the simplest and most effective ways is through regular physical activity.

All body cells can reproduce themselves except for those in the central nervous system. You cannot grow new nerve cells, so you must keep the ones you have well nourished and supplied with oxygen. Over time, the blood supply to the brain may be reduced, due to hardening of the arteries, but by exercising regularly you stimulate the circulation of blood that transports nutrients and oxygen to the brain. This helps maintain brain activity and promote health and longevity.

CHALLENGING YOUR MIND

From midlife onwards, many people stop using the full potential of their brains, and as they get older, use less and less. One reason is that you are not automatically exposed to the same degree of stimulation as when you were younger and still learning about life.

A stimulating and mentally challenging environment will keep your mind sharpened. Professor Bryan Kolb of the University of Lethbridge in Alberta, Canada, studied animals kept in stimulating environments and measured the nerve cell development in their brains. He found that they sprouted longer connecting pathways than animals in unstimulating surroundings. This comparison also applies to people.

The importance of keeping mentally active has also been researched in Japan. A study involving a survey of Japanese octogenarians found that those who continued working, or took another job after retiring, remained mentally active. It concluded that individuals who continued to work a normal day had sharper minds than contemporaries who had retired at 60. There was improved brain function even when people spent as little as an hour at work. Constant interaction forces the brain to exercise. It has to assess, question and respond to information and then assimilate it. In essence, work maintains the thinking process.

Just as practical experience continues throughout life, so too can your formal education. Older students are not only capable of studying and achieving, but they also have advantages over younger people. Their experience enables them to place much of their new knowledge in context and to see its practical uses; they do not view the accumulation of information as a purely academic exercise intended merely to pass exams.

Of course, it helps if you have laid the foundation for these mental skills in earlier years. If you learned a second language as a child, you'll find it easier to relearn that language than to study a completely new one from scratch. Skills are maintained through regular practice, and those that are used repetitively become highly developed, while those that are used infrequently become rusty, or are even lost altogether.

FOOD FOR THOUGHT

The mechanisms that control the thought processes are very finely balanced and can be easily disrupted. Stress, depression, menopause, drugs and alcohol can all upset the chemical balance of the brain. By including certain foods in your diet, and/or taking dietary supplements, you can help to restore this balance and, therefore, help your brain function more efficiently.

For instance, the brain's main chemical nerve messenger, or neurotransmitter, is acetylcholine. Not surprisingly, poor brain function is associated with low levels of

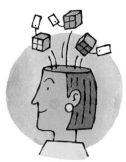

THE HUMAN COMPUTER

The brain has a huge capacity to hold new information and skills. Each of its cells can link up with a multitude of other brain cells in numerous ways in order to store data. As a result, the brain can store at least 1000 trillion pieces of data. The world's most powerful supercomputers, in comparison, can currently only store 1 trillion.

MIND CONNECTIONS

Brain mass is believed to shrink by around 10 per cent during one's lifetime. This was the case with the legendary physicist Albert Einstein, yet there is no evidence to suggest that shrinkage had impaired his massive intellect at the time of his death (aged 76). According to research carried out at the University of Alabama, brain cells (known as neurons) may shrink but do not actually die, and can be maintained far beyond your 60s.

The connections that form between the neurons are more important than the actual number of neurons in the brain. Neurons react to mental stimulation by sending out new connecting fibres, or dendrites, to link with other neurons. These hair-like filaments carry the signals that pass from one neuron to another and work like the microcircuits in a computer chip, only more efficiently. As brain mass declines, the cells become bushier as the links increase, improving your ability for lateral thought and 'seeing both sides of the coin'.

Dendrites are formed whenever you acquire knowledge, skills and thinking patterns and they continue to develop throughout life – as long as you keep your brain active. The interconnections between neurons actually become more elaborate and intricate with age. Research at the University of California shows that as your brain ages, it sends out new, longer dendrites and makes more efficient connections than a younger brain. On average, these connections are 25 per cent longer in 80-year-olds than in 50-year-olds, establishing a better environment for interconnected thought processes.

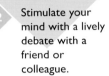

WAYS TO STRETCH YOUR MIND

1. Seize every opportunity to acquire and analyse new information.

2. Stimulate your mind with a lively debate with a friend or colleague.

3. Stay up-to-date with news and current affairs by watching news programmes and reading newspapers and magazines.

acetylcholine. Choline, found in eggs, soya, cabbage and cauliflower, is vital for the formation of this neurotransmitter, while vitamin B_5, from liver, eggs and whole-grains, is needed to convert choline to acetylcholine.

Many vitamins and chemicals can enhance brain function both directly, by improving blood flow to the brain, for example, and indirectly, by protecting the brain from the damaging effects of free radicals or other harmful agents. Vitamin B_1 (thiamin), for instance, is essential for concentration, reasoning and memory. Vitamin B_3 enhances the flow of oxygen to the brain cells.

Vitamin B_6 is needed for an efficient memory, and women taking hormone replacement therapy are often deficient in this vitamin. As you get older, the digestive system is less efficient at absorbing B_{12} and this can lead to impaired memory. Folic acid (folate) plays a part in maintaining memory, and memory lapses often occur in those with signs of folic acid deficiency.

BOOST YOUR READING POWER

One of the most important sources of knowledge is the printed word. More written information is available to you today – in the form of books, magazines, newspapers and the Internet – than ever before. Yet the ability to read is acquired in childhood and largely taken for granted ever after. If you learned poor reading habits as a child, which inhibit your speed of assimilation and comprehension, you may not realise the extent of your reading potential and have probably never tried to enhance it.

By improving reading skills you can acquire more information faster and – most importantly – understand and retain it.

Most people read a top range of 250 words per minute. They only read one word at a time and often become distracted; they lose their place and skip back over words they think they have failed to understand. This process occurs at an almost subconscious level so you do not realise you are doing it. In some cases reading speed can drop as low as 100 words per minute. Yet your brain is capable of coping with text at a much faster rate and can usually grasp the meaning of unfamiliar words from the context.

KNOWLEDGE BUILDING

Learning didn't stop when you left school – in fact you may find you have more time and inclination as you grow older to take up a new language, or perhaps you simply want to educate yourself about history.

Continually expanding your knowledge pool helps you to handle new information more easily and effectively.

Whether your reasons for wanting to enhance your knowledge base are prompted by interest or necessity, the following tips may help your studies.

Break up your study times into short periods with breaks in between. A tired brain is a less efficient one so, to keep it fresh, break the period you have set aside into small sessions. Concentrate entirely

Speed your reading

With just a little practice and concentration, most people can easily improve their rate of absorbing and retaining information. Exercise your reading skills every day for at least 20 minutes, and use the following tips to help you read faster.

Use a pointer Follow the words as you read them with a pencil or another pointed utensil. This will keep your eyes and mind focused on the line you are reading so you're less likely to be distracted.

Increase your speed Try to comprehend two or three words for every one you used to read.

Read forwards and avoid going back Concentrate so that you do not need to go over words you have already read.

Time your reading speed Try to improve on your previous performance by regularly testing your speed.

QUICK & EASY
mind workout

Brain function can be greatly improved by exercises that strengthen hand–eye coordination. Dr Paul Dennison and his wife, Gail, of the Education Kinesiology Foundation in California, have devised an exercise programme to enhance memory, coordination, learning ability and other mental functions. Originally developed for children, these exercises are said to be effective for adults of all ages. They are designed to improve connections between the creative left side of the brain and the logical right side, and they can aid reading, spelling, comprehension and mathematical skills.

THE OWL

1 Squeeze the muscles of your right shoulder with your left hand, breathing in. Breathe out and turn your head until you are looking over your right shoulder.

2 Still squeezing your right shoulder, breathe in and slowly turn your head back to the front, then over to the left, until you are looking over your left shoulder.

3 Breathing out, return your head to the centre and rest your chin on your chest. Breathing deeply, let your head and shoulders relax. Repeat with the opposite side.

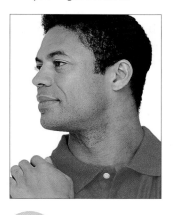
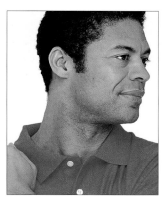
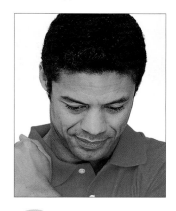

THE POSITIVE POINTS

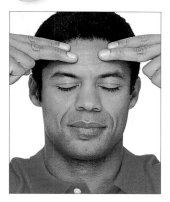

Lightly press two fingers on each side of your forehead, as shown, and hold for 3 to 10 minutes. This will relieve tension and increase the blood flow to the brain.

THE THINKING CAP

Pull the tops of your ears up and away from your head, gently rolling out the skin and pinching the inside. Work down your ear pulling out gently and pinching. Press your earlobes firmly and pull them down. Repeat the exercise 10 times, concentrating on the pressure.

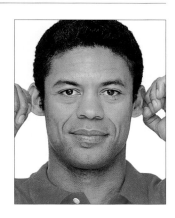

THE ENERGY YAWN

Open your mouth wide, as if to yawn. Place two fingers in the gap between your upper and your lower jaw; your index finger should be positioned at the joint. Massage the jaw muscles with slow rotations of your fingertips. This exercise relaxes your vision.

on the subject for no more than 10 minutes at a time, and then take a rest.

Take notes of your work as you go along to aid your recall, highlighting the most important points or making thumbnail sketches. The more distinctive your notes appear, the easier they are to remember. Use the 'Mind mapping' exercise on page 163 to help you organise and summarise your subject matter.

Don't get side-tracked. To avoid losing your concentration when studying, keep a separate notepad handy, so that if you suddenly remember something you must do, you can quickly jot it down and then go back to what you were doing without too much of a delay.

Know your limits and don't try to take in too much at once. Start with bite-sized chunks of information and slowly build on them.

For example, if you are learning a new language, commit vocabulary to memory in small batches of words, beginning with two or three. Keep testing yourself until you are confident you have assimilated these, then add another two and test yourself on all four. Then learn another two and test yourself on all six. With each repetition you'll strengthen what you have already learned and you will link the new words in their correct context.

Work in other ideas from other subjects or knowledge that you have. Think about your subject from a few different points of view, such as a historical angle or

THE PQRST TECHNIQUE

One learning technique that can be highly effective is called PQRST – Preview, Question, Read, State and Test. This sequence of actions can help you effectively identify and retain the key issues of a complex article or report.

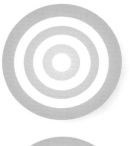

Preview – first skim through the article to identify the main thrust of the piece, taking in any side headings.

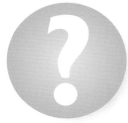

Question – ask yourself what the article is really about, and note any side issues that are raised.

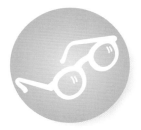

Read – now read through the article more carefully, making sure that you fully understand every point discussed.

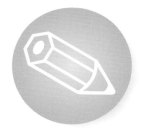

State – pinpoint the main arguments and points of discussion, and then critically assess each one.

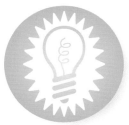

Test – finally, quiz yourself on what you have learned, and make a note of your own view of the piece.

from someone living in a different country. You can also link the new information to other subjects or interests.

Make time to revise what you have learned. Aim to go back over your notes regularly – it will reinforce the memory links.

MENTAL AGILITY EXERCISES

Crossword puzzles, chess, jigsaws and card games are bonafide brain boosters. Invite a few friends over for an evening of games, or learn the intricacies of chess. Keep a detailed diary of your weekly mental activities.

You will also extend your mental capacity by practising your observation, estimation and concentration skills, as follows:

▶ *Be observant* On a journey, instead of being preoccupied with your destination, spare a few moments to study the objects and people that you pass on the way. Is that tree's bark rough or smooth? What shape are its leaves? How old are those people, what are they wearing? Would you know them again if you saw them? When you get home, try to recall what you have seen.

▶ *Compute costs* When shopping, total the costs as you go. Estimate the bill and the amount of change you expect. Compare the prices between different shops or organisations. Try to keep an accurate estimate of your income and expenses.

▶ *Estimate numbers* If you are doing any home improvements, gardening or carpentry, estimate the amount of materials you need

FREE YOUR CREATIVE SPIRIT

Tap into your creativity with inspiring new activities. The creative side of many people is underutilised in today's stressful world – we simply don't have the time to be creative because we're far too busy being practical. Many people forget that being creative is often highly practical, bringing together the powers of logic, analysis and imagination. Research has found that those who value their individual creativity use it the best. To have faith in your creativity, you need to give it a chance – let it guide you and see how it can change your life. Take your easel to a park and sketch some wildlife, or write a short creative piece on a recent journey. With practice your creative side can help you express yourself.

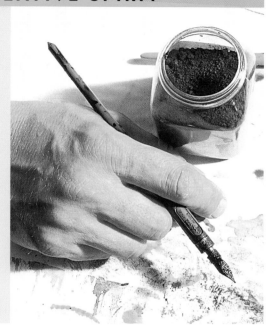

for a specific task. Estimate the sizes of items or rooms. Check these figures against the actual measurements.

▶ *Investigate new subjects* After reading a newspaper, magazine or book, write down points of interest to look into further. Discuss with partners or friends what you have read or seen on television, at the movies or the theatre. Consider joining a book group.

▶ *Inform yourself* Select a newsworthy topic each week to learn more about – maybe a political situation or an ecological issue.

▶ *Learn something new* Consider adult education courses in both academic and creative areas for a few hours each week.

PROBLEM SOLVING

Don't let small obstacles come between you and your goals; view problem solving as a challenging and stimulating exercise. Practise your skills often and keep a positive attitude to overcoming troubles. Using a simple problem-solving technique you can find solutions and work around your difficulties without letting them get on top of you.

Identify and define the problem. Before you rush into problem solving, you must spend some time developing an accurate understanding of the difficulty so that you can properly tackle it. Consider the nature of the problem, the possible causes and any underlying symptoms. For example, a pool of water on the kitchen floor may mean a leaky pipe, but this may also be symptomatic of a larger plumbing problem that could ultimately affect the whole home.

Explore the possible strategies for handling the problem. Make a list, noting even the more ridiculous options – they may appear more logical with more consideration. Understanding why one option is inappropriate may allow you to see why another is a preferable solution, or it may inspire you to find better possibilities.

Let your mind go – thinking up a solution is as much a creative process as a logical one.

Keep your thinking flexible. When you see a problem, step back and look at it from a different perspective, generate a number of responses and then decide which will work the best. It may even be necessary to try a few

3 DECISION-MAKING TIPS

1 Make a list of all the pros and cons of each course of action. Go with the one that has the most pros.

2 Alternatively, try to assess the likely success of each course of action. Which is easiest to achieve?

3 Then consider how disastrous each would be if it did not work out. You may want to choose the one with the least risks.

out. It is sometimes helpful to see it from another person's angle – how would your old school teacher sort out the problem?

Broaden your horizons to help your strategy-making skills. The more knowledge you have at your fingertips – or, better still, inside your head – the more options you will have to choose from. Find the time and energy to investigate all possible strategies and enjoy the challenge. See how you perform in creative and logical strategy building, and strive to improve strategy-making skills.

A technique used by some professionals to cover all possible strategies is known as mind mapping (see opposite). By branching outwards from a central theme, you can make sure that you cover all possibilities. This will help you to see the problem and possible solutions in a broader context. Some strategists start at the end point and work backwards; others divide the problem into subgoals that can be solved one by one. Ask for advice from people who may be able to help, or delve into books and manuals. Generate a number of possible actions and put them into an order, starting with the first that you are going to try, then the second, and so on. If your first action fails to successfully solve the problem, appraise the rest of your options before trying another.

People tend to attack a problem most efficiently if they do it in a systematic way – the greater the problem, the more time and effort they will put into finding and trying out solutions. So if you feel you are facing multiple problems, prioritise and organise.

DECISION MAKING

Throughout our lives we are called upon to make a continuous stream of decisions, with the options broadening at every horizon. The best way to make decisions is to research the facts, weigh out the costs and benefits, the possible outcomes and risks. However, in the real world, decisions are made with a less thorough analysis. People more often choose the path of least resistance and, since thinking means hard work, make decisions on hunch or intuition.

The key to solving problems is to consider all the factors and then make the best decision you can at the time. Think about the following points:

▶ **Know the facts** Of course it is impossible to know and understand every situation completely, but try to read and recall as much as you can before you make a decision. Your memory is not infallible, so ask others around you to remind you of the facts.

▶ **Understand the 'spin'** The information leading to a decision is often couched in a fashion that you are more likely to respond to in a particular way. For example, people are less likely to take risks if the information includes the potential losses, rather than the potential gains, of a situation. This highlighting of the positive is known as the 'spin', and is often used in sales strategies.

▶ **Don't take situations at face value** In many decision-making situations, the scene is often set a long time before the point at which you enter. For example, if you buy a property, the vendors will have been involved in the sale and the property long before you came to view it. Try to find out what happened before you came on to the scene. Why are they selling the property? How long have they lived there? How long have they been trying to sell it?

▶ **Be aware of your biases** Problems in decision making may arise because of false assumptions. We project our own ideas and biases onto the situation. For example, many people think that being in an aeroplane crash or winning the lottery are more likely to occur than they really are, mostly due to media coverage of such events and the emotions that these situations evoke.

▶ **Don't generalise** We all make sweeping generalisations without even realising we're doing it. Yet it's essential when making important decisions to think twice before you link what's typical with what is likely.

▶ **Remain flexible** Don't fall in love with your decisions and allow yourself to become blinkered – be prepared to admit that you have made a mistake. It is often difficult to keep an open mind to better ideas, especially if you have already put a lot of time and energy into making a decision.

▶ *Think laterally*   Try to consider all the options open to you by working around a subject laterally. This will help you to look further than the surface situation and identify the less obvious solutions to a problem. For example, two chefs working together both need an orange, but there is only one orange. The obvious solution is to cut the orange in half or spend time finding another. However, if you look for more detail you will discover that one chef needs juice and the other needs rind, and so both could actually use the whole orange together. This is where mind maps are useful in displaying a wealth of layered information, allowing you to see all the possibilities of a situation.

Mind mapping

When writing a complicated report, or planning a major event, such as a wedding or a family holiday, most people simply make a list of points to include or options to consider. But, according to Tony Buzzan, founder of the World Memory Championships, this is the wrong way to work because it goes against the natural operation of the brain.

The brain does not store pieces of data in list order, like a dictionary, but in context, with connections linking them to related words and concepts. Tony Buzzan has devised a technique called mind mapping which presents information in an interlinked way that more closely matches the brain's own system of assimilation. This technique can be used to help you learn new skills, start a study course, plan a speech, write a report and in other situations where you need to deal with complex information.

To create a mind map, draw a symbol representing the main subject in the centre of a sheet of paper. Using different coloured pens, draw thick branches radiating out to key topics. These topics are the basic ordering ideas (BOIs) and act as group headings. They should be clearly printed in capital letters and comprise striking words and images.

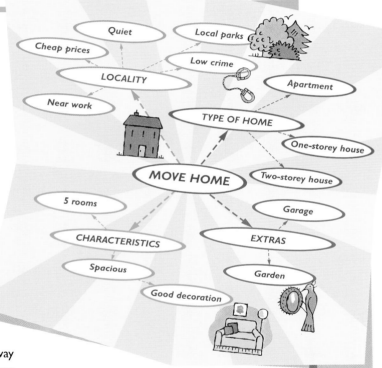

Next, draw thinner lines, radiating out from your BOIs, to related subjects. For your new skill-learning plan, you might make the skill a BOI. From this, thinner lines would be marked taught courses, friends and contacts, books and magazines, and so on, until you have covered all the elements involved.

Carry on until the map has all the salient points – including dates, times and prices, where relevant. If necessary, redraw the map, revising the plan and information and adding new symbols or lines where you think they will help you remember key elements.

Memory

You will be amazed at how much you can improve your memory skills. The technique is simple – train your memory to organise, store and retrieve information, and then practise as much as you can.

Memory is the process by which the brain acquires and stores information, and then retrieves it when needed. To get your memory working properly, you need to practise using it – the more times you store and retrieve, the easier it becomes. You can also improve your memory using specialised techniques, such as mnemonics and retrieval triggers or cues (see page 166–167).

Your memory, contrary to popular belief, has the potential to stay sharp throughout your life. If you find your memory deteriorating as you get older, it is more likely to be due to stress, poor health or a lack of mental exercise. Research from the University of Kentucky has concluded that only 5 per cent

of cases of bad memory are actually attributable to brain disorders such as Alzheimer's disease. However, recent studies have shown that memory loss in women is related to decreased oestrogen levels.

In the vast majority of cases of short memory, the problem is one of simple neglect and under-used basic memory skills.

MEMORY STORAGE

Memories are laid down as physical connections that link the brain cells, or neurons, together to form patterns. On seeing a face for the first time, for instance, the image

SENSORY MEMORY
Your brain takes a momentary snapshot of your environment. Sights, sounds, smells, tastes and feelings are registered; this reaction lasts an instant (0.25 to 3 seconds).

SHORT-TERM MEMORY
Your brain selects and then transfers important and/or relevant information to your short-term memory. The storage time is longer, about 30 seconds, but capacity is limited.

LONG-TERM MEMORY
Information is then encoded and stored in your long-term memory. The capacity for storage here is unlimited and storage is potentially permanent.

Your sensory memory is like a camera taking a snapshot – for example, of this man (right). Your short-term memory is like looking at a photographic print of him. Your long-term memory is like a photograph album storing his photo with related pictures.

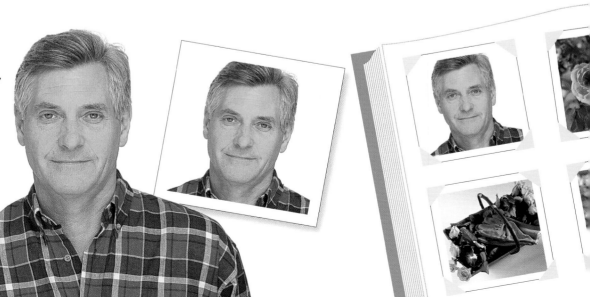

enters your eye and is converted into electrical impulses that travel along the optic nerve to the brain. The impulses pass between neurons along particular pathways, forming a pattern in the brain that corresponds with the face. For a short while you can recreate that face in your 'mind's eye'. This is part of your sensory memory.

If the face is striking in any way – beautiful or frightening – you hold the image longer, strengthening the connections and making the face more memorable.

With repeated exposure, you will store the picture permanently. Names, dates, facts, new skills – in fact, all stored pieces of information – are represented as patterns of neuron connections in your brain.

These patterns also overlap with other pieces of sensory information collected at the same time, such as sounds and smells. Not only does this provide a fuller picture, it also means that a scent, for example, can trigger a particular memory, of a person or place, that has interconnections. Many people find that they come to associate the scent of a perfume with a particular person, for example.

When learning new information, try to make the best use of the brain's system of memory storage. Go over the information repeatedly to strengthen the connections between neurons. Also, involve your other senses in the learning process to help make memory retrieval easier. Make a note of smells, sounds and even tastes if appropriate.

MEMORY RETRIEVAL

A crucial part of memory function is the ability to recall information from your long-term memory, and it is this process that suffers more as you grow older, mainly because of a lack of practice.

The memory process begins when you decide to remember a piece of information and encode it, either verbally or pictorially. A verbal memory would be a statement, such as 'I must remember to book the tickets for

RETRIEVAL TEST

Associating words, ideas or pictures with others can trigger your memory. Study the sentences below for two minutes, then cover the list and write down as many as you can. Next, use the list of retrieval cues on page 167 to jog your memory for those you missed the first time around.

A brick can be used as a doorstop.
A magazine can be used as a place mat.
A wine bottle can be used as a candlestick.
A shoe can be used to pound nails.
A rug can be used as a bedspread.
A sheet can be used as a sail.
A pair of scissors can be used to cut grass.
A newspaper can be used to swat flies.
An orange can be used as a ball.
A coin can be used as a screwdriver.
A TV antenna can be used as a clothes rack.
A boat can be used for shelter.
A pen can be used as an arrow.
A knife can be used to stir paint.
A barrel can be used as a chair.
A mop handle can be used as a curtain rail.
A sock can be used as a glove.
A rock can be used as a paperweight.
A telephone can be used as an alarm clock.
A balloon can be used as a pillow.
A lampshade can be used as a hat.
A pan can be used as a drum.
A leaf can be used as a bookmark.
A guitar can be used as a canoe paddle.
A board can be used as a ruler.
A table can be used as firewood.

the comedy show', whereas a pictorial memory may be a picture of the actors or comedians you are planning to see. You are more likely to remember the picture of the comedians than the verbal statement because, according to research, visual imagery forms a stronger impression than verbal techniques. So, try to associate anything you want to remember with a visual picture to help the memory last longer.

The brain is particularly bad at recalling abstract data such as telephone numbers or people's names. It often helps to use an association technique.

▶ **Name games** Use pictorial techniques to help remember names. The important part is to make a strong association between the name and an image when you encode it into your long-term memory, so that remembering one will bring forth the memory of the other. If you meet someone called Bill Penfield, for example, imagine a pen in a field with an electricity bill stuck on one end. Or, conjure up an object that you can link with the name or part of the name, or something that rhymes with it. For Brown, you might think of a crown – perhaps a brown crown; for Jones, choose a rhyme such as bones or phones. Next, imagine the person wearing or holding items that help you link his face with the object, such as a cowboy hat for John (as in John Wayne). The same system works for other names, such as capital cities. The capital of Ecuador is Quito so think 'key-toe' and fix in your mind the image of a foot with a key in between its toes.

▶ **Number techniques** One method is to convert numbers into letters, according to their position in the alphabet, and then make a name out of those letters. So 72 would be GB (the seventh and second letter of the alphabet) and becomes George Bush; 12 would be AB (the first and second letters) or Alexander Bell and 44 would be DD (fourth letter) or Doris Day. A mental image involving these three memorable characters could help you recall the number 721244.

It is often easier to recall numbers if you group them into singles, pairs or triples that you can associate with a famous person, object or song. Certain numbers will be particularly memorable – birth dates, anniversary dates and house numbers of close friends and relatives. Card experts use a range of number techniques to remember how an entire pack has been played. For practice, play a game of cards with a friend and try to remember all of the cards in play.

▶ **Linking** The link system, used by five-times World Memory Champion Dominic O'Brien, involves pegging new information to familiar visual scenes from the home environment. A shopping list of eggs, bacon, bread and cheese could be remembered, for example, by visualising a hen pecking on the porch, a pig rolling in the hall, a baker kneading dough in the dining room and a cow grazing in the bathroom.

▶ **Mnemonics** Named after Mnemosyne, the Greek goddess of memory, the mnemonic system is one of the oldest aids to recall. It involves creating a memorable sentence in which each word starts with the same letter as one of the words you want to remember. For example, the points of the compass

Magic number seven

Along with having a relatively short period of storage, the short-term memory also has a limited capacity – approximately seven items can be stored at a time. Important research in the United States by psychologist George Miller found that the short-term memory is limited to between five and nine items of information at one time – an average of seven, plus or minus two.

Similar research in China and other Asian countries has confirmed that this is the case. A Chinese person can store on average only seven Chinese characters at one time.

According to the findings, when your memory is filled to capacity, new information will bump out the old. So if you want to remember something, make sure you repeat it and encode it into the long-term memory to prevent it from being wiped out.

If you have a lot of things to remember, divide them into groups of seven. It is no coincidence that local telephone numbers around the world usually consist of seven digits!

(North, East, South, West) can be remembered as Never Eat Soggy Wheat. Another method is to make an acronym out of the first letters of the words you want to remember – handy when making lists. For instance, pick up Laundry, check bank Account, buy Nuts and make Dental appointment spells LAND. A recent study found that individuals who used mnemonic methods to memorise a list recalled approximately two and a half times more than those who did not.

MEMORY BOOSTING

If you have trouble remembering things, first of all don't worry about it, and, second, make an effort to improve your memory through practice and exercise.

Keep exercising your memory and use these guidelines to help day-to-day memory storage and retrieval:

▶ **Concentrate** Among the top reasons for forgetfulness is a lack of concentration. After you have chosen to remember a piece of information, spend a few moments concentrating on that memory to ensure that it is imprinted on your mind.

▶ **Be selective** Don't try to remember everything, you'll simply overload your memory. Prioritise the things you need to remember and make sure that the important ones go in first. Write lists to help keep your memory clear of everyday chores.

▶ **Be predictable** Avoid having to remember day-to-day things by sticking to a routine. If you always put your keys down in the same place, you won't lose them. If there's a note on the refrigerator door, then it must mean that you need more milk. Just think how many simple items can come off your mind if you have a routine!

▶ **Reduce your stress levels** Stress interferes with memory function. Memory efficiency appears to be linked to stress; the more stress you experience, the less you seem able to remember. It is not yet fully understood why this happens, but it is probably a

SENSE RECALL
The writer Marcel Proust found that the taste of a small cake – a madeleine – was enough to bring back a flood of memories from his childhood.

brain reaction telling you to shut down and get some rest. Your brain needs time to assimilate information in order for it to be passed to the long-term memory. Stress management enables you to store and retrieve information more easily and boosts your ability to process and assimilate data.

BRAIN FOOD

The brain is an amazingly sophisticated organ. It would be impossible, therefore, for any single therapy to provide a cure-all for failing memory. However, certain nutrients can boost or help prevent loss of brain functioning. Vitamin E, for example, can delay the onset of Alzheimer's disease and ginkgo biloba can dramatically improve alertness.

There are hormone receptors throughout the brain and, undoubtedly, many hormones have complex actions that affect your mental functioning – as said earlier, oestrogen has effects on memory. However, research into how each hormone affects specific brain functions is still in the very early stages, and much more research is underway to tap into this enormous mental potential.

RETRIEVAL CUES

Use the following words as retrieval cues to remember the rest of the words from page 165. You should be able to get nearly all of them, and if not you should try again.

table	lampshade
sheet	shoe
rock	guitar
telephone	scissors
boat	leaf
coin	brick
wine bottle	knife
board	newspaper
pen	pan
balloon	barrel
sock	rug
record	orange
TV antenna	magazine

II ways to **improve your mind**

By keeping the brain fit, healthy and active, you will enhance all your mental processes, including concentration, reasoning and memory.

CONCENTRATE

1

Play the card game Concentration by spreading a whole deck of cards face-down over a table. Turn one card over and then choose another that you think has the same number. If they match, you can pick them up; if not, you must turn them back over and try again. The game requires you to remember where all the different cards are when they have been replaced face down. You can play by yourself or with friends.

Keep working

2

Even in retirement, it is important to keep your mind occupied. Consider part-time employment, starting a business, learning a new employment skill and taking up a new career. Many volunteer opportunities are open to retired people, especially those with skills that they can teach others. If you have special skills or knowledge that you can pass on, you can also investigate openings at schools, colleges and other education centres.

FOCUS YOUR ATTENTION

3

Keep your wits about you by focusing your attention on one thing at a time. Interference causes you to switch your mind to too many things simultaneously. Concentrating on one thing at a time helps to sort, store and assimilate data faster and more effectively.

Have a good night's sleep

4

The brain is thought to assimilate and store memories while you sleep. Shortened sleep makes it more difficult to learn new information and recall it, so ensure you have sufficient sleep. However, avoid sleeping pills, which induce the wrong type of sleep for efficient memory storage.

ENCODE IMPORTANT ITEMS

5

For information to be remembered, it needs to be carefully encoded into the long-term memory. Make sure that you consciously take mental notes of where you put your keys down. You may picture your keys, or make an elaborate link that you won't forget – if you put them by the phone, you may think of the phrase 'key ring'.

STAY CREATIVE

6

Take up a hobby, craft or learn a skill such as painting, photography, writing, pottery or gardening. If you already have basic skills, find a more creative dimension, for example by branching out from carpentry into cabinet making or from sewing into embroidery.

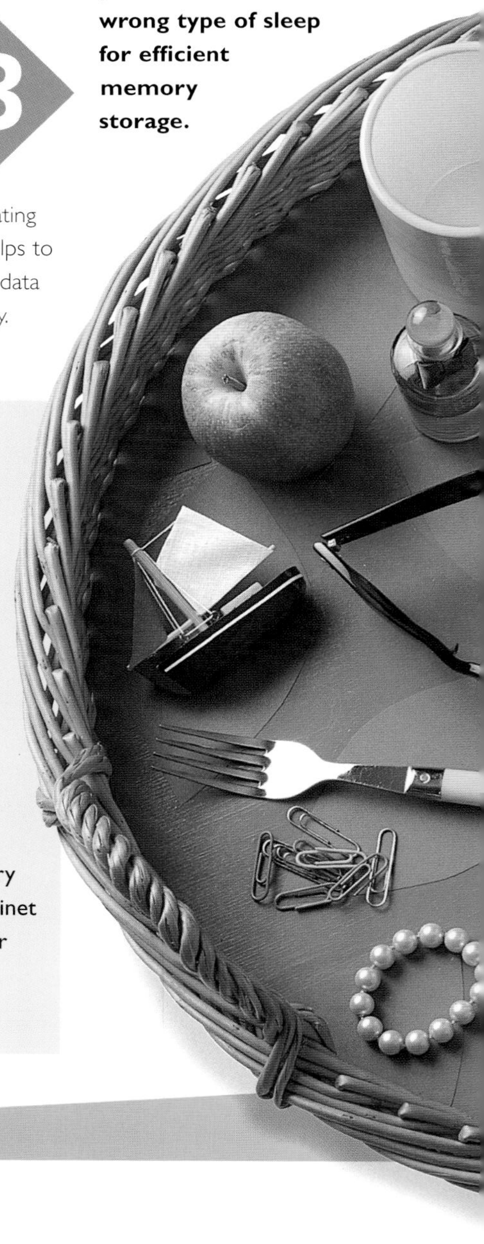

LISTEN TO CALM MUSIC

Research shows that response patterns of the brain are stimulated and become more alert after hearing the quicker melodies of Mozart, compared with slower-paced heavy rock and slow tranquil music.

7

GO TO THE THEATRE

The mental stimulation of a thought-provoking drama, particularly when enjoyed in like-minded company, has been shown to greatly enhance the brain's reasoning and intuitive functions. Research from the U.K. suggests that regular theatre-going may even increase your lifespan.

8

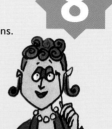

Drink sensibly

10

Keep your alcohol consumption at a moderate level (see pages 46–47). Excess alcohol, particularly in the form of weekend binges, hinders concentration, coordination and reasoning. It also interferes with the brain's ability to store and retrieve information.

FIT BODY – FIT MIND

Aerobic exercise, such as brisk walking, cycling, jogging and swimming, can stimulate the circulation of blood, which transports oxygen to the brain. Researchers from the University of Maastricht in the Netherlands ran tests on over 150 men and women of varying ages and found that, without doubt, their mental performance improved following aerobic exercise. They also found that the older you are, the more important it is that you exercise to keep your wits.

9

MEMORY WORKOUT

11

A game based on 'Kim', the Rudyard Kipling story, makes a good memory test. Get a friend to place 20 different items on a tray covered with a tea towel. Ask your friend to uncover the tray for 1 minute while you memorise the items. Then, with the items covered, try to recall as many as possible.

Sight and hearing

The senses, particularly vision and hearing, are your contact with the world at large. Keep them sharp and in tune by understanding the way they work and learning to safeguard their functions.

The eyes are often likened to twin cameras because they can focus on an object and produce an image. But in fact the eyes are much more sophisticated than any camera. They are self-cleaning and capable of working both in light levels ranging from bright sunshine to virtual darkness and in a remarkably wide range of temperatures and weather conditions. Because of this, people tend to take their eyes for granted until symptoms such as blurred vision, headaches, itchiness or even pain indicate a problem. Some eye disorders or a predisposition towards one are unavoidable and may be genetically programmed, such as glaucoma, but there is a lot you can do to protect your eyes – and maintain your vision.

The eye's focusing ability is controlled by muscles that become weak when forced to concentrate on a fixed point for long periods, as when reading or doing needlework. To avoid this, lift up your head and look into the middle distance – say, to the other side of the room; then look into the far distance, if possible, out a of window. The effect is rather like stretching your legs to relieve cramp. If you do this every 15–20 minutes, your eyes will tire less quickly.

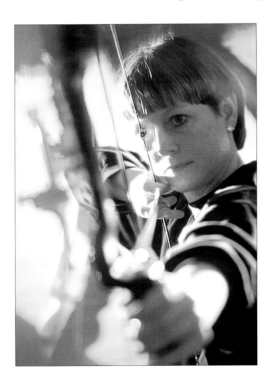

Archery is a good exercise for vision, demanding the eye to focus on both near and far points simultaneously.

Poor lighting quickly strains the eyes, so always have a good light directed on your work, either positioned overhead or behind and to one side of you. Make sure it does not cast a shadow on your work.

Television and computer screens also cause eye strain by taxing focusing muscles and reflecting glare from lights or windows, a particular problem with computer screens. Position the monitor to avoid glare – if necessary, fit an anti-glare screen. Take frequent breaks from the computer – every 15–20 minutes – and use the time to relax the eye muscles by looking into the distance.

SUN PROTECTION

Like the skin, the eyes are under attack from ultraviolet (UV) rays (see pages 73–74). Most UV radiation comes from the sun, but it is also generated by fluorescent lighting, welding equipment and lasers. UV light is invisible to the human eye and can cause eye damage and disorders. One of the most serious is cataracts – opaque patches of protein fibres that form over the eyes, reducing the amount of light that can enter the eye and eventually impairing eyesight. Another serious condition linked to UV light is macular degeneration – loss of central vision because of changes in the retina.

Your eyes are particularly vulnerable to UV damage in snowy areas and on beaches, because the light reflects off snow, ice, sand and water.

In some cases, UV light can cause a condition called actinic keratopathy of the cornea,

HOW VISION CHANGES WITH AGE

The most common vision problem facing the 40–64-year-old group is presbyopia – far-sightedness caused by aging of the eye muscles. The muscles become sluggish and less able to squeeze the lens to see near objects (the lens is flattened to see objects further away). This problem is compounded by the lens itself as it becomes thicker, less flexible and more opaque as you age. If you find yourself unable to read the phone book, then it's time for an eye exam.

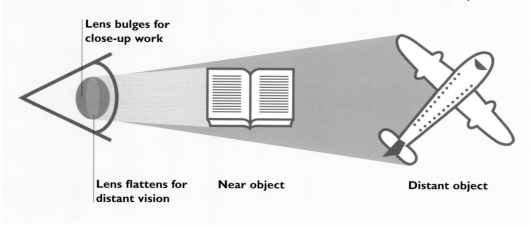

Lens bulges for close-up work

Lens flattens for distant vision   **Near object**   **Distant object**

or snowblindness. The UV rays strip off the outer layer of the cornea – the transparent area at the front of the eye – exposing nerve endings and causing severe pain. Always wear UV-protective sunglasses or ski goggles or a cap to shield bright sunlight.

SPOTS BEFORE THE EYES
Most people are familiar with the little spots that appear in the middle distance of their line of vision from time to time. They seem to float and move around as the eyes move, lasting from a few minutes to a few hours. These are the result of a temporary thickening of the clear vitreous liquid that surrounds the eye and are quite normal. If, however, you start seeing a large number of flecks or lights before your eyes, either at any one time or at close intervals, contact your doctor, as this may indicate an underlying medical problem that warrants further investigation.

VISION CHECKS
Eyesight changes subtly over the decades; around 90 per cent of 40–64-year-olds wear glasses or contact lenses to correct their vision. You may notice that as you age you find it harder to focus on the print in a book or a newspaper, although you don't have problems seeing far-away objects, such as street signs or birds in a tree (see box above). Known as presbyopia, this form of far-sightedness is easily corrected with reading glasses or, if you already wear spectacles, by changing to bifocal or varifocal lenses.

Presbyopia and other vision defects, such as myopia (near-sightedness) and hypermetropia (far-sightedness), are usually corrected with prescription glasses or contact lenses, but near-sight can also be treated with laser eye surgery (see page 176).

VISUAL AIDS
A revolution is underway in the eye glass industry. Lens technology offers a variety of new possibilities, using high-density plastics and specially manufactured glass. You can buy slimmer and lighter lenses, shatterproof and scratch-resistant lenses, and UV-protective and reflection-free lenses. If you have trouble reading because of presbyopia, new varifocal glasses enable you to see clearly close-up without needing the split-lens bifocal glasses, which bother some people. It

all comes at a price – the more 'high tech' the lenses, the more expensive the glasses.

In the last few decades there has been radical change in the way that contact lenses are used to correct vision problems. Probably the most dramatic breakthrough has been the growth in affordable and easy-to-use contact lenses.

You can choose from hard, soft, gas-permeable and disposable lenses, depending on your prescription and lifestyle. Some people like coloured lenses – now, you can dye your hair and change your eyes to match! Although bifocal contact lenses are available, they are expensive and difficult to use. A cheaper option uses one distance-vision lens in your dominant eye and one reading lens in the other. After a short adjustment period, the eyes are able to focus near and far.

MORE SERIOUS EYE PROBLEMS

Regular eye exams will ensure that your prescription – if you have one – is up to date, and will also detect any age-related eye disorders. If found early, most eye problems can be treated more effectively.

Watch out for symptoms such as blurred or cloudy vision, difficulty with or slow focusing, and unexplained headaches or eye pain – visit your doctor if necessary.

Eye disorders that are more common as you age include:

▶ *Glaucoma* Responsible for around 10–13 per cent of all cases of blindness in the Western world, glaucoma is caused by fluid

THE BATES METHOD

New York eye specialist William H. Bates developed a series of eye exercises known as the Bates Method to help prevent eyesight from deteriorating with age. Do the following exercises at least once a day. Bates also recommended we blink between five and ten times a minute to ensure the eyes stay moist.

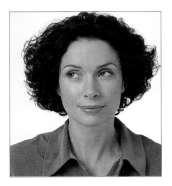

SWINGING

This exercise restores the eye's natural movement. Stand with your feet apart and quickly look from one point of interest to another. Next, swing gently from side to side and allow your eyes to swing with your eye movement.

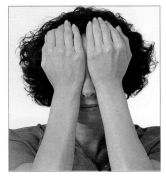

PALMING

Sit at a desk or table with your back and neck straight and head level, and rest your elbows on a pillow. Close your eyes and cover them with your cupped palms. Think of a peaceful scene, such as a beach or meadow

NEAR AND FAR FOCUSING

This exercise improves focusing ability and should be done daily. Hold two pencils out in front, one about 15 cm (6 in) away and the other at arm's length. Focus on the nearest one with both eyes. Blink, then focus on the farther one. Repeat several times.

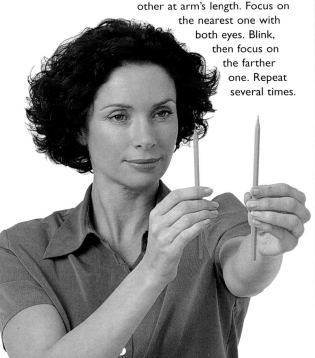

build-up in the eye placing pressure upon the delicate nerves that transmit impulses to the brain to create vision. Loss of sight gradually occurs as the pressure increases. Doctors have been unable to pinpoint the causes of glaucoma and no cure exists. It can, however, be controlled if detected in the early stages. Treatments include eye drops or pills, which can reduce the pressure on the eye. If the disease is too advanced for these to be effective, laser surgery may be used to unclog the drainage channels in the eye, allowing excess fluid to filter away. Anyone over 40 should arrange annual eye check-ups and you should be particularly wary if an immediate family member suffers from glaucoma. Also watch out if you are diabetic, have had an eye injury, have undergone eye surgery or are taking steroid medication.

▶ *Cataracts* A build-up of protein in the lens of the eye causes it to turn opaque and yellow, forming a cataract, eventually clouding over completely and blocking vision. Cataracts are usually associated with old age, but they can begin forming much earlier in life. Like glaucoma, there is some evidence to suggest that the disease is hereditary, and other high-risk groups include diabetics

and people who have had an eye injury in the past. You should also arrange regular eye examinations if you have undergone radiation treatment, chemotherapy or have had an organ transplant. Cataracts cannot be cured, but surgeons can remove the clouded lens and insert a plastic replacement. The artificial lens is unable to react to light in the same way as a healthy natural lens, but it will restore vision to a satisfactory degree.

▶ *Macular degeneration* A disease that hits people over the age of 60, macular degeneration is the most common cause of blindness in people over 55. It is not known exactly what causes macular degeneration, and it is rarely completely curable. Watch out for the most obvious warning sign – loss of your central field of vision. Laser eye surgery may help some cases if problems are caught early. Antioxidants (see pages 47–48) offer protection against this condition.

▶ *Diabetic retinopathy* The leading cause of blindness in people between the ages of 20 and 50, retinopathy affects only diabetics. The blood vessels in the back of the eye leak, causing blurred vision and preventing the proper transport of nutrients to the eye. Laser eye treatment can slow the damage to the

COLOURFUL CHANGES

As we grow older, the muscles of the iris may have more trouble opening and closing the pupil, reducing the amount of light that can come into the eye. By age 60, the amount of light entering the eye will have been reduced by half and by 80 it's down to a quarter.

The paintings below by the artist Claude Monet are of the same garden, but the one on the left was painted when he was in his 30s, and that on the right when he was in his 80s, when he had cataracts. The difference in colour is marked, although both remain masterpieces.

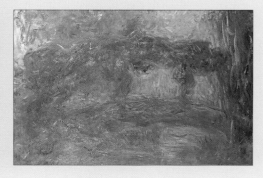

blood vessels, although it must be caught early. There is a high chance of eyesight recovery if the condition is treated while it is still mild. If your diabetes is controlled, the onset of retinopathy will be delayed.

SOUND AND HEARING

Hearing tends to deteriorate slightly with age; the eardrum loses elasticity, and fibres in the auditory nerve, which carries sound signals to the brain, start to degenerate. But damage due to disease or excessive noise exacerbates the problem.

> *Unlike the eyes, which rest*
> *when you shut them or fall asleep,*
> *your ears are open and working*
> *constantly.*

Even when you are asleep, the ears continue to receive sounds from all around you and transmit them to be processed in the brain. The brain monitors these sounds and wakes you up if there is a loud or alarming noise, such as a door slamming or someone shouting your name. Because the ears are constantly open to sound, they are vulnerable to damage from sudden or persistent loud noise.

An extremely loud noise – an explosion, for example, can cause immediate and permanent deafness. But more commonly, hearing loss is the result of an accumulation of loud noises throughout life. Up to 30 per cent of the hairs and fibres in the inner ear can be lost without impairing hearing, but losing more than that proportion will inevitably lead to some degree of deafness.

Members of rock bands, steelworkers and other people subjected to loud sounds over long periods can become deaf to high tones. Millions of workers in industrialised countries are threatened each day by extreme levels of noise in factories, construction sites and airports. Be aware of your environment – it is easy to become accustomed to noise and to forget the dangers of overexposure.

For reasons that are not fully clear, intense physical activity further reduces the body's ability to withstand extreme noise. According to recent research, a combination of exercise and noise, such as dancing to loud music or manual labour in a noisy factory, makes the ears more vulnerable to hearing loss. One theory is that activity depletes the body's supply of magnesium – it is magnesium that protects the sensitive eardrums.

Ensuring that your diet includes plenty of foods that are rich in magnesium can help protect hearing, as can taking daily magnesium supplements (see page 48). But, more

SOUND CONNECTIONS

From the moment you are born, your hearing starts to diminish, mainly due to the desensitisation of the tiny hairs in the inner ear that are responsible for turning sound vibrations into electric signals. Different cells are activated by different sound frequencies, sending signals to the brain for decoding. The cells responding to high frequencies are the first to become damaged and die off, making you less sensitive to high-pitched sounds.

If you are exposed to a lot of loud noise without protection, the hairs in your inner ear will be destroyed much faster.

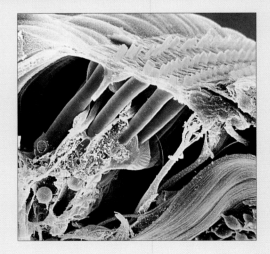

importantly, be sensible and try to avoid excessively high noise levels. Surprisingly, perhaps, too little noise is also potentially harmful to hearing.

According to research carried out by Dr Deepak Prasher, of University College London, a steady hum of low sound, such as distant traffic or quiet background music, is better for the ears than a totally silent environment, as it conditions the ears to cope with sudden, loud noises.

This idea – known as the stochastic effect – is utilised in the latest cochlear implants.

EXERCISING YOUR EARS

When you want to concentrate on a visual detail – such as a painting in a gallery – you can direct your eyes towards it and ignore everything else. But because you can't move your ears for better reception or to concentrate on a particular sound, you have to tune in using your brain.

To single out particular sounds – the music of the violin section in an orchestra, for example – you have to identify the sound and learn to block out or ignore the rest of the orchestra. We tend to take this ability for granted, but like any other skill it needs practice or it will weaken over time. To fine-tune your hearing ability, take time to listen to a mixture of sounds – orchestral music, groups of people talking, birdsong – and use your brain to separate the different sounds and concentrate on each one in turn. After a while, you will find that you become more aware of individual sounds and are better able to distinguish, comprehend and appreciate what you hear.

CORRECTING HEARING LOSS

Many forms of hearing loss are temporary and/or treatable, especially if caught in the early stages. It is vital, therefore, to seek medical help as soon as you become aware of impairment. If your hearing is lost

Protect your hearing

The best way to safeguard your hearing is to protect your ears from loud noise. Never assume that noise must be painful to cause damage – if in doubt, cover your ears.

Put safety first at work If you work in a noisy environment, use ear protectors or foam ear plugs, which mould themselves to the shape of your ear canal.

Plug out the noise If you are using a lawn mower or drill, wear ear protectors or ear plugs.

Cut down the noise Reduce the amount of background noise in your life. Turn off appliances if they are not being used, close windows to noisy streets or install double-glazed windows.

Turn down the volume If you have your music or television on at a high level, you will find that you constantly need a higher volume over the years.

Use machines one at a time When vacuuming, drilling or using other noisy household equipment, resist the temptation to turn the volume up on the radio. Try not to have too many appliances running at the same time.

permanently or if it needs boosting, you could use one of the many different hearing aids available. New technologies allow hearing aids to be made smaller. You may have to try a few before finding the one best suited to your requirements. It is essential, for the success of your hearing aid, that you visit a professional for fitting and maintenance.

In the case of total deafness, a certain amount of hearing can be restored with a cochlear implant. This device consists of a microphone, processor and transmitter that convert sounds into signals that are sent to electrodes implanted in the ear. The electrodes then stimulate the auditory, or hearing, nerve into sending signals to the brain, which are interpreted as sounds. Many profoundly deaf people have found their quality of life dramatically improved after they were fitted with a cochlear implant.

VISION CORRECTION
and laser eye surgery

Laser eye surgery is used to correct near-sight (myopia), where the eyeball is slightly elongated and so the cornea does not focus light onto the retina's light-sensitive cells, but just in front. The most widely used type of laser eye surgery is photorefractive keratectomy (PRK), which uses a high-energy beam to remove cells and flatten the cornea, refocusing light onto the retina.

Some doctors also use PRK to treat mild forms of astigmatism, in which the cornea is oval-shaped instead of round, preventing proper focusing. Some cases of macular degeneration (see page 173) can also be helped if detected early.

Laser treatment for far-sight (hypermetropia), although not common, is also performed. Laser surgery is impossible for presbyopia, the reduced vision that comes with middle age as a result of a loss of flexibility in the eye's internal (crystalline) lens and muscle.

Mild near-sight (–5 dioptres or below) has an 80–90 per cent chance of great improvement, while –6 dioptres is less certain. Some doctors say PRK is predictable only below –3 dioptres. People with very severe myopia have more success with a technique called laser *in situ* keratomileusis (LASIK) which combines laser and conventional surgery. To qualify for surgery, your vision cannot be changing rapidly, and it's not for anyone under 21.

PRK is very quick – 15–150 seconds – and is done under local anaesthetic, so is virtually painless. Around 15 per cent feel little or no pain when the anaesthetic wears off, although some may need analgesics, eye drops and painkillers for several days. You'll wear an eye patch for two to three days to prevent infection, and you must rest your eyes – stay home from work, avoid watching TV and using computers.

Vision may be blurred for three to six months afterwards because of 'over-correction'. When part of the cornea is removed, the body's natural healing response is to try to grow it back. To allow for this, the eye surgeon removes slightly more tissue than the prescription requires. This makes driving and reading difficult until the eye adjusts. Only when the first eye has settled down should the other eye be treated. Most eyes stabilise within a year, but it can take two years or longer.

Older patients may take longer to adjust because the muscles of the lens that make fine adjustments to vision are not as strong. But long-term results are the same for all ages. Over 80 per cent report a dramatic improvement, and 60 per cent no longer need lenses.

There is a risk that patients will sense no improvement, or end up far-sighted instead of near-sighted, or that their vision will be worse than before. However, a six-year study by eye surgeons at St Thomas's Hospital in London concluded there is no serious risk in the case of mild to moderate myopia. The study found some corneal scarring, making vision slightly hazy, but this usually disappeared after a year.

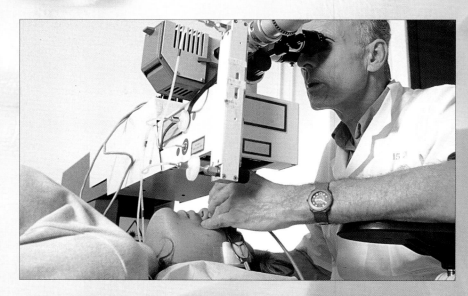

Chapter 6

Feeling good

Emotional health

A positive mental outlook can do wonders for both your physical wellbeing and your social life. So keep happy and stable by staying on top of any emotional problems as and when they arise.

The link between emotions and health has been fully established since the 1970s, when psychologists in North America found that the body responds physically to how you feel emotionally. So, for example, if you are depressed your immune system will be lowered and there will be a ripple effect throughout your entire body.

KEEPING ON AN EVEN KEEL

No matter how you live your life, there will be times of joy and times of difficulty and sadness. In order to remain on an even keel during these highs and lows, you need to maintain a rational perspective, not getting too carried away by the good times or feeling too bitterly disappointed through the bad. Keeping sight of the ups and downs and looking back on the changes through time can help you retain some control over your emotional state and, as a result, maintain your physical health.

There is evidence to suggest that some people have a fairly constant level of happiness throughout their life and that the most important factor influencing individual happiness actually appears to be personality. If you are naturally happy, outgoing and optimistic then you are likely to be more content than someone who is naturally pessimistic. But the good news is that, with a little training, even born pessimists can learn to brighten their outlooks. Expectations also play a major role in how you feel about your life. If you got the pay rise that you had been waiting for, you would be happy until you felt that you needed another pay rise, and so on.

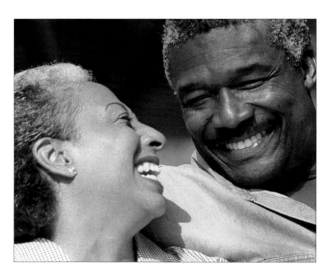

Smiling and laughing encourage your brain to release endorphins, which improve your mood, reduce stress and boost your health.

Understanding the factors that contribute to your all-round contentment and distinguishing them from the superficial anxieties and stresses can help you to work towards a happier, healthier life.

MAINTAINING A POSITIVE OUTLOOK

To remain contented, you need to think positively about life in general and about yourself in particular. It is important to make positive thinking an integral part of your outlook and behaviour, even if it demands a certain amount of conscious effort. By overcoming a natural cynicism or pessimism, you can eventually train yourself to be naturally quite positive and outgoing, believing in yourself and your own capabilities.

Dr Bernie Siegel was one of the first to isolate the use of positive thinking in health care. In 1978 he started the Exceptional Cancer Patients programme, a form of individual and group therapy utilising patients' dreams, drawings and images. His work with cancer patients is based on 'carefrontation' – a loving, therapeutic confrontation that facilitates personal change and healing. Helping people in group therapy and stress sessions helps them to 'resist' cancer and live longer. The success of his 'mind over matter' programmes is proof that emotional wellbeing plays a great part in physical health. He is now working to involve emotional therapies in conventional health care and believes that the effects of consciousness on health will become a scientifically accepted fact in the near future.

Louise Hay's work, published in the book *You Can Heal Your Life*, focuses on altering your beliefs to change the course of your life. The secret to success is to tell yourself that you can change your life, believe that you can change your life and then watch your life gradually changing to keep in line with your new view of yourself and of the world around you. Her theory is that our inner beliefs steer us towards certain courses of action or patterns of behaviour. For example, if you believe you should have a higher position at work, then you will easily find the confidence and assertiveness to strive continually for a promotion. People are all ultimately driven by their inner beliefs and subconsciously fulfil all that they privately expect from themselves and from life.

You are guided by your backgrounds and the messages you received from a young age. But relying on and following this course is often inappropriate.

Using positive thought, you can develop your own belief patterns and slowly change your life as a result. If you were told as a child 'I want doesn't get', then you may want to change this to 'I can get what I want'. Can you hear the difference?

Many people have successfully used positive thinking to turn around their lives, renewing their energy and zest for life. The methodology is very straightforward. First, decide what you would like to change or achieve; for example, you may want to be more assertive. Second, compose a statement reasserting this belief; for example, 'I am a very assertive person'. Say it over and over in your head. Write yourself notes with the statement large and clear and stick them onto your refrigerator, bathroom mirror, front door and so on. These reinforce your new belief throughout the day. When you are in situations where assertiveness is needed, you must visualise the words and think clearly to yourself 'I am a very assertive person'.

Seek out enjoyable, positive activities to elevate your sense of wellbeing; avoid stressful, negative situations that drag you down.

UPPERS:
Socialising
Enjoying a good book or show
Exercising
Relaxing
Playing games
Romancing
Having fun
Helping others
Making things
Dancing
Laughing
Living life for today

UPPERS & DOWNERS

DOWNERS:
Complaining and complaints
Feeling guilty
Being lazy
Feeling bored
Always seeing the negative
Feeling isolated
Being overly pressurised or stressed
Taking life too seriously
Worrying about the future
Dwelling on the past
Feeling sorry for yourself

You can make up your own mantra or use one of those below to believe yourself happy. Repeat it to yourself as often as you can.

I can achieve anything I want.
I am superbly fit and healthy.
I am successful and happy.
I am good company and likeable.
Good things happen to me.

BUILDING SELF-ESTEEM

Self-esteem is perhaps one of the most important contributors to good self-perception and emotional health, and it is amazing how personal perception can affect an individual's motivation and behaviour. Research suggests that self-esteem has a collective as well as an individual aspect to it. We often evaluate ourselves based on the groups we belong to, wishing to win our friends' approval and to feel at ease in social situations. Individual self-esteem may be boosted if you perceive that others view your social groups favourably. Disapproval of your social circle can undermine and lower self-esteem greatly.

All research agrees that much of the groundwork of good self-esteem is laid down in childhood. The memories of approval and disapproval from your parents lay the foundations of the self-critic within you. Although you may have taken steps to compensate in areas in which you have felt failure and, in part, restored your sense of self-worth, the inner critic can continue to nag.

Self-esteem needs to be reinforced regularly, which is why those with a strong, supportive network of friends and family have better self-esteem and fewer related health problems than those who do not. As an adult, you have control to choose the social group that you identify with, value and are valued by. You can also work on improving and reinforcing your self-esteem in many ways (see pages 188–189).

EMOTIONAL PROBLEMS

The mental health of adults in the United States was gauged by a survey carried out in the mid-1990s by the National Comorbidity

How do you feel?

How emotionally healthy and well rounded are you? Do you have a positive and stable state of mind? Do you feel in control of your emotions and supported by those around you?

Honestly answer the questions below, then count up how many As, Bs and Cs you have at the end. Read the corresponding advice below to see how your emotional health rates and what you can do to improve it.

How ready are you to express your emotions?

A As often as possible
B It depends on the emotion and if the other person asks
C Rarely or never

Do you feel valued by society, including your family and friends?

A Most of the time
B I sometimes feel undervalued
C I never feel valued

How many people do you think know the real you?

A More than six
B One to five
C None

Are you satisfied with your achievements?

A Yes, but I still have more to achieve
B The more I achieve, the less substance it holds
C I never achieve anything worthwhile

How would you best describe the way you deal with worrying?

A I deal with worries when I can, and put those I cannot out of my mind
B Worries get on top of me sometimes
C I cannot control my worrying

Do you have a supportive family unit?

A Most of the time
B There are some strains but we get over them
C Family relationships are difficult

How would you describe your frame of mind?

A I am an optimist
B I like to think of myself as a realist, and that bad is an inevitable part of life
C I am a pessimist

As a child, were your feelings paid attention to?

A Usually or always
B Often or sometimes
C Rarely or never

How frequently do you review and reset your goals and ambitions?

A At least every month
B About once in six months
C Never or rarely

How would you describe your satisfaction with life?

A My life is essentially complete
B There are things I cannot improve
C My life is unsatisfactory, but that is inevitable and I cannot change it

How far are you able to let yourself depend on someone?

A I can depend on most of my good friends and family
B I am cautious and trust only a few
C I cannot let myself depend on anyone

How would you describe the way that you cope with depression?

A Talk to others and remember the good things in life
B Time heals all
C Depression is a usual way of life

MOSTLY As

You have good emotional health and a positive outlook on life. Keep up your good score by working on the subjects for which you scored Bs or Cs.

MOSTLY Bs

It seems that you do not pay enough attention to the state of your emotional health, simply letting it control you to a large extent. You may find that this policy lets you down in times of trouble – an actively positive attitude is often necessary to lift yourself out of depression and raise your self-esteem to fulfil your ambitions.

MOSTLY Cs

Your negative outlook is holding you back from living a happy and healthy life. Insisting on seeing the bad side of everything is eroding your self-confidence and *joie de vivre*. Ask yourself why you are negative: do you have any unresolved problems?

Survey. The results were surprising – almost one-half of the representative adults surveyed had experienced the symptoms of psychological problems at some point in their lives, and one in three had experienced them within the last 12 months. Of the latter group, only 20 per cent had sought professional guidance or treatment of any kind. Only 3–5 per cent had very serious conditions, usually as a response to a build-up of several problems over time. The main problems experienced included depression and anxiety.

DEPRESSION

To a lesser or greater degree, depression is a common human experience, ranging from a case of the blues to a serious life-threatening condition that needs medical attention.

A variety of symptoms are caused by depression, and it is generally considered that if you feel more than five of the following symptoms for over two weeks, you are probably suffering from some kind of serious depression:

► Feelings of sadness and a loss of interest in pleasurable activities including sex.
► Restlessness and an inability to sit still.
► Feelings of worthlessness and guilt.
► Thoughts about death and suicide.
► Difficulty in concentrating, remembering, and making decisions.
► Changes in appetite and fluctuations in weight.
► Insomnia and troubled sleep, or sleeping more than usual.
► A loss of physical and mental energy, even to do simple chores.

Most mild bouts of depression pass over in a week or two, although more serious cases can last for extended periods of time. Women are twice as likely as men to be diagnosed as having major depression, although it is still unknown why this gender imbalance exists.

Depression is often triggered by a negative event or stressful situation. Events outside of your control can easily make you feel helpless

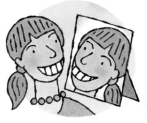

HO HO HO!
Laughing is among the simplest, cheapest and most powerful health boosters. Medical research has found that laughter lowers blood pressure, exercises the lungs and massages the heart. Laughter also releases stress-relieving chemicals in the brain, helping us to stay calm and feel great. Psychologists have found that people who laugh frequently have better self-esteem and a more positive outlook.

and undervalued. The loss of a job, failing an exam, not living up to your own and others' expectations can all initiate depression. Bereavement (see page 182), divorce (see page 209) and loss of sexuality (see pages 214–215 and 218) can leave more painful wounds that may continue for long periods.

Developmental crises may also trigger depression due to the difficulties associated with change. Even a positive transition, such as moving home or a promotion at work, can be stressful. Major role changes can cause depression, such as a shift from mother to grandmother, or wage-earner to retiree. Particular transition periods associated with depression include menopause (see pages 131–133 and 139–140), retirement (see pages 244–247) and middle age (see pages 186–187 and 247). Depression may last while you adapt to your new circumstances, but if it continues, do visit your doctor. It may occur for all of the above reasons, a combination or for no apparent reason at all – whatever the trigger, it can seriously affect your health.

According to many specialists, people who are depressed suffer from a decrease in immune function due to a redirection of natural killer cells.

The extent to which this occurs has yet to be specified, but one thing is sure – chronically

GOOD COMPANY

Keep in touch with your friends. Having a successful social life can help ward off depression. Isolation is the most frequent social cause of or contributory factor in depression. Dozens of studies have shown that socially isolated people are more prone to depression and suicide than those with regular social contact. Married people — even when the marriage is faltering and difficult — experience less depression than those who live alone. Research is currently focusing on social isolation within marriage and other situations where people shut themselves off from dealing with the outside world. Some experts believe that depression can be initiated by failing to express feelings and emotions to those around you and can be prevented through self-expression.

depressed people are more prone to disease, especially viruses. Chronic depression has also been found to aggravate heart disease, rheumatoid arthritis and muscle weakness. The result is a downward spiral of illness and further depression.

If you have a simple case of the blues, pushing the dark clouds out of the way to see the light can be a hard task, but most people find their way out within a few days. If it takes longer than two weeks, you may find it necessary to seek professional help and your doctor may recommend therapy (see pages 190–191) or suggest that you take antidepressant pills, such as Prozac. These work by increasing the number of neurotransmitters in the brain, which has the effect of dulling emotional feeling and response. In combination with psychotherapy or counselling, antidepressants can relieve the symptoms of emotional disorders and allow you to retain some perspective for a more thorough investigation of the underlying causes.

BEREAVEMENT AND GRIEF

The loss of someone very precious inevitably results in grief. It is a difficult time, often full of complex and contradictory feelings, explosions of guilt and anxiety mixed with disappointment and huge sadness. It may lead you to think about religion and your own life, or you may find yourself reliving past experiences in your mind and becoming withdrawn from the present. The psychological and physical effects of bereavement can be overwhelming. Stress and its physical manifestations are common results of bereavement, and sleeping difficulties may lead to lethargy (see pages 192–197).

Grief is a natural response to bereavement, and most people see it as a therapeutic release of emotional pain. Grief is an active

Busting the blues

Altering your attitude slightly will help you to feel more positive about life:

Think positive Forcing yourself to think, say and repeat positive statements makes you see the good side of things, and your body reacts accordingly with more energy. You may want to tell yourself 'People like the way that I am and are supportive of me', or simply 'I am a wonderful and happy person'. Write it down on a piece of paper or in the front of your diary so that you can look at it during your day.

Indulge yourself Too often it is easy to shun the happier elements of life when you are depressed. Make a point of watching your favourite comedy show, read a funny book or visit someone who you know will remind you how to laugh.

Express your feelings Self-expression is an important element of emotional health, and depression itself may result from keeping feelings too close to your chest. Ask a friend or relative if you can talk about your problems; most people are more than willing to help.

Get some routine in your life A routine will help you through the bad times and encourage you to move back to normal living.

Exercise A great way of boosting your spirits, exercise raises your brain activity and increases the supply of adrenaline and endorphins – the body's natural painkillers and feel-good drugs. Put aside 20 minutes each day for an aerobic activity, such as swimming, cycling or jogging.

Avoid negative escape mechanisms Drowning your sorrows in alcohol or spending extra money on yourself are unlikely to tackle the underlying problem. If you are not facing your depression, you may delay its resolution.

process rather than an event; it involves the expression of feelings and an adjustment to the loss. In this way, grief is actually an inbetween stage – the journey between losing something and actually coming to terms with that experience.

In the 1980s, Ross Mitchell, a psychologist in the United States, separated the grieving process into nine main stages, although not everyone will experience all of these or in the same order:

▶ **Anticipation**   The process of waiting for someone to die is the first stage of bereavement. Although often painful, this period of years or months can give you plenty of time to come to terms with the idea of death. It may come as a relief when death finally arrives after a long period of suffering, and you should not feel guilty if this is the case – you have probably done a great share of your grieving already. However, death can still come as a terrible blow, even after a protracted illness, although death without warning is often a greater shock.

▶ **Loss**   The feeling of loss encapsulates all that the person meant to you – the companionship, friendship, security and comfort. Suddenly a gaping empty space exists where that person used to be and this is often felt as a physical ache. Even negative emotions create an empty space: you can still feel a real sense of loss after the death of someone with whom you had a love–hate relationship.

▶ **Numbness**   A period of numbness follows in which you shut down your emotions as a means of self-protection. Vital functions become depressed in order to exclude pain.

▶ **Anger**   Feeling indignant and resentful because you have lost someone precious, you may believe that you don't deserve it and that you have been unfairly treated. You may want to grab back the person who's gone, and feel angry and frustrated that it is beyond your power to do so. You may feel like taking revenge on someone else because you want to put the blame somewhere.

▶ **Searching**   You begin to look for the person you have lost in the places where he or she used to be, hoping they'll still be there and praying that it never happened.

▶ **Denial**   The searching episode culminates in a period of total denial, where you make up reasons why the loved person is not there and pretend that everything is normal. This is a difficult time for you and for those around you. You are playing a desperate game to avoid the terrible realisation that your loved one is gone.

▶ **Acceptance**   Eventually the feeling that the loved person will not come back grows into an acceptance. Anger and denial burn themselves out and you face up to reality.

▶ **Letting go**   At last you accept the death and feel ready to move on, burying the person properly in your own mind. Hope predominates during this phase, where you seek new life after the loss.

▶ **Regrowth**   In time you will start to return to normal – changed by the event or growing in a different direction. During this phase you may return to previous stages of the grieving process, but movement is mostly forwards. This stage can last a number of years and it is important during this time that friends and

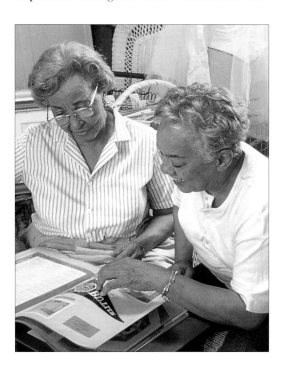

The grieving process can take a number of years. Although it may be painful, talking about your bereavement and looking over old pictures can help you to come to terms with the loss.

3 WAYS TO COPE WITH LOSS

1   Commemorate your loved one by planting a tree – see new life grow.

2   Visualise your loved one in your mind and discuss any unresolved problems that you had together.

3   Have your own intimate get-together with a few friends to remember the loved one.

family support your positive moves and decisions – even if they are a little unexpected. A lot can be learned through death and can lead to a new way of living.

The flow of these processes varies from person to person, and obviously depends upon individual circumstances, such as the relationship to the deceased. The first three stages can take a few days to pass through, or they may take a number of months; the whole process may take a number of years. If you are close to someone who is bereaved, remember that grief does not go away overnight and may still cause pain and repercussions long after the event itself.

Above all, it is important to grieve the loss fully and realise that the feelings you are experiencing are both normal and natural.

If you feel anger, let it out. Guilt is also a common response – try to work through it so that you don't waste too much emotional energy on self-recrimination. Talk to others about how you feel and do not cut yourself

off. Get out and about and make sure that you assert your independence. Maybe you could take a break or give yourself a treat and acknowledge fully that you are in a kind of emergency state for a while. Don't try to carry on as normal – you need to regain your identity and start looking at life from a new perspective. But remember: don't make any major decisions hastily. Take control of your grief; it is crucial that you take your own time to grieve properly and do it in your own way. Do not let others deny your grief by telling you to snap out of it.

While grief is a natural and healing response to bereavement, denial of grief is distressing and abnormal, and can have serious physical or psychological repercussions. Your grieving process may take you on a pilgrimage of your life with the loved person: it may involve months of looking over old photographs or reliving past memories. On the other hand, it may necessitate a gradual disposal of all the loved one's personal items, or a ritual affirmation of loss and sorrow. However your grief takes you, follow it as you feel necessary.

You may need professional help and your doctor will be able to give you advice and contacts. Counselling can help you talk through your grief honestly and can provide much needed support during the difficult period of mourning.

WORRY
Most people, both men and women, spend about 5 per cent of their waking day worrying – that's 48 minutes. For the average person, worrying is a temporary anxiety about life and the events encountered, but for some people it takes up a disproportionate amount of time – up to 100 per cent of their waking hours may be spent feeling anxious.

According to a study in the United States, over 30 per cent of women and almost 20 per cent of men surveyed had suffered anxiety disorders of some kind in their lives.

A friend in need

If you have a friend who is mourning the loss of a loved one, don't be scared to talk about it. Most people welcome the opportunity to talk about their sadness without feeling they are being a burden. But take your cue from them: broach the subject gently; if they seem unwilling to open up, it may be that they are still in a very private phase of mourning. Once they reach the stage of wanting to talk, chat together about the person who has died. Be honest: discussions that acknowledge the deceased's qualities – both good

and bad – promote healing. Ask how the loss has affected your friend, encouraging him or her to grieve. If your friend had unresolved problems with the deceased, he or she may be feeling a great deal of guilt and regret. Talking this over and allowing the bereaved to express these emotions is an important step in accepting death. It is easy to confuse grief with depression: do not try to cheer up your friend as this impedes the natural process of mourning. Also, avoid discussing future plans until the initial stages of grief have passed.

Excessive worry primarily has psychological effects, such as poor concentration, difficulties in facing problems and sleeping disorders. In many cases, these can lead to physiological symptoms and illness. Feelings of helplessness often trigger excess worrying, and if you were raised by worriers, research has shown that you may be prone to excess worrying yourself. If you feel that you lack control over a particular situation, your only option is to worry that the worst will happen. University students with worry problems were found to over-react greatly to ideas of difficulty or failure. If they got bad grades, they said that they would end up as failures, addicted to drugs, physically ill or may even die or go to hell. On the other hand, students without worry problems said that although a poor grade might eventually lead to a less satisfying job, they felt that they could limit the extent of any negative effects.

You can stop worrying, or even rechannel your worry into positive energy, with a change of attitude and a few helpful tips. First, seriously think through your worries. A recent study has shown that people who try to put worries out of their minds are more likely to become obsessed with them.

Think your worries through carefully and thoroughly. What is it that you are worrying about? Can you do anything about it? If your worry is beyond your control or simply unrealistic, you are wasting your energy worrying about it.

If a worry is more legitimate, such as a genuine concern about your physical health, you can channel your worrying energy into more exercise, better eating habits and a healthier lifestyle. Try to work actively on a solution.

Second, don't let worrying stop you from doing the things that you want to do. Susan Jeffers suggests repetitive positive feedback in her book, *Feel the Fear and Do It Anyway.* Worrying is a natural human response to a challenging situation, but you must take control of it and not let it control your life.

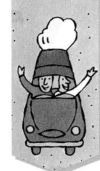

PROBLEM
My partner is unusually distracted and uncommunicative.

THE WORRY CYCLE
My partner may have doubts about our relationship.

GETTING OFF THE WORRY WHEEL
Instead of getting stuck in a cycle of self-perpetuating anxiety, put your energy to more positive use by thinking your problems through calmly and thoroughly. Be as objective as possible, formulate a solution, put it into action and bring an end to your worrying.

There is tension between us when we are alone.

I am too worried to broach the subject with my partner.

THINK IT THROUGH
The problem could well lie outside the relationship.

RESOLUTION
I will talk to my partner and find out what the problem is. If it involves our relationship, we can address it together; if it is something else, I will offer my support.

Are your worries realistic? Some psychologists contend that 99 per cent of things worried about never actually happen. Stop being unrealistic and create positive endings to your internal narratives. Express your feelings to those around you. You may only need someone else to tell you that you are worrying unnecessarily to lift you up. Keeping it inside is more likely to make you become obsessed with worry.

Serious worrying becomes a clinical condition known as generalised anxiety disorder. Anxiety sufferers worry about multiple problems simultaneously and often about things that they have no control over, such as earthquakes or war. This kind of psychological disorder develops commonly during people's 20s and 30s and may last for the rest of their lives if they take no action to stop it. The main differences between normal worry and more serious pathological anxiety conditions are that the latter are irrational, uncontrollable and can be very disruptive to normal life. If you are having problems concentrating on your work or escaping from a particular worry and it is interfering with your relationships and performance, you should make an appointment with your doctor.

Set up a worry centre

Psychologists who practise behavioural therapy recommend combating worrying by means of a worry centre. Set aside a small room or area in your home or workplace where you can deal with all of your worrying at scheduled times throughout the day. It is hoped that by limiting your worrying to these places and times, the rest of your day will be worry free. It is easy to set up.

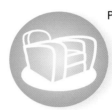

Pick a place Choose somewhere that you won't be disturbed – a particular chair or a spare room. Then select a time to set aside each day for solid, no-nonsense worrying – about 15 minutes is all you need.

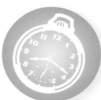

Limit your worrying Do not allow yourself to worry at any other time than your worry periods. If you feel the need, write a note of the problem and keep it for your next worry period.

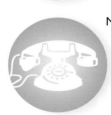

Make positive associations After each worry period give yourself a reward, such as a snack or a call to a friend. This will create an association in your mind between finishing worrying and feeling good.

When anxiety is a severe, temporary state of acute arousal, it is known as a panic attack. Sudden episodes of extreme anxiety usually appear quickly, often out of nowhere, and rapidly escalate in intensity. The most common symptoms include a pounding heart, choking, rapid breathing and breathlessness, although you may also experience hot sweats, trembling, light-headedness, chills or hot flushes. Feelings of terror accompany the intense physical arousal, possibly becoming an acute fear that you are going to die, go crazy or lose control. Panic attacks typically subside within ten minutes, although they can cause considerable strain on the body.

A panic attack may be triggered by a stressful period, although after one attack,

the body may become conditioned to respond in a similar way to stress and anxiety, leading to a panic disorder. The best way of treating panic disorder is to avoid stressful situations and use relaxation exercises to ease the panic (see pages 152–153 and 198–199). Ask your doctor for information on the many drug therapies to treat panic disorder – they are effective and non-addictive.

MIDLIFE CRISIS

It is estimated that around 10 per cent of people go through a serious midlife crisis. It can happen at any time between the ages of 35 and 55, and is characterised by varying degrees of anxiety, depression and insecurity at getting older. Typically, people suffering a midlife crisis report that they feel insignificant and powerless. Many also believe that they are failures.

If you answer yes to more than ten of the following questions, you may be entering or already in a serious midlife crisis. If you answer yes to more than five, you may be suffering a midlife crisis, too, only not as severely.

► Do you feel that your future looks less positive than it did ten years ago?
► Do you find your life less rewarding than you expected?
► Is security increasingly important to you?
► Do you feel that your life is dull?
► Are you less flexible in your values than you were ten years ago?
► Do you get angry about the struggle to find satisfaction in life?
► Do you feel like time is running out?
► Is your life too stressful?
► Are you less certain of the person you are today than ever before?
► Do you find it hard to balance your work and family life?
► Do you feel tired of trying to 'make it'?
► Do you find it hard to accept your age?
► Do you miss the challenge and excitement of your earlier years?

▶ Do you find your work less satisfying?

▶ Are you more concerned about your health as you get older?

Midlife crisis is often triggered by a negative event that challenges your view of yourself, such as divorce, loss of job, death of a parent or friend, or illness. Your reactions, usually with other contributory factors, result in a great questioning of your life, your values and your self-worth.

Women who suffer a midlife crisis usually start to experience it between 45 and 50, whereas men begin between 40 and 45. Some researchers believe that a midlife crisis is exacerbated by hormonal imbalances both in men and in women. The onset of menopause may play a large role in midlife crisis since losing the ability to give birth can be devastating to some women.

Dealing with midlife crisis is not easy, and many people find their own ways to cope.

It is important to view midlife crisis as a transitional period that allows you to readjust and reset your goals and ambitions. It is an opportunity for a new beginning and a chance to focus on the dreams, passions and hopes that you haven't had time for before.

Talk about your feelings to your close friends and family members. Challenge your existing lifestyle and endeavour to realise how it needs to change to get you on track. If you have friends who have been through midlife crises, they may be able to give insight into your own situation, offering you advice and reassurance that the confusion will pass.

Remembering your goals from childhood will remind you of some of the other things in life that you wanted to do. Contact some old friends, perhaps from university, and discuss how your values and ambitions have changed over the years. It may help you to put your life in perspective.

Stay positive about your life and think of the good things about being your age – a better understanding of life, a larger salary,

a secure family and greater independence. For some people, life really does begin at 40; and it is easy to understand why, when all the plus points of maturity are considered. Many people have turned their lives around after 40, finding new prosperity and fulfilment.

Helping those younger than yourself to learn the skills that you have acquired over the years can be extremely rewarding. You may not have the ability, time or motivation to become a world famous sportsperson, for example, but you may get a great deal of pleasure from teaching another person your skills and watching them learn.

Most important, don't make any rash decisions in an attempt to 'quick-fix' the confusion – you'll probably end up in a greater crisis.

Take things slowly – make long-term plans rather than sporadic and impulsive ones. Welcome your birthdays and celebrate them with pleasure. Take time out to feel and express anything you need to.

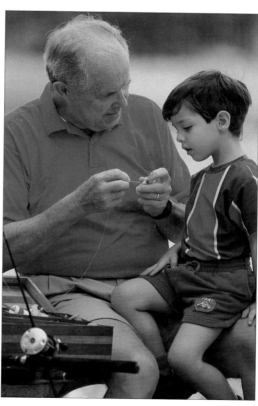

Sharing your skills with others reinforces your value in society.

5 WAYS TO TAKE COURAGE

1 Tell yourself you will succeed.

2 Don't let fear of failure keep you from achieving your goals. Always keep your goal in mind.

3 Call to mind similar situations in which you've been successful.

4 Get it in perspective. Will the world stop turning if it all goes awry?

5 Play the situation through in your mind, gauging your feelings and reactions.

10 ways to **boost your self-confidence**

Self-esteem is essential if you want to achieve your goals and live a happy and healthy life. Believe in yourself and you will find many of your worries slip away. Here's how to give an instant boost to your confidence.

1 MAXIMISE YOUR TALENTS

Each of us has a special talent – something we can do better than most of the people around us. It may be a practical skill, such as furniture making or cooking, or it may be a gift for teaching or making people laugh. Jot down a list of your talents. You don't have to be a champion at golf or tennis – if you can win more often than you lose you should regard it as a talent. Think back to moments when you've been at your happiest or most fulfilled – this will help you remember what you're good at. Focus on these talents when you're feeling low; it will help you to feel good about yourself again.

MAKE YOUR OWN MISSION STATEMENT

What is your life's purpose? Do you want to make the world a better place? Are you anxious to raise consciousness about environmental or social issues? Do you want to bring up your children to be good people? Do you want to make people laugh and feel good about themselves? Reiterate your mission statement, starting with your purpose on this planet, what you wish to achieve and why this is important.

3 FOLLOW YOUR HEART

Nothing instils confidence as much as the strong force of motivation. When you really want something, you will usually muster the necessary confidence to get it, so if you find yourself constantly lacking courage, it may be that you are seeking the wrong goals. Take time to determine your true desires and you will increase your ability to make things happen.

Just be yourself
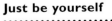
Forget your fears for a moment and remember all those quirks and foibles that make you unique. After all, you are a well-rounded human being with much to offer. **4**

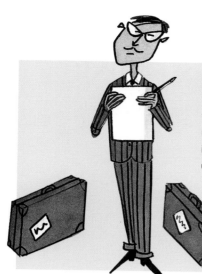

SEND YOUR INNER CRITIC ON HOLIDAY

Everyone has an inner critic – the voice inside you that tells you off all the time and makes you feel like you're never good enough. Learn to recognise this voice and ignore it; what it wants of you is unreasonable and unrealistic. Don't be your own worst enemy!

5

Take action

Find new ways of putting fun and joy into your life. Make new friends and broaden your horizons. Stagnation never did anyone any good, and psychologists believe that boredom is one of the main causes of depression. Don't let go of life.

6

BE ENCOURAGING AND POSITIVE WITH OTHERS

Supporting others will have a positive effect on your relationships. People like being with someone who looks at the bright side of life, so keep cheerful. Encouragement is catching and, with luck, your friends will soon be returning the compliments.

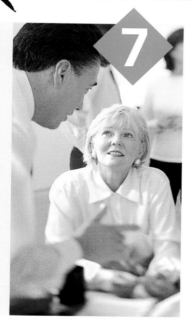

7

IDENTIFY YOUR BEST QUALITIES

Make a list of all your good qualities, just to remind yourself how great you are. You can use the following list to help you: good company, gentle and kind, responsible, practical, talented, honest, loyal, generous, creative, hard-working, witty, meticulous, wise, fun-loving, charming, intelligent, caring, interesting, thoughtful, romantic, respectable, agreeable. Then make a list of all your bad points. Try to be honest, and if you have difficulties, think of yourself from someone else's viewpoint. Your character is complex and balanced; on the reverse of every bad point there is usually a good point. Take each of your bad points and match it with its opposite good point, like this:

I am obsessive, but that also means I am meticulous and attentive.
I am impatient, but that also means I am creative and full of energy.
I am intolerant, but that also means I know what I want.

8

Spruce up your image

Take a good look at yourself – not just your appearance, but also your attitudes and lifestyle – and decide how you can improve them. The effort will result in a boost to your self-confidence.

9

PAT YOURSELF ON THE BACK

Positive thinking, such as 'I can achieve whatever I want', can fuel you on to fulfil your dreams and goals. Reminding yourself of your good qualities can help to boost your confidence. Remember how someone told you that you were fun to be with the other week, and how you were praised for your sharp thinking a few months ago. Recalling positive feedback can help to remind you that you are master of yourself and have much to offer others.

10

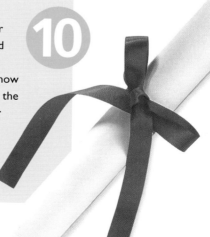

UNDERSTANDING
psychotherapy

Psychotherapy can help you deal with a range of problems, from a rocky relationship to post-traumatic stress disorder. But don't expect to simply lie on the couch: changing your thinking and behaviour takes hard work.

Since the 1950s, the number of people in the Western world who visit trained therapists has rocketed, and the figure is continuing to rise. Attitudes towards psychotherapy have changed; resolving emotional troubles and sharing inner feelings are no longer taboo. It is now known that psychotherapy can improve psychological conditions, but it may not work for everyone.

Choose a therapy that is right for you and the problems that you want to resolve. Discuss from the start what you aim to achieve with your therapist and put it into a time-frame. This will give your therapy a goal and help you stay on track. Feeling comfortable with your therapist is an important factor in the success of psychotherapy – you must establish a mutual respect.

Ask for advice from your doctor or local clinic, or visit one or two therapists to see whether they have the appropriate manner and treatment. Always check that your therapist has the correct qualifications and a licence.

Common therapies explained

You should consider undergoing psychotherapy if you have a problem that you can't solve simply by talking to your friends and family. Common reasons include troubled relationships, midlife crises, bereavement, phobias, addictions and eating disorders. Therapy gives you space to address problems with someone trained to help you in a confidential setting.

TYPE OF THERAPY	PROBLEMS TREATED	WHAT HAPPENS IN A SESSION
PSYCHOANALYTIC THERAPY		
The founder, Sigmund Freud, believed that psychological problems come from repressed, unconscious conflicts stemming from early childhood experiences. The goal is to recognise and resolve conflicts and to analyse and master subconscious desires.	Psychoanalysis is most suited to help those with chronic neuroses, such as phobias and relationship or sexual difficulties. Its use in tackling immediate or dangerous problems is very limited, and most treatments remain open-ended.	The person spontaneously reports all images and feelings that come to mind (free associates), which are analysed by the therapist, who also interprets his or her dreams. The person transfers to the analyst some of the emotions felt towards others in his or her life.
PSYCHODYNAMIC THERAPY		
A popular modified version of psychoanalysis, psychodynamic therapy puts less emphasis on inner conflict and more on current ego functioning. The goal is similar to psychoanalysis – helping people gain insight into hidden motives and conflicts.	Psychodynamic therapies attempt to treat a broader range of problems than psychoanalysis and aim for a more satisfactory practical end. However, some therapists can overemphasise practical results to the neglect of self-understanding and deeper reflection.	The therapist takes a more active role than in psychoanalysis, directing and advising rather than merely listening. The main goal is investigating and altering the way that the ego acts as a controlling agent. The person's social environment is also analysed and adjusted if necessary.

TYPE OF THERAPY	PROBLEMS TREATED	WHAT HAPPENS IN A SESSION
BEHAVIOUR THERAPY		
The second most influential therapy after psychoanalysis, behaviour therapy helps people to unlearn bad habits. It deals with changing behaviour rather than analysing the root of the problem.	It tackles a range of disorders, such as compulsive eating, addictions and phobias. However, treatment needs a focal negative behaviour pattern to work on.	Techniques include creating an unpleasant conditioned response to a bad habit, learning a more appropriate conditioned response in its place, and reinforcing good behaviour.
ROGERIAN THERAPY		
Developed by Carl Rogers, this humanist approach views an individual as essentially whole and good. Psychological problems occur due to a person's distorted self-concept.	Based on self-perception problems commonly experienced, Rogerian therapy has been able to help a range of problems, from mild neuroses to severe schizophrenia.	Creating an empathetic and psychologically safe environment, the therapist encourages people to resolve their inner crises by expressing their emotions and challenging self-concepts.
ADLERIAN THERAPY		
Developed by Alfred Adler, the therapy is based on the theory that birth order and early memories formulate a set of beliefs, which continue to operate in later life.	This is a short-term, common-sense therapy, gaining in popularity because it is cost-effective yet can be extended to long-term work.	Adlerians see clients as equals who need help in interpreting their own story. Extra therapy is offered in the shape of regular group work.
GESTALT THERAPY		
Developed from psychoanalysis, Gestalt therapy stresses feelings rather than mental and verbal analysis. It places the body, with its movement and sensations, on the same level as the mind.	It helps minor problems to moderately severe neuroses. However, the lack of analysis can hinder treatment of certain problems, and many therapists adapt Gestalt to tackle this problem.	Gestalt relies heavily on dramatisation, largely using group sessions; group members re-enact situations (often employing chairs to represent people) and express their pent-up feelings.
FAMILY THERAPY		
Family therapy treats a whole family rather than focusing on individuals and enables people to focus on those closest to them and to help bind the family unit together.	Originating 20 years ago, family therapy is expanding particularly in the public health sector. It is used to resolve family conflicts, children's problems and families living with a schizophrenic.	Roles and beliefs are identified and problematic patterns are challenged. Therapists may be limited to basic counselling if people have difficulties with a particular family member.
GROUP THERAPY		
Group therapy is extremely popular. Using a combination of different methods, it treats several people with a common problem simultaneously.	It has been successful in a range of problems, notably addictions and phobias. It is, however, not as intense as individual therapy and success rates vary according to the problem.	Members express their experiences and are challenged and guided by the leader and other members. This adds a social dimension that provides support and can be very helpful.
COUNSELLING		
Aimed at treating personal problems rather than psychological disorders, counsellors encourage clients to express their feelings and guide them in resolving problems.	Counselling can help people with emotional traumas, such as relationship breakdown, bereavement, terminal illness and post-traumatic stress syndrome.	Counsellors ask questions, allowing people to talk openly and express their feelings, and help them understand and resolve any underlying problems.

Stress management

Stress – the accumulated pressures of everyday life – can goad you into action or stifle you with frustration. Positive stress helps you to feel in charge of events; negative stress makes you feel that events control you.

Constant stress causes a host of disorders, from chronic headaches to high blood pressure. It can diminish quality of life and lead to destructive behaviour such as smoking, heavy drinking and violence.

There's a positive side to stress. Competition, motivation and excitement are forms of positive stress, stimulating the mind, aiding concentration and helping you to work efficiently and effectively.

Stress boosts your heart rate to send extra oxygen and nutrients to the brain and body tissues. It enables you to stay in control and direct your life the way you want it. High-flying business executives thrive on the stress of making big decisions. Some people become addicted to the adrenaline rush that comes from placing themselves in dangerous situations, and seek out stress. Not everyone can tolerate such a high level of stress, but you can increase your capacity to cope with stress, so that it becomes more of a positive factor in your life.

Stress factors tend to increase with age, although you may become better at handling stress and managing your life. Throughout your 40s and 50s, you may face the pressures of increasing work responsibility, an expanding family, more financial commitments and less free time. It is important during this time to relax properly and prioritise the work and responsibilities that you take on. Many people find that with each passing decade they cope better with the obstacles that life throws them – yet unexpected or protracted stress can still knock you sideways.

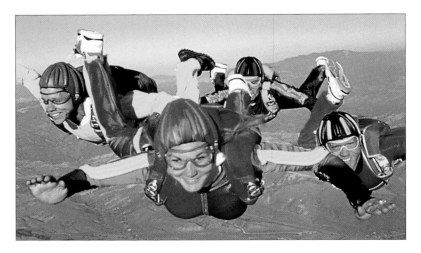

Feel the buzz – positive stress puts you on a natural high.

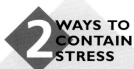

WAYS TO CONTAIN STRESS

1 Try to isolate stressful situations. For instance, leave work problems at the office.

2 Relax properly after a stressful period to prevent it from affecting your health and relationships.

THE 'FIGHT OR FLIGHT' RESPONSE

Stress is not new. It is a primitive reaction inherited from our prehistoric ancestors – the 'fight or flight' response. When you are faced with a life-threatening situation, your body is flooded with booster hormones, such as adrenaline, to spur you into action. Blood flows to the brain and your breathing rate speeds up to increase the availability of oxygen, and the liver releases stored sugars and fats for extra energy. Your heart rate rises to pump these nutrients around the body, and your blood pressure also increases.

These physiological effects ensure you are fully prepared to deal with the threat, either by standing your ground and fighting or by running away. In a threatening situation, such as a steep ski run, you will experience these effects as a racing heart, shaking hands, dry mouth and tightness in your stomach.

In the 1930s, a study by a Canadian endocrinologist and pioneer researcher of the effects of stress in the human body, Hans Selye, showed that the body cannot distinguish between physical danger and psychological distress and reacts to both in the same way. Difficult, emotionally charged situations trigger the stress response but frequently stay unresolved. Consequently, your body remains in a constant state of tension.

The result is pent-up tension that causes serious side effects. This type of stress increases the risk of ulcers, heart attacks, stroke, liver and lung disease; it can also lead to accidents, violence and suicide. Negative stress may depress the immune system, leading to increased risk of infectious diseases and even cancer. It is an underlying cause of premature death in Western society.

Many different events can trigger stress, including divorce, job change and money worries. Even happy occasions such as weddings and birthday parties cause stress.

Stress is cumulative, so if you are unlucky enough to face several stress factors over a short period, you are more likely to suffer health disorders. Watch out for the physical signs of stress, in yourself, your partner, friends or relatives. Common warning signs include tiredness, appetite or weight change, difficulty concentrating, sleeping problems and irritability. The more signs you notice, the more likely it is that stress is the cause.

EFFECTIVE TIME MANAGEMENT

Now that you've resolved to reduce the stress in your life, start by learning to use your time more efficiently. Set aside enough time to finish tasks. If you have several jobs piling up, tackle them individually, rather than feeling overloaded. Deal with unpleasant tasks right away so they don't prey on your mind and reduce your effectiveness in other areas.

Taking on too much, at work or at home, is a sure cause of stress and it means you will be less efficient at what you do. It is better not to do a job at all than to do it badly. Rather than taking on more work, keep your workload manageable to ensure that the work you do is of a high standard. Similarly,

STRESS AND PERFORMANCE

Get the right balance between positive stress and negative stress by organising and prioritising. Excessive stress saps your productivity: have you ever noticed that the more you have to do, the less you get done? However, too little stress can also have a negative effect on your productivity, leaving you lacking motivation and excitement in your life.

When you take on a new challenge, decide whether it is providing too much stress, too little or a productive middle ground.

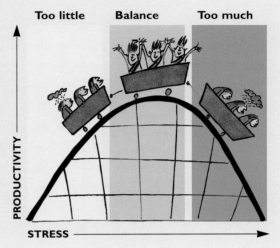

learn to delegate tasks and have faith that the other person can achieve the goal you set. Don't hesitate to ask for support. Rather than just floundering, seek out information and advice to consider your options. Discuss things with your friends, family or co-workers and never try to carry all the load yourself.

USING YOUR BODY CLOCK

Your body has its own in-built clock (see page 148), which copes best with particular demands at set times of the day. In general, the body favours catabolic (energy-releasing) functions in the day and anabolic (energy-storing), recuperative functions at night.

By planning your timetable around your body clock, you'll be better able to cope with life's ups and downs. For example:

▶ *Early morning* As you wake, levels of the feel-good hormone serotonin and the stress hormone cortisone have peaked to galvanise

STRESSFUL EVENTS

The stressful events in life have been rated by two psychologists in the United States, Thomas Holmes and Richard Rahe, to help you measure your stress load. If your total score in a year exceeds 200, you have a 50 per cent chance of suffering serious health problems. If you score 300, this risk rises to a staggering 80 per cent.

EVENT	STRESS SCORE
DEATH OF SPOUSE	100
DIVORCE	73
MARITAL SEPARATION	65
JAIL TERM	63
DEATH OF A CLOSE RELATIVE	63
PERSONAL INJURY OR ILLNESS	53
MARRIAGE/PARTNERSHIP COMMITMENT	50
LOSS OF JOB	47
RETIREMENT	45
ILLNESS IN FAMILY	44
PREGNANCY	44
SEXUAL PROBLEMS	39
CHILDBIRTH	39
CHANGE IN FINANCES	38
DEATH OF A CLOSE FRIEND	37
CHANGE OF JOB	36
TAKING OUT A MORTGAGE OR LOAN	31
MORTGAGE FORECLOSURE	30
INCREASED RESPONSIBILITIES	29
OFFSPRING LEAVES HOME	29
FIGHT WITH IN-LAWS	29
PERSONAL ACHIEVEMENT	28
PARTNER STOPS OR STARTS WORK	26
CHANGE IN LIVING CONDITIONS	25
FIGHT WITH BOSS	23
CHANGE IN WORK CONDITIONS	20
MOVING HOME	20
CHANGE IN SLEEPING HABITS	16
HOLIDAY	13
MINOR CONVICTION	11

you into action. The metabolism is most active in the morning, so eat a carbohydrate-rich breakfast to kick-start your day. Vitamins are absorbed best now; take a vitamin B complex supplement to strengthen the nervous system and fight stress.

▶ *Mid-morning* This is the best time for a dental appointment as the painkilling properties of the hormone adrenaline are at their highest mid-morning. Your back and neck muscles are least susceptible to injury now so you could do weight training or work involving heavy lifting.

▶ *Late morning* Your brain is at its most logical and creative in the late morning. This is the best time for clear-minded forward planning, problem solving or activities involving art and design.

▶ *Early to mid-afternoon* Have a lunch high in complex carbohydrates, fruit and vegetables, to give you energy, vitamins and minerals. This will help get you through the afternoon's tasks. The brain is at its most sluggish after lunch, and mistakes and accidents are more likely. Put off complex tasks, driving or operating machinery until later. Studies conducted in Greece suggest that taking things easy at this time reduces the risk of a heart attack.

▶ *Late afternoon* The body is now at a physical peak, and temperature, strength and suppleness are at optimum levels. So this is the best time to tackle jobs requiring great physical effort – most Olympic records are broken during the late afternoon. Hand–eye coordination is also at its best now, so try to schedule tasks requiring manual dexterity for this time. Ideally, you should plan a daily exercise routine or some kind of sporting activity at this time of the day.

▶ *Evening* At this time your body is less capable of handling negative moods such as loneliness and depression, and you should make this a time to socialise or talk on the phone to friends and family. The liver is able to deal with alcohol best at this time, and your senses of smell and taste are at their most acute, so treat yourself to a good evening meal with friends.

▶ **Night**   The body gently winds down in preparation for sleep. If you have difficulty falling asleep or staying asleep, you can find helpful advice on pages 149–150.

SET YOUR OWN GOALS

Get your life organised and reduce worry and time-wasting. Stress can come out of not doing enough, especially if you worry, lack purpose or feel that you are not being used to the full. People who set goals for themselves – both short- and long-term – tend to perform better than those who don't.

> *By setting yourself a goal, you will strengthen your ability to cope with stress and experience fulfilment, gaining a sense of achievement when you succeed.*

Your goals should stretch you or you will lose motivation and become bored. But be realistic or you will set yourself up for failure. Decide what exactly you want to achieve, so that you have a definite aim, and set yourself a practical schedule.

Break the work up into several shorter deadlines so that you can measure your progress as you go along. For example, if you are decorating a room, set different times for cleaning the walls, painting the ceiling and finally painting the walls. As you successfully meet each of the deadlines you will be spurred on to reach the next.

TAKE A BREAK

Regular physical exercise is especially beneficial during times of stress. Exercise gives your heart, lungs and muscles the workout your stress hormones prepared them for, allowing your body to dissipate stress through physical activity. Exercise also releases endorphins, the body's natural mood enhancers, which help to counteract stress.

Relaxation therapies, such as aromatherapy, reflexology, hypnotherapy, yoga, the Alexander technique and t'ai chi, can help to relieve stress. Some methods, such as meditation and visualisation, can be adapted to almost any situation where you feel under stress (see pages 152–153).

Allow yourself time to relax properly and take the opportunity to get away from stressful situations. Use your lunch break to relax and pursue other activities. Set aside time in the evening to read an absorbing book, or

Assertiveness training

People who have trouble asserting themselves often suffer from stress as a result. Assertiveness training helps you to identify what you really want – as well as what you don't want – and get it.

The assertiveness Bill of Rights   I have the right to:

▶ judge my own behaviour and take responsibility for it.
▶ change my mind.
▶ make mistakes and be responsible for them.
▶ deal with tricky problems in my own way.

Just say yes   Each week say yes to three things that you want, and say no to three things that you don't want. This will help you to prioritise your goals.

Take it slowly
List the ten problems you want to overcome and label them one to ten in terms of difficulty. Starting with the easiest, work your way up the list. Success builds on success.

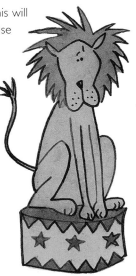
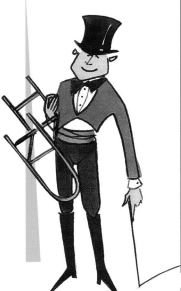

listen to your favourite music, and put work and family worries from your mind. Socialising with one or two friends is a great stress reliever, and talking over your troubles can help calm you down immensely.

A change is as good as a break, and taking up a hobby or other pastime can help you to put stressful problems to one side.

Active hobbies or chores, such as decorating, gardening or cooking, are particularly good for stress relief as they combine physical exercise with a methodical skill that demands little concentration, allowing you to think through your problems.

ASSERTING YOURSELF
Don't allow your needs and wishes to take second place to those of others, and don't be pressured into doing favours or extra work. Learn to assert your rights in the face of another's unreasonable demands. Remember that you have your own rights, which include the right to say no. Being assertive is not the same as being aggressive. There is no need to resort to violent words or gestures to make your feelings known. Simply stand your ground and state your views clearly.

CHANNELLING YOUR ANGER
When you're angry, do you ever wonder if you're taking it out on the right person? Recent research in the United States suggests that people tend to let anger build up inside and release it inappropriately on to those close to them. If your boss blames you for something that wasn't your fault, for example, you are more likely to come home and be furious at your partner or kick the dog – neither of whom are to blame for your anger. Psychologists and counsellors suggest that anger is best dealt with by facing the matter in hand; if you are angry with your boss, you should address the problem there and then.

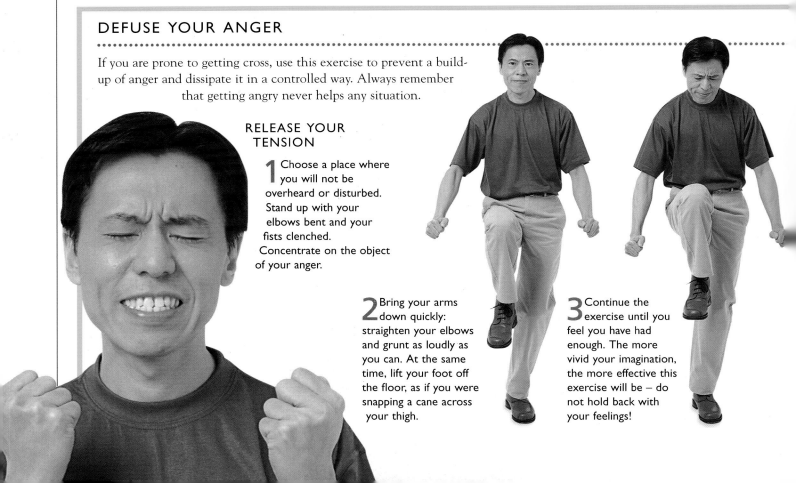

DEFUSE YOUR ANGER

If you are prone to getting cross, use this exercise to prevent a build-up of anger and dissipate it in a controlled way. Always remember that getting angry never helps any situation.

RELEASE YOUR TENSION

1 Choose a place where you will not be overheard or disturbed. Stand up with your elbows bent and your fists clenched. Concentrate on the object of your anger.

2 Bring your arms down quickly: straighten your elbows and grunt as loudly as you can. At the same time, lift your foot off the floor, as if you were snapping a cane across your thigh.

3 Continue the exercise until you feel you have had enough. The more vivid your imagination, the more effective this exercise will be – do not hold back with your feelings!

Don't take it home with you. Take a few long, deep breaths, calm down and decide how best to tackle the situation (see below).

PREVENTING BURNOUT

All work and no play can lead to burnout. Unrelieved stress at work and little or no time for pleasure or relaxation are the main culprits, resulting in fatigue, poor concentration and a variety of aches and illnesses.

Burnout is most often the result of trying too hard at one thing to the exclusion of all else, and is a sign that you need change.

Overwork is the most common cause, especially when other aspects of your life, such as socialising and hobbies, are neglected. Many people suffering from burnout are highly ambitious and perfectionist – heading for that promotion taking priority over everything else in their lives. A lack of support and appreciation by others is another common characteristic of burnout, often because the sufferers have cut off social links in an attempt to stay on top of the situation.

Prevent burnout by becoming aware of your stress levels and balancing work with pleasure. Get away from it all for a few days, take up a new hobby or simply get some exercise. Having other interests in your life will help to put things in perspective. Recognising your personal and emotional needs is important; you need support and feedback and must make socialising a priority. Stop being a slave to your goals – you will never achieve anything if you don't allow time for relaxation. Be more realistic about what you want – ask yourself whether achieving that goal will make you happy, especially if you are giving up a lot to get there. By re-evaluating your lifestyle and setting your sights a little lower you may lead a more contented, healthier life.

CALM YOUR ANGER

Count to 10 slowly and evenly until you calm sufficiently to think straight – you can think and feel at the same time. Focus your emotional energy into improving the situation.

▶ You may need to address your own part in the problem. Have you been too quick to jump to a conclusion? Are you asking for too much? Is a confrontation appropriate? Remember that assertion is meant to reduce stress, and anger is a passion that can be used to initiate change in your life.

▶ Calmly address the situation in the way you think best. It may be telling your neighbours they are upsetting you and requesting that they stop their troublesome behaviour. Complain politely about another's actions – standing your ground until you have a satisfactory answer.

▶ Make sure that you relax after the episode. Don't carry your anger around with you for the rest of the day. A relaxation technique such as meditation (see pages 152–153) may help.

AROMATHERAPY
and relaxation

Once regarded as an exclusive treatment for royalty, aromatherapy can now be enjoyed by everyone as an aid to relaxation and stress relief. Use in a base massage oil, a burner or add a few drops to make a luxuriously relaxing bath.

TAKE CARE

Essential oils can be very potent: never use more than 5 drops of oil at one time. If you are pregnant, you should take special care to limit your exposure and avoid certain oils completely (see table opposite).

Aromatherapy is an ancient treatment dating back at least to the age of the Egyptian pharaohs. It involves the use of highly aromatic oils with medicinal properties, derived mainly from the seeds, stems, bark and leaves of fragrant plants. These aromatic oils – known as essential oils – can be absorbed through the skin or warmed to emit healing vapours, which can then be inhaled.

Aromatherapy is claimed to relieve a wide variety of symptoms including skin disorders, sinus problems, chest coughs and headaches, but it is particularly recommended for alleviating the tension, anxiety and depression brought on by chronic stress. This may be because of the link that exists between the body's olfactory sense and the limbic system – the part of the brain that controls emotional responses.

Aromatherapy essential oils are highly concentrated and are therefore too potent to be applied, undiluted, directly onto the skin. There are many ways in which they can be used, including room sprays, candles, bath, body and facial oils, perfumes, warm compresses and footbaths.

Swedish massage strokes

There are three main strokes used in aromatherapy, derived from Swedish massage techniques. Professionals often use massage techniques derived from Thai massage and Indian massage in addition to the strokes below. Although massage is good for aches and pains, check with your doctor first if you have a more serious complaint.

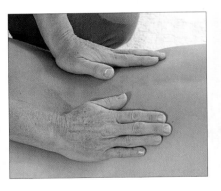

EFFLEURAGE
Smooth, sliding strokes soothe the skin as they distribute the oil. Always stroke towards the heart to enhance blood circulation and lymph flow.

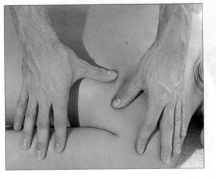

PETRISSAGE
These kneading and rolling actions stimulate the deeper layers of tissue and ease tense or tired muscles. Avoid painful areas or varicose veins.

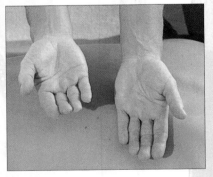

TAPOTEMENT
These are light percussive pummelling movements carried out with the outer edges of the open hand, a loose fist or the knuckles.

The following methods are popular for relieving stress:

Massage Mix up to 5 drops of one or more essential oils with 2 tablespoons of a natural carrier oil – almond, olive, sunflower or wheatgerm oils are good – and rub into the skin. The oils, mainly absorbed through the pores of the skin, and the relaxing massage action combine to alleviate stress symptoms.

Bath/jacuzzi/hot tub Add up to 5 drops of essential oil to your bath. Agitate the water to disperse the oils. If you have a warm aromatherapy bath after a stressful day, the oils will be absorbed into the skin and also inhaled, supposedly aiding relaxation.

Fragrancers Also known as diffusers or vaporisers, these devices are designed to release aromatherapy vapours into a room and are particularly popular as an aid to meditation and for creating atmosphere. Candle fragrancers and electric models are easy to use.

Inhalation Fill a bowl with hot water, add a few drops of essential oil and breathe in the water vapour. Place a towel over your head to increase the concentration of vapour. This is a decongestant, using oils such as eucalyptus, hyssop, lavender and pine.

Aromatherapy essential oils

ESSENTIAL OIL	THERAPEUTIC QUALITIES	USES	SAFETY
FRANKINCENSE (regulating)	This soothing and warming oil has been used for centuries in religious ceremonies and as an aid to meditation.	Massage, bath, fragrancer and inhalation.	No specific safety precautions.
JASMINE (stimulating)	A highly aromatic oil, it eases anxiety and depression; it has long been regarded as an aphrodisiac.	Massage, bath, fragrancer and inhalation.	Avoid if you have kidney problems or are pregnant.
LAVENDER (relaxing)	Versatile and relaxing, lavender alleviates headaches and boosts the immune system. It can combat sleeplessness when added to a bath or mixed with a little water and lightly sprinkled over a pillow.	Massage, bath, fragrancer and inhalation.	No specific safety precautions.
NEROLI (relaxing)	Also known as orange blossom, this calming oil is particularly effective for stress relief. It soothes, relaxes and alleviates tension and anxiety.	Massage, bath, fragrancer and inhalation.	Avoid exposure to ultraviolet light.
SANDALWOOD (relaxing)	This has a sweet, woody fragrance that aids relaxation and meditation.	Massage, bath and fragrancer.	No specific safety precautions.
YLANG YLANG (uplifting)	A general tonic for stress, depression and overwork, this oil is also reputed to be an aphrodisiac.	Massage, bath and fragrancer.	Avoid if you have sensitive skin.
BASIL (stimulating)	This oil has a licorice-like fragrance that acts as a refreshing nerve tonic. It works best when combined with lavender and clary sage.	Massage, bath and inhalation.	Avoid if you are pregnant or if you have sensitive skin.
CLARY SAGE (uplifting)	A soothing and uplifting oil, clary sage relaxes the muscles, helps alleviate depression and has hormone-balancing properties that can aid premenstrual and menopausal symptoms.	Massage, bath and inhalation.	Avoid if you are pregnant or if you are taking the contraceptive pill.
ROSE (regulating)	Regulating the system, rose is good for menstrual problems, including PMS and menopause, and can boost your sex drive. It is also used to treat insomnia.	Massage, bath and fragrancer.	Carry out a skin test beforehand if you have sensitive skin.
CAMOMILE (relaxing)	The calming effect of camomile has been used for centuries to soothe and relax fraught nerves, and to counteract anger and tension.	Massage, bath and fragrancer.	No specific safety precautions.

10 ways to **relieve stress**

Don't let stress wear you down. Here are some techniques you can use, singly or in combination, to alleviate stress and help relax mind and body.

Take a deep breath

1

When you feel yourself becoming stressed, take a deep breath and calm down. Research in North America and Europe has been focusing on the link between breathing and the release of neuropeptides in the brain. Neuropeptides are chemical messengers that stimulate good feelings and the sensation of pleasure. The part of the brain stem responsible for breathing is also thickly endowed with neuropeptides and neuropeptide receptors, and it is thought that this is how deep breathing can result in a calming and happier mindset.

ARE YOU A 'TYPE A' PERSONALITY?

2

Are you always on the go, working like a superhuman? Are you competitive, with a strong need for recognition and advancement? If so, you are probably a 'type A' personality. Research from Harvard Medical School found that 'type A' personalities have a 50 per cent higher chance of suffering a heart attack than the mellower 'type B' personalities. Define and prioritise your aims, and remember to pace yourself.

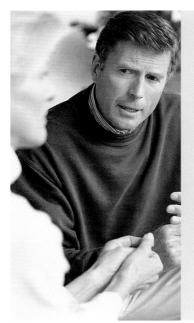

COMMUNICATE

3

Don't bottle up your problems. Share them with a friend, partner or co-worker and listen to what they have to say. The act of telling someone else your concerns helps you to put them in perspective. Talking things over has been shown to alleviate stress by reducing the sense of isolation and hopelessness that results from stressful situations. Lack of communication is itself a cause of stress. If you feel aggrieved or angry, talk it over with the person you feel has upset you – but be prepared to listen to their explanation and, if justified, accept some blame yourself. Talking not only eases stress but also stops minor disagreements from turning into major feuds.

Write it all down

4

Writing down your problems can help relieve stress and improve your health, according to several studies. Put aside about 20 minutes every day to write down your deepest thoughts and grievances – it will help you sort out your life.

STOP USING STIMULANTS

Stop smoking and limit caffeine and alcohol consumption. People often turn to cigarettes,

5

coffee and alcohol to help them through stressful times. There is a general misconception that these props can alleviate tension and anxiety, but in fact they are stimulants that increase stress levels and exacerbate symptoms of stress.

GET ORGANISED

Lack of organisation is a common cause of stress. These guidelines can help you to keep your life in order.

6

▶ Keep a day planner and make a point of recording all important events, tasks and deadlines.

▶ List all your commitments in order of priority. Be realistic about what you hope to achieve.

▶ If possible, delegate tasks or shelve them until you have more time.

Take a hike
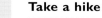
Exercise is one of the best remedies for stress. A brisk walk or hike will increase the amount of endorphins in your brain, helping you to relax, calm down and remember the good things in life.

7

LOSE YOURSELF IN A DAYDREAM

Stress often occurs because you are so engrossed in day-to-day troubles that you lose sight of the pleasant parts of life. When you feel stressed, take ten minutes out to daydream – imagine yourself on a golden beach fringed with palm trees, or bathing under a waterfall. You may prefer to remember a place that makes you feel calm: your childhood home, a friend's country house, a cosy restaurant. Try to recall the actual feeling of calmness you experienced and remind yourself that there is more to life. A daydream can be a first rehearsal for really making things happen.

8

GET A PET

Pets offer unconditional love and loyalty to their owners, which can be especially beneficial during times of stress. A pet can also help to reduce stress in other ways. The physical act of stroking a cat or a dog has a relaxing effect, reducing anxiety and tension, and has been shown to lower blood pressure. Caring for a pet offers the opportunity for play and interest. Walking a dog provides valuable exercise and gives you time to yourself or an opportunity to meet other owners.

9

STAND UP FOR YOURSELF

10

By asserting your rights you enhance your self-esteem and relieve stress. Whether you are at work, at home or making a complaint in a shop, make your point politely but firmly.

▶ Prepare what you want to say in your mind.

▶ Maintain steady eye contact, without staring.

▶ State your case firmly in a steady voice without shouting or sounding apologetic.

▶ Avoid seeming confrontational by showing that you are prepared to listen to the other person's viewpoint and to compromise.

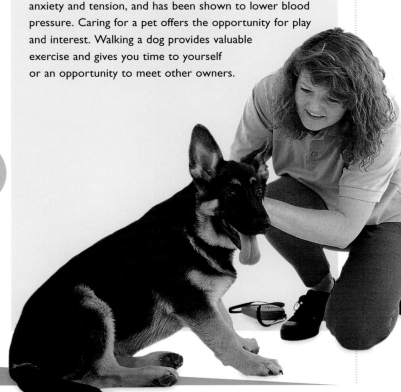

Friends and friendship

Most people need friends for relaxing, going out and, at times, emotional support. Making friends and looking after them are important skills that can enhance your life in many ways.

Friends are often rated as highly as or even higher than lovers and marital partners, according to two recent surveys. In this transient world, where men and women move far away from blood relations, a friend is a lifeline. Friends are especially valued during times of personal crisis – separation or divorce, illness or bereavement. Friends listen when you need to be heard; they comfort when you need comfort. Most valuable of all, your friends are simply there for you.

Friends have a profound effect on your wellbeing; they're a source of fun and support.

Openness is a key factor in establishing friendships, so too are humour, and good conversation and listening skills. The more you divulge about your feelings and experiences, the more vulnerable you become and so the more confidence you place in your friends. Honesty and modesty are both attributes that we admire in others, but bear in mind, friendship is a two-way street – it's give and take. Try to instil the qualities that you look for and respond to in a friend into your own personality. Get tips on meeting potential friends on pages 204–205.

The importance of friendship is now so widely recognised that it has become the subject of thorough study. A British psychology lecturer, Steve Duck, has spent several years researching friendship.

Steve Duck's findings offer a fascinating picture of how friendship works and what makes it remarkable:

▶ *Interests* For friendship to survive you and your friends need a broad base of interests – one shared hobby will not be sufficient to provide a stable platform.

▶ *Friendship skills* Some people may think they aren't good at friendship. But friendship skills can be improved; training and practice will make you more fluent.

▶ *Need for friends* Not everyone has the same drive for friendship. Some self-assured people can do without friends. The drive for friendship seems to decline after the age of 30 except where there is a serious disruption to life, such as divorce. Retirement brings on a new need for friendship.

▶ *Bad experiences* It's harder to make friends if you've been previously hurt by one.

▶ *Changing friends* Friendships may change through time in accordance with your experience and self-esteem. If, for example, you spent several years of your life abroad, you may not have as much in common with friends in your home town. This is why we grow out of friends.

▶ *Critical number* Friendship needs are influenced by a critical mass phenomenon: once we have a certain number, we don't seem to need any more.

► *Loneliness threshold* There is a critical threshold before we feel motivated to do anything about loneliness and isolation.

MAINTAINING YOUR FRIENDS

Fairness is the buzzword in keeping friendships alive and well. Quarrels between friends are usually caused by feelings of imbalance. But if conflicts are managed well, they can further develop the relationship. In this respect, it's like marriage: the more openness there is about differences, the more things can improve and evolve.

The rules of equity dictate that you have to put as much into a friendship as you take out – no one likes feeling that the work is one-way. If you have a friend who always contacts you, why not try taking the initiative next time round? That friend will be delighted that you made the first move and you will have the pleasure not only of suggesting the activity but also of demonstrating that you do indeed value the friendship.

Everybody needs somebody

Friends help you maintain emotional stability, which influences your physical health. Here are some ways in which friends can offer support.
► Having friends helps prevent loneliness and depression.
► Friends provide anchor points for opinions, beliefs and emotional responses. They help you form a picture of your 'self'.
► As well as averting loneliness, friends stave off panic at the great unknown, and therefore the need for friends may possibly be a survival mechanism.
► Friends can provide help and physical and emotional support.
► A good friend values your opinion, and that show of respect boosts feelings of self-worth. This is especially important for older people who may feel unappreciated.

Interestingly, putting too much effort into a relationship can also unbalance things. Over-attentiveness may lead to the friend on the receiving end feeling pressured or suffocated. He or she may subsequently retreat.

With your main circle of pals, only minimal effort is required to maintain friendship. Social activities are probably spontaneous – little planning is necessary. However, keeping in contact with old friends, from school or university or a previous job, for example, who now have their own separate social circles usually takes more effort. Because you no longer see them in the course of everyday activities, it is easy to lose touch. If you haven't spoken to an old friend for a while, make that call and arrange to meet for coffee or lunch. It can be fun to share memories or catch up on news. This sort of friend, whom you see only once in a while, can enhance your social life by providing an occasional alternative to your core social circle.

Look after your friends and make them feel special. Listen to what they have to say and show them that you care about their thoughts and feelings. The more you put into a friendship, the more you will get out.

TAKING FRIENDSHIP FURTHER

We all spend some of our happiest and most secure times with our friends, so it is no surprise that friendship can lead to love. Some very successful relationships start off as friendships, but making the transition can initially be rather awkward.

The advantages are that you already feel relaxed in that person's company and probably have knowledge of his or her likes and dislikes when it comes to relationships. If you feel uncertain about stepping over the borderline of friendship to sex, however, it may be that you sense, unconsciously, that sexually the friend may not quite suit you.

It appears to be difficult to stay on friendly terms with a friend-turned-lover if the relationship goes sour, whereas many people find it easy to stay friends with someone who started off as a lover. Think carefully before taking that step.

4 WAYS TO KEEP YOUR FRIENDS

1 Suggest trying an exciting new social activity to give your friendship a boost.

2 Make your friends feel good about themselves.

3 Give them enough space to see other friends and take pleasure in their interests.

4 Let them know that you are always there for them.

8 ways to **meet new people**

**Love and friendship can blossom when you least expect it –
even during the spin cycle at the laundrette – so be open to
new opportunities and seize the moment.**

VISIT PUBLIC PLACES: CAFES, GALLERIES AND EXHIBITIONS

1

When was the last time you sat in a café and a woman at the next table struck up a conversation, or someone met your eye from the opposite table? Public places are packed with chances for new friendships and relationships. Galleries and exhibitions hold special appeal in that there's always plenty to talk about, and the people around you are likely to be interested in the subject matter. An open-minded approach to meeting new people may lead to many new and exciting friendships.

2

Surf the Net

The Internet chat rooms, the newest and easiest way to talk to strangers worldwide, provide excitement and interest for everyone. The technology is straightforward and this may be your ticket to finding a lifelong partner or, at the least, a pen pal.

MAXIMISE YOUR CHANCES

3

Many marriages and friendships have originated from people using personal ads and dating agencies. Placing a personal ad in a local paper can be far less expensive than a dating agency, and answering someone else's ad is cheaper still. First meetings are easiest in a public place: if the chemistry isn't there, you can say farewell after a quick cappuccino.

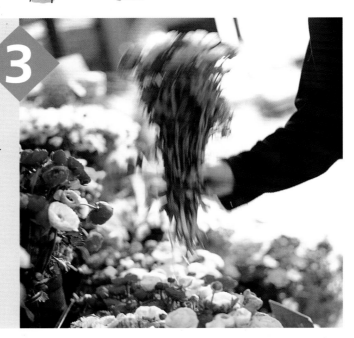

Volunteer your time

4

Many people give up time to widen their experience and help others. There are many types of activities, some needing only a few hours a week, others virtually a full-time job. Libraries, hospitals and retirement homes always need volunteers, as do many charities. Or if you fancy being outdoors, find out about a local conservation group and see if you can help your environment.

5

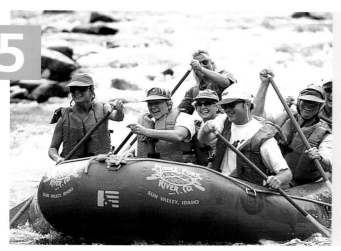

GO ON HOLIDAY

If you travel with a large group, such as on a cruise, you're bound to meet half of your fellow passengers by the time you get home. Many travel companies cater to singles. Be outgoing and remember that people want to make friends just as you do – after all, you're all in the same boat!

6

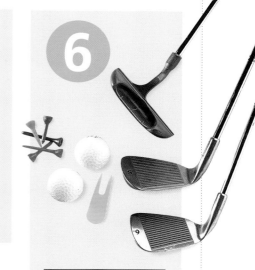

ENROL IN A CLASS

Join an adult education class to expand your knowledge and meet new people. You could learn to re-upholster old furniture or master Thai cooking. Then again, learning a language offers many opportunities to strike up a conversation. Find out about the courses taught locally – you will soon discover there are limitless options.

7

Network, network
....
Encourage your friends and family to introduce you to their friends. More couples meet through mutual friends than through any other channel and studies have shown that they are more likely to stay together if they meet this way, too.

8

JOIN A CLUB – SPORTS OR SOCIAL

Get fit, get active and get friends – sports clubs are great for meeting people. You may enjoy tennis or golf, or seek a bit of adventure in biking or mountaineering; if you like more action, try squash or skiing. Many clubs arrange trips, which are especially good for building new friendships. If you're not into sports or prefer something more sedate, you could join a bridge club or a lunch club, where a group of like-minded individuals take turns preparing delicious food for one another. The goal, whatever club you join, is the same – expanding your circle of friends by meeting people with similar interests.

Relationships

Rejoice in your relationships – they are among life's greatest pleasures and essential for your mental health and wellbeing. But care and energy are needed to ensure that you and others always find them meaningful.

People learn about relationships during infancy and childhood. Perceptions of relationships differ from person to person – moulded by their youthful observations of parents and relatives. This can mean that your partner has surprisingly different views on things you expected to agree on, particularly traditional roles for men and women and how and when to show affection. Cultural and religious differences can also add pressure to a relationship, but many couples find that learning about each other and growing together to a state of understanding and compromise strengthen their love and friendship.

Rejoice in your love, and strengthen your bond with passion and intimacy.

LOVERS AND FRIENDS

Friendship is the cornerstone of every relationship – it is virtually impossible to have a meaningful relationship with someone if friendship is lacking. It enables two people with different views, ideas and backgrounds to appreciate each other and work as a team rather than against one another.

True friendship is where both parties are equal and each respects the individuality and opinions of the other.

For friendship, you need to be able to talk, laugh and communicate with each other. A good relationship is one where both partners can express their dreams, fears and joys. Naturally, this involves trust on both sides and a deep confidence in the relationship.

Good friends support each other, offer advice and praise, give constructive criticism and share intimacies. They engage in constant communication – if there is ever a problem they talk it through. They do not set impossibly high standards for each other, nor do they compete. They try to keep the relationship alive with new sources of stimulation and by finding different ways to make each other happy.

DEALING WITH ANNOYANCES

If you spend a lot of time with someone, you will be familiar with those little things that every now and again really get on your nerves – annoying eating or personal habits, always being late, wearing awful clothes or leaving a mess in the bathroom. Many people find it difficult to deal with these annoyances without becoming resentful and often finally blowing up.

The ideal solution, of course, is to compromise, because, like it or not, you probably have a number of habits that really irritate your partner. Sit down together and talk about the things that drive each of you mad – remember to be sensitive to your partner's feelings. Some people would sooner give up an annoying partner than a comforting habit. Discuss the things about each other that bother you and try to trade them off – you can promise to be tidy if your partner stops wearing that awful cardigan. If nothing else, you can each gain an understanding of what annoys the other and give up the easy things.

Other ways to deal with annoyances include using shock tactics. If your mate is untidy, don't clear up for a while and see if the accumulating mess inspires a clean-up from him or her. Encourage your partner to wear the awful cardigan as much as possible until boredom sets in or it becomes too worn. Alternatively, take your partner shopping and buy a replacement jumper that you both like as a special present. In return, think about what you can do about your own irritating habits to keep things fair.

Five ways to keep love alive

1 Music and laughter Play the song that you first danced to, make love while playing a sensitive piece of classical music or a fast and furious pop song. Have a quiet night in with extravagant food and love songs.

2 Holding hands Closeness, care and empathy can all bring romance into your relationship. Spend time together enjoying a starry sky or a magnificent sunset, or share a treat such as a lobster or your favourite dessert.

3 Making love Physical expression is an important aspect of every sexual relationship. Try to be relaxed about your sex life. Talk honestly to your partner about concerns you may have.

4 Keeping your life inspired Ensuring that your life is full will help your relationship stay healthy. Think of a novel thing to do each week; take a trip, go for a walk with a picnic, cook a *cordon bleu* meal together, catch an opera, take a dance class or invite some friends over for dinner. Avoid boredom and stagnation – they can make you miserable, overcritical and, ultimately, bad company.

5 Romance You don't need to be extravagant, but a little bit of effort can keep a partnership fresh – in fact, the most romantic gestures are those that rely more on imagination than money: a single rose, wild daisies picked from a field, a poem that you composed yourself, a card, a small gift or an intimate candlelit dinner for two at home.

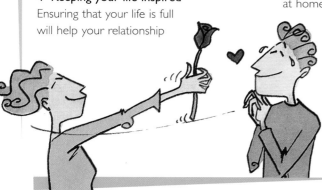

HOW FEAR TRIPS YOU UP

Some people become so immersed in a relationship that they develop a deep fear it might end. As a result, one partner continually looks for reassurance and the other has to provide it. Perversely, it is when people love like this that they become their own worst enemies – sabotaging relationships so that they have no real chance of survival.

Fear of losing someone can manifest itself in different ways, including giving too much of yourself. The more you do for your partner, the more you think your partner will stay.

But, in fact, your partner is more likely to feel burdened and lose respect for you. Needing someone is positive, but neediness is not. Needing is about trust, reaching out for support and knowing that your partner is there to help. Neediness is the desperation of someone who has no faith in the partnership.

Many psychologists suggest that you try to keep some of yourself independent from your relationship – give 90 per cent, not 100 per cent. Retain friends and interests for yourself, such as a regular golf partner or old university pals who meet up without their partners. This way, if the relationship sinks you still have a lifebelt to keep you afloat. You will also be doing wonders for your relationship – a partnership is always much healthier if it consists of two separate individuals rather than two halves of a couple.

Fear of failure also undermines relationships. If you recognise this feeling, you probably suffer from low self-esteem. Remind yourself that if your relationship doesn't work out it is neither your fault nor your partner's. If you have faith and confidence in yourself, you will be open to new experiences and, most importantly, you'll always bounce back if things do go wrong.

A close relative of fear is jealousy, which also results from low self-esteem. Jealous people feel that everyone else is superior to them and may believe that a partner has

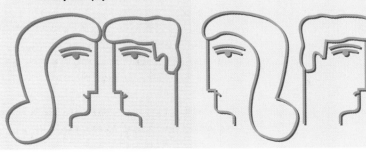

Everyone has bad habits. Some of your partner's habits may be highly amusing but others may become sore points in your relationship. Try diplomacy before launching an all-out attack.

found someone better. They see everyone as a potential threat to their relationship, and become increasingly possessive. To gain control over jealousy, you need to realise that the problem is within you and to do with your own feelings of self-worth. With more self-confidence, you would find interesting things to do yourself rather than worry about what your partner is doing. Your partner would also have far more respect for you if you had respect for yourself.

HANDLING RELATIONSHIP RUTS

Once the passion of the first few years has passed and routine sets in, relationships can flounder. Each partner may wonder what has happened to the excitement and the romantic bliss of earlier years. They may start to question their relationship, which can, if undertaken in the right spirit, allow a healthy assessment to take place. With good communication, both partners may emerge with a better understanding of their relationship. If you find yourself in a similar situation, take time to consider your feelings of discontent rationally. Talking it over as a couple can be surprisingly helpful, although it is vital that you both stay calm and remain considerate of each other's sensitivities.

Psychologist John Gottman at the University of Washington has deduced, after working with couples for 20 years, that difficult relationships can be rescued by using a special formula of what he calls 'good strokes'. For every bad stroke (behaving badly in some way) you offer your partner five good strokes (praise for achieving something or sending some flowers or a funny card).

Any number of situations, often out of your control, can lead to problems. Financial difficulties, job-related travel, addictions and family illness are prime culprits.

FIGHTING FAIR

A certain degree of fighting is good for a relationship. But the dangers mount when things get out of control. Learning to calm down is, therefore, a prime element in healthy fighting; some find this more difficult than others.

When you are flooded with emotion it is almost impossible to think straight. So, one extremely simple way of dealing with the situation is to ask for a short truce – time out to cool off and calm down. Here are some other tips:

▶ **Pick your battles carefully** Don't simply criticise – try to solve problems.

▶ **Acknowledge the other point of view** In doing so, you have shown a form of respect; to show respect is to combat contempt.

▶ **Moderate emotions** Too much fighting may erode the foundation of the partnership.

▶ **Be positive, not negative** Don't tell your partner what you can't or won't do; instead say what you can and will do.

▶ **Trust your partner's judgement** It has been pretty good in the past.

▶ **Be direct and honest** But also learn to back off when directness becomes too much.

MAKING IT WORK

Positive communication	Negative communication
▶ Show interest	▶ Criticise
▶ Be affectionate	▶ Show contempt
▶ Give compliments	▶ Be defensive
▶ Be appreciative	▶ Refuse to cooperate
▶ Show your concern	▶ Close your mind
▶ Display empathy	▶ Blame your partner
▶ Be accepting	▶ Tease
▶ Have fun together	
▶ Share your joys	

▶ **Be careful about teasing** Even when intended as harmless, teasing can be hurtful.
▶ **Don't allow a fight to get physical** Lashing out at your partner means that communication has truly broken down.

TAKING TIME OUT FOR EACH OTHER

Stress and overwork can put a huge strain on relationships, possibly paving the way for depression. Talk about your work problems together and help each other out. To recharge your emotional batteries, take weekend breaks with your partner to give yourselves some quality time in a completely different place or environment, such as a health spa or a hotel in the country. Another idea could be for you both to enrol in a weekend course or sign up for a couple's workshop if your church offers one.

GOING THROUGH SEPARATION AND DIVORCE

Once a couple decide to break up, they are frequently in a hurry to get it over with, believing subconsciously that this will get rid of the pain faster. What gets lost in this notion is the real possibility that there is still something left to rescue. Many couples, for example, find it impossible to stop fighting once they have separated. Therapists often interpret this as the couple's need still to feel connected and the continued fight as their method of staying in touch. It is precisely those circumstances that make it worthwhile to think hard about your decision to divorce.

It is not the end of the world if you postpone your split for a week, a couple of weeks, or even a month. At the very least this pause allows you to finish your relationship with some maturity and dignity.

Each partner needs to feel that the end of the relationship is fully worked through and that there are no questions left unanswered and no explanations pending.

If one person is leaving the other, the reasons must be clearly spelled out, or the person who has been left cannot fully mourn. This is a particularly bleak feeling and sometimes leads to an emotional breakdown years later.

If you have children, the first principle of separation and divorce must be to put your children's welfare first, over and above any emotional issues between you and your estranged partner. If this proves difficult, there are first-class, child-orientated mediation services available that can help so that the youngsters experience as little disruption as possible. Try to ensure continuity in your children's lives by keeping them in the same house and neighbourhood, so that they can still attend the same school and continue to see their friends.

It is also important for them to have access to their relatives. A stay with a grandparent or aunt who lives nearby may be a temporary solution while the two of you work out the terms of your separation or divorce. Wherever the children stay, they must have easy access to the other parent.

TAKING TIME OUT FOR YOU

Be kind to yourself. A separation or divorce can mean that you're living on your own for the first time in years, or perhaps the first time ever. You can expect to feel confusion,

Trying out something new together can strengthen and revitalise your relationship.

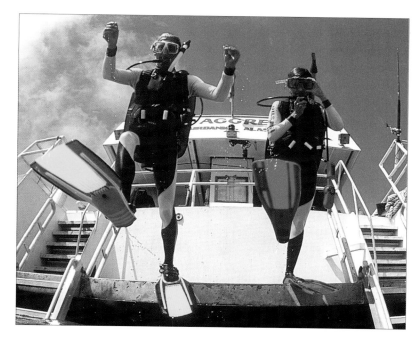

loneliness and a sense of being cut off initially; it takes time to adapt to your new situation. Do your utmost to turn such emotions into something positive. View the preparation of a new home (or the renovation of an existing home) as an exciting challenge and ask friends to help. If you think you'll be lonely, consider inviting a friend to share your quarters. If you want the adventure of living alone, treat the first occasions you stay home as special events. Put some effort into decorating so you have a place you really want to come home to. You may find it a refreshing change living on your own and being single again; your life could be busy and full – you now have the opportunity to do those things you always wanted to do.

Only if and when you are happy with yourself should you think about seeking a soulmate to share your life with. If you prefer to be single and are fulfilled and content, it is far more important to please yourself than to respond to social pressure to form a couple. Some of your married friends may even be a little envious of your new independence.

GETTING BACK IN THE DATING GAME

Get organised, get romantic and get yourself out there – once you've decided the time is right to find someone new, you need to summon up your courage and jump in.

> *Think positive and boost your self-image – you are more likely to attract other people if you feel good about yourself.*

Take a long, hard look at yourself and work out what you like and what you don't like. Decide how you can bring out your best attributes, and then invest a little time and money improving yourself.

REACHING THE PEAK AND STAYING THERE

Charles Handy, a business guru, believes that every relationship, every project, every business eventually suffers from entropy. In other words, what goes up must come down, be it ever so gradually. Marriage, he argues, is no exception. His antidote is the idea of The Sigmoid Curve. He visualises marriage as rising gradually in the growth and satisfaction stakes, topping out in a graceful curve and then slowly subsiding again.

The trick, he argues, is to predict when it is about to peak and to start a new activity or enterprise – taking up golf or organising a trip – to initiate new growth and energy, so that you stay at the peak. You also need to learn to recognise the critical point, below which you don't want to fall. The result is a curve with much shallower ups and downs, based around the peak of happiness.

You have embarked on a new relationship and are falling in love...

Plan an exciting weekend away for two...

While on holiday, make plans to start a new hobby together on your return...

First, tackle your appearance. Do you need a new haircut (see pages 102–104)? Or maybe a trip to the dentist? Could you lose a little weight (see page 61)? Remember, you are looking for a result with which *you'll* be happy – don't do it for anyone else.

Second, you may need a change of image (see pages 90–97). Maybe you should splurge on a full make-over (see pages 80–83)? Look at your clothes: are they dated? Do they still fit and flatter you? What do they say about you? You may want to buy something new simply to boost your confidence, or may even want to visit a colour or image consultant.

Third, get something to talk about. Read the papers or watch a new film or some comedy programmes to learn a few jokes. Remember, too, to be charming – no one wants to hear you moan about your last relationship, but they may enjoy a funny story about something else that happened to you.

Finally, you've got to get out there and find people. Don't allow yourself to become cynical. It may not have worked out the last time around but there is nothing to stop you from succeeding this time – give it a go.

FALLING IN LOVE AGAIN

It's happened. You've sworn you'll never have anything to do with the opposite sex again and then bam – you are kissing someone.

If you're half lucky, you'll have fun with a new partner. If you're really lucky, you'll discover yourself in the throes of a wonderful love affair that is deeper than you could ever have imagined.

It can be hard to start from scratch again with a new relationship. If you haven't been in the dating game since you were a teenager, you may find it difficult to judge how quickly or slowly to take things. Finding out about each other can be exciting if you just let it happen and allow yourselves to make mistakes.

As the relationship grows, you may find yourself comparing your new boyfriend or girlfriend to an ex-partner and this may bring

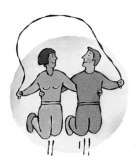

HEALTHFUL MATRIMONY

Get married if you want to stay healthy – married people eat better, exercise regularly and are more relaxed. Studies in North America and Europe have concluded that marriage results in less illness and a longer lifespan.

Romantic gestures use imagination and show heartfelt love.

back painful memories. Don't block out those feelings, but do give your new lover the benefit of the doubt. Enjoy this new, exciting chapter in your life.

As you rejoice in the passion of a new relationship, you naturally expect the whole world to share in your ecstasy. So it can come as a shock if you discover that they don't. Family members might fear that you will neglect them, friends may worry that you won't have time for them, and children (the grown-up ones) sometimes find it hard to stomach the thought of a parent enjoying a free, full love life. It's essential to consider the impact any new partner may have on any young children you have. For advice on how to deal with this, see pages 239–240.

Don't allow others to dissuade you from pursuing this second chance for happiness. Some friends and relatives may disapprove at first, perhaps hoping that you will be reconciled with your ex-partner. But if you feel this new relationship is right, then you should grasp the opportunity with both hands and go for it – you deserve it.

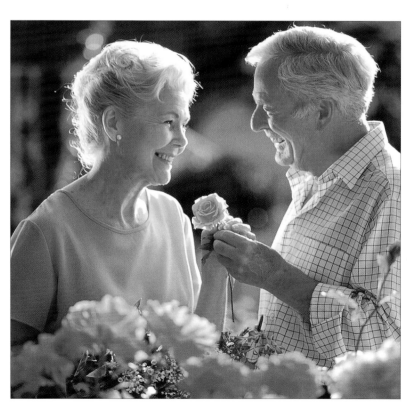

Enhancing your sex life

A satisfying sex life is a key ingredient in a strong marriage or relationship. Although desire and excitement may wax and wane, people never lose their need for intimacy and affection.

The importance of intimate physical contact and touch cannot be overestimated, although many relationships get by just fine without actual intercourse. Whether you are part of a loving long-term partnership or involved in a brand new 'friendship', sex can make your relationship sparkle with delight. A fulfilling sex life brings a special intimacy between two individuals, thereby bonding a couple and creating a unique alliance.

Communication and self-expression are among the most important requisites for emotional wellbeing. Because a healthy sexual relationship involves both, it can help many find fulfilment and happiness.

With the experience, confidence and open-mindedness of age, many people over 40 enjoy the best sex of their lives. The lifestyle changes that accompany middle age usually bring more spare time to enjoy sex, and many people take the opportunity to explore new avenues and refine the art of lovemaking.

WOMEN'S SEXUALITY

Rarely in history have women been so free to express and appreciate full sexual pleasure as now, and more is becoming known all the time about female sexual anatomy and responses. Women's sexual responses change throughout life, from the onset of puberty, through menopause and right into old age. Under-standing and accommodating these changes can make sex an enjoyable and

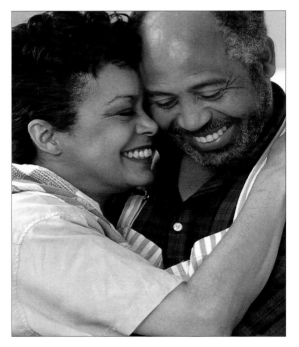

Expressing your feelings through touch and intimacy is vital for your sexuality.

ever-evolving voyage of discovery. As she grows older, a woman learns what type of stimulation she likes and what will arouse her to orgasm. She also acquires expertise in keeping her partner happy. She expresses her needs and desires openly, especially within a long-term relationship, and capitalises on the freedom to enjoy sex as a creative pastime.

During and after menopause (see pages 130–133), the complex hormonal changes that occur can sometimes boost a woman's sex drive. This is because oestrogen levels decline in relation to testosterone, the hormone largely responsible for sex drive in both sexes. However, you will not benefit from this effect if you are having hormone replacement therapy (HRT, see pages 137–139), although gynaecologists occasionally prescribe testosterone treatment to increase a woman's sex drive if HRT depresses it.

Each woman responds differently to menopause. Some enjoy a sexual renaissance as they discover new freedom from the restrictions of contraception, while others have a more difficult time and may benefit from HRT. Some women, for example, find that as their ovaries slow down and eventually cease to release sex hormones, sexual drive and response slow down, too. Without HRT, the capacity for orgasm may diminish and orgasmic sensation may lessen.

Many women find their sexual identity difficult to come to terms with as they cast off their role as fertile woman and potential or actual mother. But this natural reaction passes with time, making way for a new era full of different aspirations and challenges, and liberation that dispels sexual inhibitions.

MEN'S SEXUALITY

Men can be expected to enjoy sex and remain fertile throughout their lives. Many of those interviewed in Shere Hite's *The Hite Report on Male Sexuality (1981)* said that sexual enjoyment reached a peak at age 40–49, because they had gained an intimate knowledge of both their own and their partner's sexual responses.

This knowledge increased their sexual confidence, enabling them to shed their inhibitions and express their sexual needs and desires more openly and honestly than they had in the past. Some men said that the connection between love and sex had become more important to them and lovemaking had become more of an art form. From a woman's perspective, this often means that a man will spend more time on foreplay and listening to her needs.

Like women, men go through a slow, although less well-defined, change in their sexual behaviour as they get older.

The emphasis shifts from the hectic, hardworking father and husband towards a more relaxed, enjoyable role. Many men, nevertheless, find the middle years a testing time for their sexuality, although this soon passes as they find fulfilment in their new maturity.

SHED YOUR INHIBITIONS

One of the best lessons to learn about sex is that there are no rules. Sex can be many things: fun, a show of affection, recreational, stress-relieving, exhilarating and tranquillising all at the same time. The media's preoccupation with sex is testament to its power, but it is easy to lose the pleasure of lovemaking under the growing pressure to perform and fulfil. You are not going to lose your partner if you can't make love every night. Your partner won't leave you if you don't always achieve orgasm. You both may actually enjoy sex more if you are honest about likes and dislikes, making way for new experiences and forms of expression.

Shedding your inhibitions takes courage, but by starting with small steps (see pages 214–215), you can gradually entice your partner into your sexual pleasureland. Naturally, it is a two-way thing, so be prepared to listen, appreciate, participate and open your mind.

Sex benefits your health

Maintaining a regular sex life can be good for your health, especially for its stress-reducing qualities.

▶ Sexual intercourse is an aerobic exercise, benefiting your heart and lungs and exercising a range of muscles.

▶ Research has shown that for women regular sex increases oestrogen levels, which can improve the condition of skin and hair and redress menopausal hormone imbalances.

▶ Regular sex (with ejaculation) has been shown to decrease the risk of prostate problems in some men.

▶ Sex boosts the immune system; it has also been found to counter breast cancer development.

▶ The sexual act results in the release of endorphins in the brain, the feel-good chemical that acts as a relaxant and a painkiller.

▶ Probably the most powerful health benefit from sex is the emotionally soothing quality of touch, helping us to relax and feel good about ourselves.

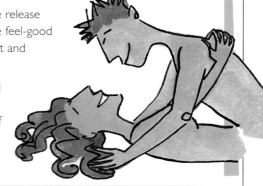

THE SEXUAL MIND

The mind has been described as the most important organ of sexual pleasure, and many sex therapists promote sexual fantasies to enhance excitement during sexual activity. Letting your mind go can be difficult though, partly because you may not be ready to admit

WOMEN'S PEAK PERFORMANCE

According to the landmark study of sexual change, the *Janus Report*, 88 per cent of women in the 39–50 age bracket reach orgasm always, often or sometimes, compared with only 79 per cent of 18–26-year-olds. This proportion remains high in those over the age of 50.

AGE	18–26	27–38	39–50	51–64	65+
ALWAYS	18	16	14	21	8
OFTEN	39	51	52	44	42
SOMETIMES	22	18	22	22	37
RARELY/NEVER	21	15	12	13	13

that certain thoughts turn you on. People may feel that they are being disloyal to their partners by imagining things they have never experienced, such as contact with someone of the same sex. They may even feel excited by situations they would never want to occur, such as forced sex. Sexual fantasies can enhance masturbation or sexual activity with a partner. Some people prefer to keep fantasies secret while others share them, and even act them out.

MALE SEX PROBLEMS

Of all the sexual problems men experience, impotence is by far the most common, and its effects often ripple into other areas of a man's life. As men age, it takes longer to get an erection and requires more physical and psychological stimulation to sustain one. This sometimes becomes a source of great anxiety, leading to psychological impotence.

A better understanding of impotence has occurred as a result of the development of Viagra (see page 219). Causes of impotence are many and varied, including diabetes, circulatory disease, alcohol-related disorders, hormonal disorders and certain medications (notably antidepressants, antihypertensives and diuretics). Psychological factors can also play a significant role, particularly stress,

REDISCOVER YOUR SENSUALITY

The following plan is especially good for longtime partners who want to improve their skills in lovemaking, but could equally be used simply to discover more about a new lover. The purpose of this exercise is for both people to acquire a contour map of their partner's body, so that each learns very precisely where the other's erogenous zones are.

PHASE 1: LEARN HOW TO PLEASURE YOUR PARTNER

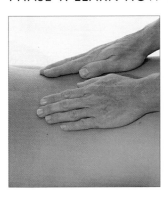 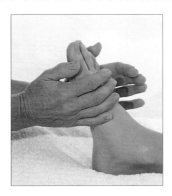 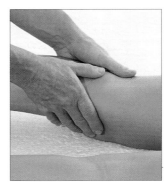

1 One partner sits on the floor or lies in a relaxed position. The other strokes specific areas of the skin.

2 Strokes are not more than 5 cm (2 in) long and start at the head, working down the body to the soles of the feet.

3 After every stroke, the partner on the receiving end rates how the strokes feel on a +3 to –3 scale (see box).

HELPFUL HINTS

► Rate responses as +3 for sensational, 0 for ordinary and –3 for bad or painful.

► Don't carry out all phases in the same session. Stagger them.

► Always slow down strokes for maximum impact.

► Use a massage oil for ease of movement.

► Keep your hands warm and clean.

► Throw away preconceived ideas of your partner's likes and dislikes.

severe depression, guilt or anxiety. The emotional side effects of impotence are a great trauma for most men.

Physical impotence can now be treated with drugs; some can be taken as a pill, others as an injection. Yohimbine – a natural treatment, originating from an African tree – has had some success. Alternatively, a vacuum sheath can be used to bring the blood mechanically into the penis and then a penis ring is attached to keep the erection.

From the age of 49 onwards, men may suffer from testosterone-related disorders, such as reduced libido, caused by low testosterone levels. Hormone replacement has proved successful in almost all cases.

Inability to ejaculate is another problem. In younger men, it may be a result of nerves or guilt about the sexual act. In older men, it more likely results from taking medication, including certain commonly prescribed antidepressants. This problem can be treated with sex therapy or a change of medication.

MEN'S PEAK PERFORMANCE

The 1993 *Janus Report* discounted the widely held notion that men peak sexually in their teens. The survey showed that there was no decline in ability to reach orgasm, and that the highest proportion of men (77 per cent) who always reached orgasm were in the 51–64 group.

AGE	18–26	27–38	39–50	51–64	65+
ALWAYS	68	68	60	77	55
OFTEN	25	26	34	18	38
SOMETIMES	3	3	4	1	4
RARELY/NEVER	4	3	2	4	3

FEMALE SEX PROBLEMS

Menopause is responsible for most female sexual difficulties experienced in later life. Happily, however, many of the symptoms can be remedied: dry vagina (with topical oestrogen cream or lubricating jelly), pain on

continued on page 218

PHASE 2: NEW TOUCH ROUTINES

1 One partner lies down with eyes closed. The other massages all over the body. It is vital to tell each other if a stroke feels good and if it could be better.

2 Experiment with varying levels of touch. With age, your partner may have become less sensitive, so find out how much pressure works and what feels erotic.

3 Using your new knowledge of your partner's erogenous zones, deliberately stimulate them (genitals excluded).

PHASE 3: FOCUS ON GENITALS

The aim here is to further expand your knowledge of your partner and learn much more powerful methods of stimulating him or her by hand.

1 Repeat phase 2 but this time you want to stimulate and concentrate on the genitals. You are not deliberately trying to achieve orgasm, although it's OK if this happens.

Sex is one of the primary ways of expressing love in a relationship. A good sex life means adapting techniques so that your lovemaking is always exciting. Here are some simple suggestions to keep sex satisfying and fun.

GREAT LOVING
techniques

As you grow older there are many reasons why sex should remain good or even get better – you have privacy, more time and energy, a need to enjoy sexual pleasure and the freedom to do so. Furthermore, you've probably shed many of your inhibitions by now and so are much more open and honest about sex.

To be a good sexual partner, you must keep sex vital and interesting, not only by regarding it as the best way of expressing your affection for your partner, but also by experimenting with a variety of techniques. Don't let your love life wane. If you notice changes in how often you have sex or the amount of energy and enthusiasm involved, realise that you may need to make small adjustments to find a pattern that you are both happy with.

Getting older can mean your body changes in some unusual ways. It may mean that a favourite sexual position is no longer as comfortable or as stimulating as it once was. However, you and your partner can have great fun discovering some new ones. When trying out new positions, remember that it should be comfortable, allowing freedom of movement and expression.

Here are some techniques and positions you can try to maintain active and enjoyable lovemaking throughout your life.

Intimacy without intercourse

Lovemaking via oral and manual techniques is a marvellous and inspired way of enjoying sex without intercourse. Most women and men enjoy this time for intimacy, and some even prefer it to penetrative sex. Discuss with your partner exactly what each of you would like – just cuddling up, touching or massaging all over or direct genital stimulation. Couples often engage in masturbation as part of sexual foreplay. Stimulation using fingers, sex toys, the mouth or tongue are popular alternatives to sexual intercourse. Fun elements, such as food, can also be introduced.

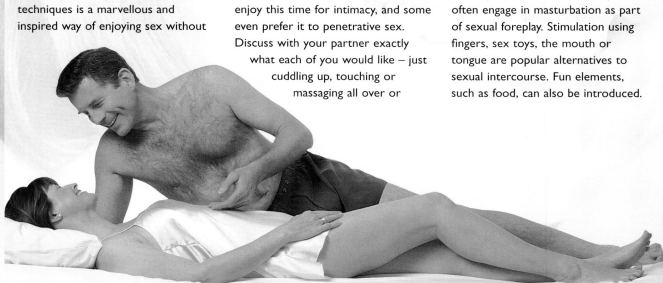

TECHNIQUES FOR HIM

As men grow older, their sexual response slows down, which brings with it great advantages: the premature ejaculator suddenly finds that he can sustain intercourse for 'long enough'; the older lover can please the woman who finds it hard to climax in a much more sustained manner than a younger man. Set against this is the fact that an older man needs longer and stronger stimulation. His penis needs firm handling but so too does his imagination. The subtle use of sexual fantasy, or the opening of the mind to erotic material, may provide that extra thrill that you or your partner need in order to feel the sort of sensations achieved effortlessly in your youth. Men often first experience multiple orgasms in middle age.

By choosing any position that gives his partner access to his penis and/or testicles, the man will achieve heightened arousal and stimulation.

The clamp position can offer the firmer handling often required by an older man's penis. The man lies on top of the woman with his legs outside hers; she can then grip his testicles and penis by squeezing her thighs together. In this face-to-face position, kissing and caressing adds to closeness and excitement.

Mutual masturbation can help men who, in later life, experience problems ejaculating inside a woman. The couple could mutually masturbate each other while the woman straddles the man. When he is close to ejaculation, he can then insert his penis inside her and thrust once or twice.

A woman-on-top position can be especially exciting for a man because the man has full view of both his and her genitalia and her breasts. The woman can control him and vary the pace – moving hard and fast is best for him. Sexual fantasy can be heightened, too, if the woman faces away from the man – it can let his imagination conjure up sexual situations that bring about his greatest arousal.

Rear-entry offers the sight of a woman's buttocks, which can be highly exciting, while also enabling the man to caress her breasts and clitoris. It also offers the option of changing the angle of entry, which can benefit lovers whose erections may not be quite so upright.

TECHNIQUES FOR HER

By their 40s, most women have developed a good degree of sexual self-knowledge, which is reflected in their enjoyment of sex and their ability to achieve orgasm. Although it may take longer to climax as you grow older, when you do so, it is likely to be powerful and deeply satisfying, especially if it's given adequate time to build up. At this time of life, a woman needs to take her own time as well as receiving plenty of tender touching, caressing and kissing from her partner.

Older women can sometimes experience pain during intercourse caused by vaginal dryness, which is common during and after menopause. If this is the case, the man should slow down and take more time over foreplay; a vaginal lubricating gel may also be helpful. Women over 40 often find that they lubricate more slowly than they used to. Preferred positions to help overcome this problem are those in which your partner can offer prolonged manual clitoral stimulation before penetration.

During rear penetration, the angle of the woman's pelvis is just right for stimulating her G-spot (the front wall of the vagina receives intense stimulation) and gives her partner manual access to her clitoris. This position could be performed lying down (on your stomach or your side), standing up or on all-fours, whichever suits you best.

A side-by-side position, both facing the same direction, allows tender lovemaking and the man can stroke all over her body and then include her genitals. She can thrust forwards and backwards for maximum sensation. This position is favoured for its comfort and intimacy; it offers lots of skin-to-skin contact, applies plenty of pressure to the vulva to heighten excitement and lovemaking can be maintained for a long time.

Use pillows if, for example, you have joints that are affected by arthritis. Placing cushions under stiff knees or hips during lovemaking will prevent further discomfort and enhance your enjoyment. Avoid certain positions, such as woman-on-top or standing up, which will place extra stress on painful knee joints.

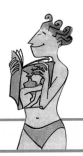

What kind of a lover are you?

Have you fallen into a rut with your lovemaking, always doing the same things? Maybe it's time to be more adventurous or to consider your partner's point of view for a change.

Take this brief questionnaire to gauge your attitudes towards sex and discuss the results with your partner. You may make some interesting discoveries.

Which do you prefer? To:	**Do you:**	**Are you more comfortable with:**
A be wooed in advance?	**A** like your partner to take the lead?	**A** familiar patterns of lovemaking?
B be taken by surprise?	**B** like to take the lead yourself?	**B** something unexpected and new?
C both?	**C** both?	**C** both?

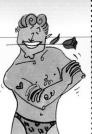

Do you prefer lovemaking:	**How many sexual partners have you had during your lifetime:**	**If your partner wanted you to look at some erotic material, would you:**
A in the bedroom?	**A** 1–3	**A** say you'd rather not?
B in the garden?	**B** over 10?	**B** produce your own?
C both?	**C** 4–10?	**C** say you'll give it a go?

MOSTLY As	**MOSTLY Bs**	**MOSTLY Cs**
You have strong feelings that sex is a private matter between you and your committed partner, sex being merely one pleasurable activity among many others that make up a relationship. You are reluctant to take sexual risks perhaps because you fear some kind of failure/humiliation. Sexual styles evolve, so be sure to keep the dialogue open and your love life fresh.	You're supremely self-confident when it comes to sex and unafraid to explore its outer reaches. You are a terrific mate for an adventurous partner but possibly overwhelming for someone more conservative. Your advantage is that you have great fun with life but you would be wise not to go overboard to a point where your judgment is impaired and you get into deep water.	You are well balanced sexually and unafraid to take occasional risks or give new ideas a try. You are a marvellous mate for an adventurous partner and sensible enough to keep him or her in check should he or she propose something you're not comfortable with. Keep in touch with your own desires so that you don't miss out in your efforts to be a good companion.

intercourse (with topical oestrogen cream) or persistent pain on intercourse (also get a pelvic exam to rule out a medical condition).

Reduced libido is a more complex subject and there are no quick and easy answers, although testosterone is emerging as a possible solution (see page 140). Sex therapy or a simple change in prescription drugs might also bring lust back into your life. These are also possible remedies for decreased sexual sensation, as is longer and more dedicated lovemaking from your partner. Recent research has focused on the similarities between male and female sexual reactions, to investigate whether Viagra is suitable for women, and for which conditions.

It is normal, in both sexes, for sexual expression to slow down with age.

Remember that you are still the same person, with or without sex, and that even if you miss the intensity of sexual feeling, you can still gain pleasure and contentment from intimacy. You can express your feelings for your partner and experience physical closeness just as meaningfully without sex.

THE SINGLE LOVER

Being single can be great, allowing you the freedom to follow your dreams and ambitions on your own. It may be a new start for you, opening new doors, taking up new interests and hobbies. Or it may be a long-term way of life – not everyone is suited to being part of a couple and the ease and independence of single life appeals to many. Whatever your situation, remember that you may still need physical touch and sex in your life.

If this is the first time you've been on your own in years, your reaction may be to panic. But try to stay 'cool' and cultivate a little self-sufficiency. You are fine; you are going to enjoy some space and time to yourself. This could be an invaluable learning experience.

If you are grieving for a former partner it may take time before you are emotionally ready to consider another. When they do get to that stage, many people find that their first dates don't feel or go right. This is often because they are used to the partner they've recently lost or have 'forgotten' how to be with someone new. Given time, you may want someone for your own sake and not because you want to fill a hole in your life.

You may feel awkward discussing HIV with a new partner, but it's advisable to do so. You could ask if your new partner has had an HIV test; although, unless he or she is in a risk category, the answer will probably be negative. The best option is to be honest and to practise safe sex.

If you are nervous about being sexual at all, don't be frightened of being honest. You might say: 'It's a while since I did this and I feel a little nervous', or 'I really want to make love, but would you mind if on this first occasion we took things very slowly'.

Above all, forgive yourself if things don't work out perfectly the first time. When you are used to one style of lovemaking, it can come as a shock to discover that other people do things in other ways, so keep an open mind. Relax and let this be an enlightening and potentially satisfying period for you. Not every journey is successful, of course, but it can be a great deal of fun finding out.

Released in the United States in 1998, Viagra quickly became the world's best-selling pill. Revolutionising all understanding of sexual response, Viagra is an important advance in treating impotence.

Viagra

Viagra works in two ways: first, by relaxing the muscles in the penis that allow blood to flow in and form a solid erection; and second, by stimulating the brain to produce a certain neurotransmitter that tells the penis to become erect with erotic thoughts. It can treat an estimated 60 per cent of impotence cases with great success. However, the rave reviews have also led men to use the drug just to prolong intercourse and improve their sex lives, rather than as a serious treatment for impotence. Although Viagra is strictly a prescription drug, difficulties in defining or proving impotence have allowed these 'joyriders' to obtain it. Other pleasure seekers buy it illegally.

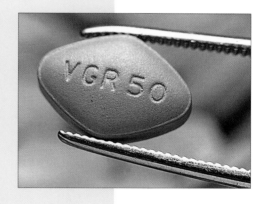

The now well-recognised blue, diamond-shaped Viagra pill.

However, doctors warn against the indiscriminate use of Viagra. A healthy sexual reaction may be impaired if Viagra is taken too often. But, more worrisome, using Viagra can lead to serious heart problems and in a few cases results in death. It is not recommended for those with a history of heart or circulatory problems.

9 ways to **boost your sex life**

Look for new ways to keep the passion alive in your relationship. Enhance your sex life by experimenting with new possibilities and ideas.

Watch a sexy video

There are many erotic videos available at video rental shops. Some are better than others – some can be highly erotic, and others may seem ridiculous. But regardless, they're always interesting, often highly amusing and usually fulfil their purpose. Erotic magazines can also titillate.

1

FEED YOUR SEXUAL APPETITE

Licking or nibbling food off someone else's stomach or other part of the body can be wonderfully erotic. The mouth plays an important part in lovemaking, so use food to stimulate more than just your tastebuds. Also, the sensations of hot, cold, sticky and runny on your skin can be exciting and slightly funny; the licking and sucking of different foods off your body may also give rise to touch sensations you've not experienced before. When selecting foods, try a range of different tastes and textures – honey, strawberries, wine, whipped cream, chocolate sauce, peanut butter, fruit jelly, ice-cream and salsa.

3

INDULGE IN SENSUAL MASSAGE

Dim the lights, put on some gentle music, take off all your clothes and shut the bedroom door. A full body massage with erotic massage oils will put you in exactly the right mood for lovemaking. Massage each other for about half an hour, avoiding the sexual parts of the body, and then gently introduce them. You may want to finish with a soothing bath.

2

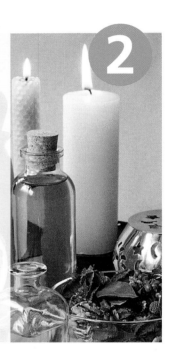

BE SPONTANEOUS

Ever done it in a shop changing room? Or have you followed your lover to the toilet in a crowded bar or café? Or maybe you've stopped the car on a hillside for a cuddle in the back seat? Many people haven't thought about having sex in a car since they were a teenager, missing all the thrill and excitement of spontaneous sex. The risk of being caught can add a special eroticism and feeling of togetherness. You can still be spontaneous at home, too. Don't always go to the bedroom; try out other rooms (and even the garden).

4

5

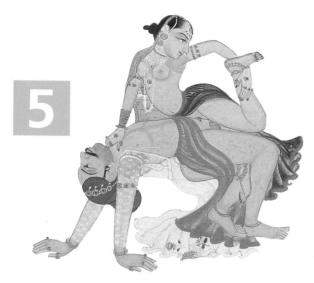

Experiment with unusual positions

Splurge on a sex manual – the *Kama Sutra* is a good one – with plenty of different sexual positions. Many may not suit you, and others may seem downright impossible, but you'll have plenty of fun trying them out together.

HAVE A SECOND HONEYMOON

Why not take yourselves away from the routine of everyday life and celebrate a new start in your sexual life with a second honeymoon. Rekindle earlier feelings and passions and explore new ones. Being in an exotic location or luxurious resort can add extra sparkle to the occasion.

6

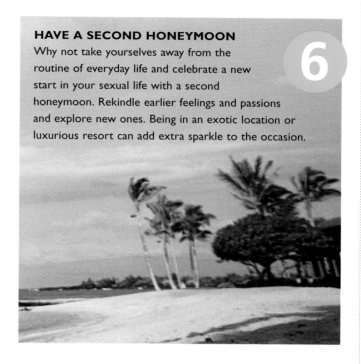

PLAY GAMES

If you have a stable relationship with a long-term partner, you may want to bring an extra challenge into your sex life by playing games. As a surprise while watching TV, pull your partner's clothes off and use a feather to tickle him or her all over. Or blindfold your partner, tie the hands gently with a cloth cord and tease.

7

ACT OUT A FANTASY

Buy some sexy new underwear, either for yourself or for your partner, and bring an extra dimension to your lovemaking. Play-acting different roles in complete costume can be tantalising and good fun. Discuss your preferences with your partner, let your imagination go and become someone else for the night. Your sex life may be improved even beyond your dreams.

8

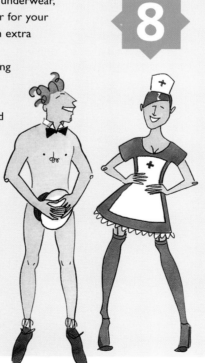

SEX TOYS

If you live close to a sex shop, why not live dangerously and visit it together? Shocking, innovative or just plain funny, the merchandise is bound to surprise you. Choose one or two toys that you feel comfortable with trying at home – many are relatively inexpensive. You can use dildos and vibrators to enhance your lovemaking, or simply for a little fun in bed. Some couples enjoy using hand-cuffs to add a subtle element of 'bondage' to their lovemaking. Experiment and decide what works for you.

9

Psychosexual therapy

It is rare for a couple in a long-term relationship not to experience some problem with their sex life. And any difficulties that do arise will always involve both of you. Because of this, honest and clear communication is essential; if you don't discuss a concern openly and frankly, a serious problem might never be solved and a minor one could grow out of all proportion.

The most common sexual problems, or dysfunctions, are not normally due to physical reasons but psychological ones. Common dysfunctions include consistent disturbances in sexual desire, arousal or orgasm, which can result in emotional suffering and psychological distress within interpersonal relationships. Physiological dysfunctions can usually be treated medically (see pages 214–215 and 218). If you have a problem that you cannot overcome between the two of you, it may be worth investigating other options, such as professional help, to sort out worries as soon as possible.

Sexual dysfunctions that may be treated by psychosexual therapy include a lack of sexual desire (hypoactive sexual desire disorder); extreme fear or anxiety about sexual intercourse (sexual aversion disorder); pain during, before or after intercourse (dyspareunia); inability to achieve or maintain an erect penis (male erectile disorder);

inability to or delayed orgasm during intercourse (orgasmic disorder); involuntary contractions of the vaginal muscles (vaginismus) and premature ejaculation for men.

A number of psychosexual therapies are available (see right). You may want to ask your doctor to suggest a therapist best suited to your needs. Sexual therapies that use a hands-on approach remain controversial, mostly because of potential difficulties in the client–therapist relationship.

As with any type of therapy, the investment in terms of time is large. Such therapies are usually medium to long term, and require visits at least once a week. Most work with couples trying to improve their sexual confidence, attitudes and performance.

Different therapies

Counselling Talking through problems with a professional counsellor can give you personal insight, enabling you to explore solutions. It's often useful for individuals or couples with minor and temporary sexual problems.

Behaviour therapy Any problematic attitudes you have can be transformed to produce more positive patterns of behaviour using association, reward and punishment techniques. It's used to overcome minor to serious sexual disorders.

Sexual/marital therapy Based on the results of the American pioneers Masters and Johnson, this is a combination of counselling and behavioural therapy. Couples talk through their problems with the therapist and then do touching exercises in the privacy of their own home.

Working together as a couple through therapy should help resolve problems sooner.

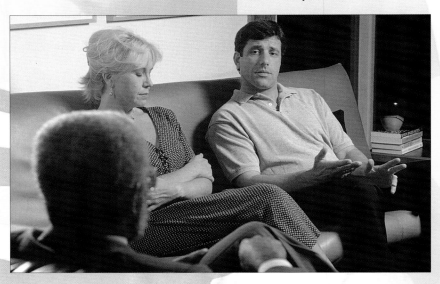

Chapter 7

Positive outlook

Work life

With so much of your time spent working, it is important to enjoy your job and maintain a healthy attitude towards it. It is not essential to stay in the same line of work; change can offer new opportunities.

Choosing a job or career is not a random act; most people deliberate about what they enjoy doing, where their aptitudes and skills lie, and whether or not money is a key issue before embarking on such decisions. But your interest and priorities change over the years, so you may find a periodic reassessment of your work habits and goals useful.

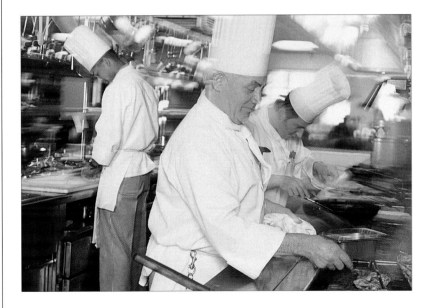

Your working environment should challenge you with new skills and quick thinking without being stressful.

POSITIVE ATTITUDES

For a healthy life it is important to take a sensible approach to work. Identify when a task is insurmountable on your own and ask for help or delegate. Be proactive, not reactive; identify potential problems and try to sort things out rather than ignoring them and simply responding when you have to.

Research has shown that a happy worker may be a long-lived worker. Although it seems to help if your work involves physical activity, in the increasingly mechanised

world this is unlikely, and so the keys to satisfaction are to enjoy working and give it all the effort and enthusiasm you can.

Being conscientious doesn't mean slogging away for hours at a time and ignoring the other parts of your life. It means focusing your energy during work hours, concentrating fully on the tasks at hand and getting things done.

With increasing pressures, it sometimes seems the only way to advance is to work above and beyond the call of duty. This may mean regularly working weekends and late into the night. Laptop computers, cellular phones and pagers keep us working even while we travel and may put us 'on call' 24 hours a day. Not only does such a lifestyle lead to burnout (see page 197), but it is also hazardous to your health. Symptoms of workaholism and burnout are fatigue, sleep disturbances, headache, chest pain, back pain, digestive problems and skin disorders.

You need to take time out for yourself and to keep up your social life; friends and family are important balances in life and can spot problems you may not be able to. Although burnout is basically overwork, it is often the lack of variety in your job, not just the volume of work, that causes it. Setting yourself impossible goals can also lead to burnout – for instance, trying to be the perfect wife, mother and professional.

If you are working too hard and for too long, talk to your boss and see if you can negotiate extra staff or different work hours; it may be that your manager doesn't realise that you're under such stress since you seem to be coping. If you cannot resolve the situation, perhaps you should look for less-exhausting employment elsewhere.

Always keep an eye out for opportunities, both within and outside your company. Read your trade magazines or professional periodicals to keep up with business moves within your field. It is also a good idea to keep your CV current; try to update it every three months – it's easy to forget all your projects, responsibilities and achievements when writing your CV after several years.

SETTING TARGETS
Having goals at work is just as important as it is in other areas of your life (see page 195).

Identifying goals means that you are forward looking, optimistic and motivated.

Goals sustain a sense of well-being and purpose, and give you a focus. Each time you achieve a goal, no matter how small, you feel a surge of pride.

To account for changing circumstances, it is a good idea to identify new work goals and review your performance every six months. Look at why you didn't meet a particular goal, see if there was anything you could have done differently and set a new deadline. The more carefully you shape your goals, the more likely you will transform your dreams into reality.

AGE AND WORK
As you approach middle age, you may start having doubts about your choice of career or job. This is natural. Sit down and focus on what you want from work and what you are currently getting. If the two don't match, consider what other options you have. You may be ready for a change of scene, redeveloping your role at work or

Setting yourself goals

Use these few simple ideas to help shape your goals at work:

Write them down Seeing them written in black and white makes them more tangible. List your goals (don't set too many) in order of importance. Discuss them with your manager; this may already form part of an established appraisal system.

Carry out a SWOT analysis Sit down with your boss and analyse your strengths, weaknesses, opportunities and threats. This will highlight a range of specific goals for you to aim at, such as delegating work to a junior colleague or improving your computer skills. Agree to a deadline to review them again, say in six months.

Be assertive Ask for the things you want, don't simply expect to be offered them – a promotion doesn't arrive on a silver platter.

Keep your goals in perspective Achieving your goals at work shouldn't interfere with your family or social life.

Reward yourself When you win that sought-after promotion, treat yourself. This serves as an incentive for setting more goals in the future.

side-stepping in your field. Take the time to research your options thoroughly to see if making such changes is financially feasible or realistic.

Throughout the last few decades the work environment has become much more competitive in many job sectors. As a result, people in their 40s, 50s and 60s may find themselves surrounded by ambitious and aggressive youngsters, treading on their toes. So, it's vital to be able to adapt to changes in the workplace. You may have to learn to deal with much younger and more aggressive employees; some may even take positions senior to yours.

Try not to think of younger people as having nothing to offer. Use their presence to concentrate on improving your own skills so that you are in a position to compete on a professional basis. Remember that all age groups bring their own unique approaches to work; a successful team is made up of people who complement each other in terms of skills, creative ideas and approach – regardless of age. It is up to you to make your employer aware of your value and potential in terms of your adaptability, enthusiasm and commitment, as well as your experience.

Experts say that to help compete in the ever-younger working environment, you should concentrate on some of the following:

▶ *Keep abreast of situations* Staying up-to-date is crucial; it shows that you are capable and right for your position. Inform yourself by learning about any new technologies introduced into your industry.

▶ *Stay competitive* Don't rest on your many years of experience; learn more and try to improve your knowledge base and ability to work.

▶ **Make your voice heard** Remind others that you have a valuable opinion and your finger on the pulse through talking, sending memos and leaflets, and by being seen in the right places at the right times.

▶ **Make the most of your strengths** List your good points and draw attention to them in your day-to-day routine.

▶ **Don't take it personally** It is easy to take someone trying to step into your shoes as a challenge. Don't be dragged into a negative personal feud. Instead, focus your energy on bettering your knowledge and position.

BACK IN THE JOB MARKET

If you've been out of the workforce for a period of months or years, re-entry may present some hurdles. You must be positive and adopt an assertive, confident approach.

Women who have been out of the work scene for years often think they have no marketable skills – this is not so. You simply need to analyse what you do already and apply those skills to a work situation. For instance, a wife and mother teaches the kids, balances the finances, plans, budgets and buys food, clothes and other necessities. The PTA president is probably a valued negotiator; and the scout leader has organisational skills.

The job market is tight for those without prior work experience, so if you don't have the necessary skills, volunteer. Although you won't be paid initially, you can build workplace experience and make useful contacts for a trouble-free transition into the professional world of your choice. Various work options exist to ease you back into the world of work, such as part-time work, flexitime, job sharing, telecommuting and short-term contract work. As you investigate the options, you might find the perfect solution.

Whether you opted to stay home to raise a family or were forced out of your job, use your time wisely. Keep up with any new and emerging technologies in your field and keep in touch with ex-colleagues – they may come in useful for a bit of networking for future job opportunities. Use your free time to explore other job interests as well and look at how you can hone your existing skills, or acquire new ones, so that you are equipped to walk into the job of your choice.

Working safely at a computer

Each day, millions of people arrive at work, turn on a computer and spend the next eight hours focused on their monitors. As a result, computer-related problems, such as repetitive strain injuries (RSIs), plague an increasing number of people. RSIs are caused by excessive keyboard or mouse work without rest. Follow these tips for safer computing:

▶ Rest your eyes by looking away from the screen into the distance once every 20 minutes.

▶ Take regular breaks and don't sit at your desk all day. Walk around, stretch and do some simple exercises.

▶ Adjust your desk height and seating. You should be able to sit up straight at your desk (good posture is vital) so that you look straight ahead or slightly downwards at your monitor.

▶ Avoid repetitive movements. If you can't, then switch to a different task. If your job involves repetitive work, regular hand and wrist exercises can help prevent an RSI.

▶ Regulate room temperature. It should be comfortable; use a fan to adjust your personal environment.

▶ Adjust lighting. Ensure your desk lamp is not too bright and is positioned so that light comes from behind you. Avoid fluorescent lighting if possible; it can trigger headaches.

UNDERSTANDING
body language

What you are saying with your body may speak louder than your words; your gestures and facial expressions can help or hinder you at work. Clear communication is important, especially if you manage staff, negotiate with clients or participate in a lot of meetings. Learn to perform better at work by controlling your body language. Keep a relaxed, confident stance, with your arms uncrossed to signal that you are open to suggestions and new ideas. Remember to make and maintain eye contact. Negative body language shows low self-esteem and an unwillingness to listen to or to adopt new proposals.

POSITIVE BODY LANGUAGE

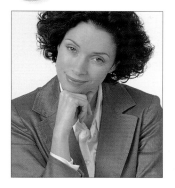 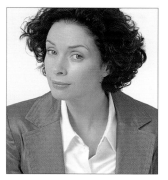

Slightly tilting the head shows approving listening, combined here with friendly eye contact.

The body is alert, shown by leaning forwards, and the eye contact shows keen interest.

Using a hand gesture while keeping eye contact adds emphasis.

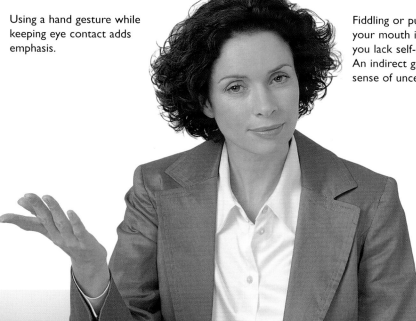

NEGATIVE BODY LANGUAGE

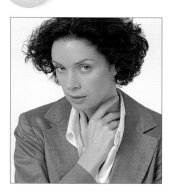 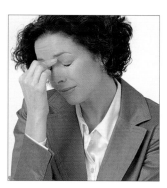

Putting your hands around your throat and waist shows you need reassurance.

Closing your eyes and pinching your nose reveals confusion and doubt.

Fiddling or putting things in your mouth is a sign that you lack self-confidence. An indirect gaze adds to a sense of uncertainty.

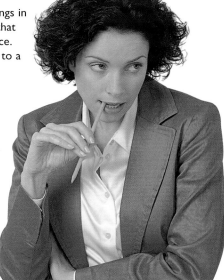

9 ways to help **choose a vocation**

For much of the twentieth century, people chose a job or profession and stuck with it, often for life, whether they enjoyed it or not. Today, however, it is not unusual for men and women to sample two or three careers in a lifetime.

EXAMINE YOUR VALUES

1 To avoid moving into a career in which you like only one aspect of the job and hate the others, try not to be too specific in what you want. Don't, for example, say that you want to be a *Vogue* columnist or a farmer, think instead that you want to get involved in women's magazines and journalism or want to make things grow.

▶ Think about the sort of environment you'd like to work in. Do you visualise yourself working in a plush corporate office, outdoors or at home?

▶ How important is financial reward? Is it crucial or is job satisfaction or helping others more important?

▶ Finally, write down all your values, dislikes, likes and skills together; they may point you to a career to which you are completely suited.

ACQUIRE MORE SKILLS

2 Taking a course that complements your career is not only enjoyable, but will also add another useful string to your bow. If you work in the field of design, for example, a part-time course in photography will expand your knowledge and allow you to consider projects from a fresh perspective. Colleges and universities now offer various flexible programmes of study – evening classes, weekend or correspondence courses. You could inquire at work to see if your company would pay for (all or part of) tuition.

RESHAPE YOUR EXISTING JOB

3 If lateral moves within the company are not possible, you could look for ways to make your job more interesting and develop in a different direction. For instance, if you are interested in becoming a teacher, can you train or teach junior people within your team or department? If this proves successful, you may be given leeway to expand and train other teams in a field outside your own.

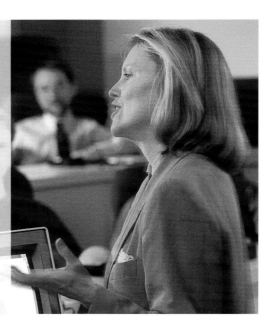

EXPLORE IN-HOUSE OPPORTUNITIES

4 Is your company large enough to offer you a transfer to a different department? An internal move allows you to keep some of your old colleagues, which can be a valuable support when starting out on something new. It also makes it easier to explore new possibilities and makes you more valuable to the company.

FINDING COMMON LINKS

Do you have experience that will allow you to transfer easily to another field? Most companies are interested only in what you can do for them based on past experience, not on what you hope to be able to do in the future. So, you have to make a case for yourself. Do you have any experience, even if done voluntarily, that you could use to get your foot in the door? It may be worthwhile putting off seeking work until you have some relevant experience.

5

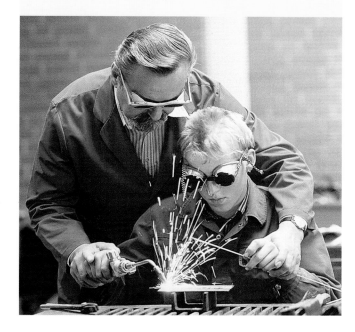

LIKES AND LOVES

Find out what you really like. What is your passion? What do you like to read about? What activities do you enjoy? Make a list and use it to decide what you really want to do.

7

Be positive

Don't run away from a career you don't like; instead make positive moves towards one that motivates and interests you. Identify what you want from a job and go for it.

8

Job change or career change?

6

Before deciding on a change at work, you must consider whether it's the job or the career you want to change. To help you decide, make a list of everything you like and dislike about your present work. If it turns out that you hate travelling so far to work, despise your manager or want different hours, then it's your environment that needs changing, not your career. However, if you find the nature of the work causes the main problems, you may need to change your career path instead.

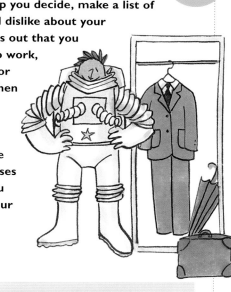

MAKE A CAREER OUT OF YOUR HOBBY

A hobby you started in your 30s may be your career by your 50s. An active interest in environmental issues may lead you towards a challenging career as a campaigner. Playing with your computer could land you your next job. Your love of flower arranging could be just the ticket for a new start. If you make good biscuits and cakes, have you thought about selling them?

9

Your leisure time

Making time to enjoy leisure pursuits is vital for your health and wellbeing. Learn some basic time-management skills so that you can fit more of the things you love to do in your life.

Leisure is critical to your overall health. If you don't allow enough time for 'play', you can start to feel tired, grouchy and depressed. Your free time offers you time for renewal – without it you could be heading for burnout.

Has your life become staid and boring? Can you predict what you will be doing most nights of the week? Now could be the time for you to get up, get out and try something new. If your children have grown up and left home, you'll probably have more free time than you once did and can use this time to explore new opportunities. If you have young children, book a baby-sitter once a week and put some pizazz into your life.

You've heard the saying 'Variety is the spice of life!' Well, incorporating a variety of interests into your life can reinvigorate you and expand your circle of friends. Although a certain amount of routine provides needed stability in life, you should always try to make room for experimenting or making each week different from the last. Without that, you'll become bored and unadventurous. Imagine how dull life would be if everyone enjoyed the same hobbies and sports!

Some people find it difficult to create leisure time or use it properly; they see play as just another chore. If this is a feeling you recognise, it may be that the leisure activities

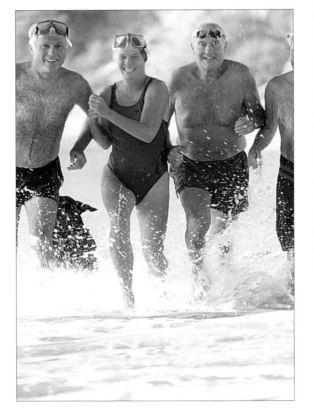

Seek out pleasure-giving activities and go for it!

you choose are too task orientated and packed with pressure. So, instead of enjoying your free time, you risk further depleting your energy reserves. Choose a hobby or activity solely because you love it; this doesn't mean that you have to excel at it or perform it to perfection – it's about the thrill and pleasure you derive from taking part.

FINDING MORE TIME FOR LEISURE

Having trouble finding 'free time' between work, household chores and family commitments? Most of us have more free time than we actually think. By analysing how you spend your time, you can pinpoint how much time is spent working or doing chores and how much is left for pleasure; in addition, you'll be able to spot how much you waste.

Use streamlining strategies along with sensible planning and control to buy extra time for your leisure pursuits. Try some of these tips:

▶ *Keep a time diary* To identify your free time, start a diary and write down what you do and when (see box opposite).
▶ *Plan ahead* Use lists of goals to help you manage your time effectively. Break down your list into 'to do today' and 'to do this

week'; some people also like to draw up a long-term schedule. Work through your goals, starting with the most important, and aim to get through the list every day. If a particular item keeps getting put off, either do it immediately or scrub it off your list. Alternatively, you can allocate a certain time for domestic chores each day. Be strict with yourself and don't go over your chore time – the rest is your free time.

▶ *Draw boundaries* By setting limits to your work and your personal lives, you let everyone know that both are important to you and that they both need your attention. You may find that being firm is a great time-saver in both areas. Some tips: as far as possible, keep overtime to a minimum; realise that it is often better to finish a task competently than to take twice as long to do a perfect job; and don't accept an invitation or take on charitable work if you don't have time or don't want to do it.

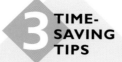

3 TIME-SAVING TIPS

1 If you find shopping a bore, try buying by phone, fax, mail order or the Internet instead of trudging around stores.

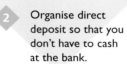

2 Organise direct deposit so that you don't have to cash at the bank.

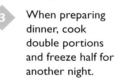

3 When preparing dinner, cook double portions and freeze half for another night.

▶ *Delegate* Don't try to do everything yourself. For household chores, involve your partner and any children over five years old. If, for example, you can delegate to three people and their tasks take 20 minutes, then you've saved yourself an hour already! People can find learning to delegate difficult, so don't expect miracles – it will take time to get used to this new chain of command.

▶ *Learn to change pace* Shift down a gear at the end of the day to be alone with your thoughts and to make the transition between work and home. For some people, a simple change of clothing – from smart suit to track-suit – does the trick, whereas others read a newspaper or listen to music.

It's very easy to fall into the trap of spending all your free time at home, and especially easy to lounge in front of the television. Try to develop leisure interests that are balanced between activities in the home and those that get you out.

Draw up a time diary

Where does the day go? To find out how much time you can devote to yourself and your leisure pursuits, you first have to identify how you spend your time. A time diary can help highlight wasted time, such as too much TV watching or unnecessary late stays at work. Pinpoint how many things could have been delegated and how many you didn't want to do. Decide on an action plan of how you are going to maximise your free time and stick with it!

ACTION PLAN

✗ **Don't stay late just because everyone else does.**

✔ **Finish work promptly. Resist the temptation to stay to finish a job that could be done tomorrow or could be delegated to one of your colleagues.**

✗ **Don't sit in front of the TV as soon as you get in; it's too easy to spend the whole night there.**

✔ **Arrive home and catch up with the latest news or your favourite radio show while you prepare dinner.**

✗ **Don't spend your evenings doing all the housework; sharing your chores will make quick work of them.**

✔ **You've got at least three hours of quality leisure time so get out there and enjoy it.**

✗ **Avoid falling asleep on the sofa; you'll awake in the middle of the night feeling groggy and unrefreshed.**

✔ **Enjoy having the time to relax so sleep comes easily. Set your alarm to get up at the same time every day.**

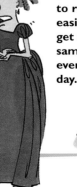

ENJOY YOUR OWN HOME

Cutting down on your TV watching might free up time for quality activities. Look over the following ideas; you may find some inspiration for things to try in your free time.

If you enjoy cooking and entertaining and are a natural host/hostess, have a party or invite friends over for dinner or for a weekend. Inspire your guests with some innovative table decorations, home-made candles and party games. There are a whole host of games on the market for a themed dinner party, such as a murder mystery game, in which everyone plays a different character – try out something new, make it unusual.

If you love being around your home but prefer to be outside in the fresh air, why not develop your garden or patio? Features you might want to include: a herb garden – use home-grown herbs to enliven your cooking; a water garden – relax in a calm, secluded corner; a wildflower patch – use the blooms for indoor arrangements. If you enjoy growing vegetables, plant a variety so that there's something new in the garden each month.

Your home is a great place to express yourself, especially if you enjoy handicrafts, decorating and home improvements.

Making decorative items for your house can provide hours of fun. Whether you are interested in paper making, model making, experimenting with different painting techniques or trying your hand at photography, be patient – it takes time to perfect a new skill.

If you like to keep your mind, body and spirit in shape but prefer to do so in the comfort of your own home, why not practise yoga? Although you may prefer to take a class to acquire the basic techniques, once you feel confident in your skills, you can build a session into your daily routine. If you find yoga difficult, you could consider another Eastern mind–body technique, such as t'ai chi.

When was the last time you relaxed with a good book or reread an old favourite? Turn the TV off and read a book instead – it encourages relaxing alpha brain waves. If you love language, you may already be an avid writer. So find out if there are any opportunities to help run a neighbourhood newsletter or write for a local newspaper or charity pamphlet – it could be a great outlet for your creative talents.

GET OUT AND ABOUT

Involving yourself in a variety of activities and spending time with different people will expand your horizons and keep your mind stimulated. A good idea is to combine activities to save time. For example, invite friends to accompany you to that exhibition you've been meaning to go to for ages. Cultural activities are stimulating and enjoyable, especially with friends or family.

Keep your mind open to new opportunities.

When was the last time you browsed in a book shop and bought a new book? Why not organise tickets for an author's book signing or an evening of readings at a local shop?

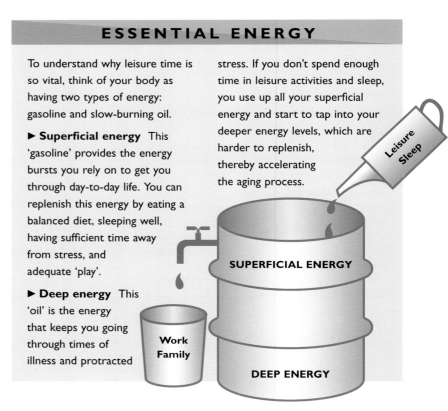

ESSENTIAL ENERGY

To understand why leisure time is so vital, think of your body as having two types of energy: gasoline and slow-burning oil.

▶ **Superficial energy** This 'gasoline' provides the energy bursts you rely on to get you through day-to-day life. You can replenish this energy by eating a balanced diet, sleeping well, having sufficient time away from stress, and adequate 'play'.

▶ **Deep energy** This 'oil' is the energy that keeps you going through times of illness and protracted stress. If you don't spend enough time in leisure activities and sleep, you use up all your superficial energy and start to tap into your deeper energy levels, which are harder to replenish, thereby accelerating the aging process.

Leisure
Sleep

SUPERFICIAL ENERGY

Work
Family

DEEP ENERGY

Find out if your local book shop runs a book club, and investigate other clubs or interest groups where you can get together with like-minded people; if you can't find one that suits you, think about starting one yourself. If you love the arts and theatre, consider joining an amateur dramatic society. If actually treading the boards is not for you, there are all sorts of opportunities in other departments, such as lighting, set design and building, and costume making.

Being a sports enthusiast, whether as a participant or spectator, is great fun. Some fans of team sports go to every game; others prefer to watch the games on TV, perhaps inviting a group of friends to join them. When considering a new sport to play, decide whether you want to play outdoors or indoors, in a team or on your own and how much time you will have to devote to training and so on.

Do thoughts of bungee jumping and hot-air ballooning thrill you? There are companies that cater to daredevils like you, with these and other activities such as tandem skydiving and white-water rafting. If this type of activity appeals to you, sign up now for the adrenaline rush.

Putting your name down for an adult education course is a great way to cultivate your knowledge – you never know where it'll take you. Investigate the options available to you at local colleges and schools; most offer flexible learning programmes nowadays.

Could you be a teacher or trainer? Pass on your own knowledge and skills to other people – by helping them you'll gain a great deal of satisfaction.

If you have experience in a specialised field, there may well be opportunities for you to teach part-time or evening classes. Even if you have no special skills, you can still get involved; charities and other volunteer-based organisations are always on the lookout for willing helpers. Whether you help out by

TOP 10 LEISURE ACTIVITIES

WALKING

SWIMMING

GARDENING

CYCLING

SNOOKER/POOL

FOOTBALL

DARTS

GOLF

KEEP FIT/YOGA

JOGGING

The chart shows the ten most popular leisure pastimes in the West.

A bicycle ride can be a relaxing and enjoyable way of getting from A to B.

teaching children or illiterate adults to read or write or by organising the office administration, the important thing is that you enjoy it – helping others is a great way to make you feel better about yourself.

TRAVELLING AROUND

You don't have to embark on a globe-trotting tour or a spectacular voyage to enjoy travel – it could mean taking a long weekend skiing, going on an annual holiday abroad, attending a weekend course or taking a few days off to visit relatives. The most important aspect of a holiday is the 'time out' it offers from your normal routine.

You don't have to go far from home to get the benefits of a holiday: explore your own neck of the woods and stay in local guest houses. If you want to slow down the pace, you could try walking or cycling.

Take a relaxing beach holiday, or, if you prefer, look into one of the many special interest tours available which provide a focus for your holiday. Whether your interests run to gardens, cooking, wine-tasting, art, golf or just about any other activity, you are sure to find a local or overseas tour to suit you. Look for advertisements promoting organised trips for small groups. Why not go for something you've never done before, such as scuba diving or horse riding?

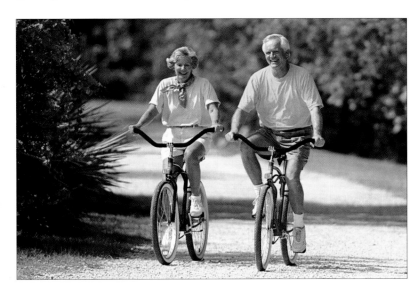

9 ways to **liven up your lifestyle**

Your lifestyle encompasses the way you live, your tastes, your personality and your passions. Making a few changes and doing things a little bit differently from time to time can really help you to get the most out of your life. Here are some ideas.

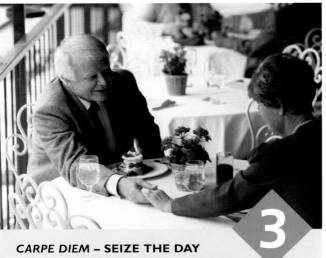

1

Become an explorer

Set up your own expedition. Decide on your destination, your objectives and your means of exploration. It needn't involve travel; you can investigate your own area or your family tree. You could also explore yourself through psychotherapy (see pages 190–191).

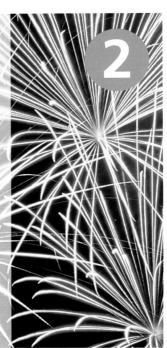

2

FIND OUT ABOUT LOCAL EVENTS

Plan your leisure time by keeping in touch with what's going on. Read the local papers, look on the notice boards of shops and cafés, listen to the radio and remember to make a note of anything that interests you. It may be the opening of a new shop with entertainment, fireworks, a new show at the theatre, a charity function or a sporting event. Ask your friends if they're interested in joining you.

CULTURE VULTURE

Arrange a night of poetry or dancing for your friends and family at home. Having a creative focus to an evening is unifying and can be stimulating. If you are musical, why not plan a trip *en masse* to see a recital or concert. Instead of sticking to the cinema, treat yourself to a night at the theatre. Getting out and sharing cultural experiences is inspiring. You can discuss the show afterwards with the group.

4

3

CARPE DIEM – SEIZE THE DAY

If you had a month left to live, what would be your three priorities? What would you say to who? Where would you go? What would you do? Make a list of all the things that are important to you and try to tick them off – you'll feel more fulfilled.

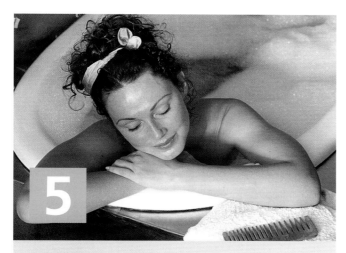

5

INDULGE YOURSELF

Can you remember when you last had a really long, relaxing bubble bath? Make an effort to spend an evening thoroughly pampering yourself. Lock the bathroom door, run a hot, fragrant bath, put on some soft music, maybe even pour yourself a glass of champagne, and immerse yourself in your own little world. Regular evenings of such sheer indulgence will cleanse your mind and body.

Colour your life

Rejuvenate your home with a little redecoration. You don't need to repaint every room; a flash of colour from a picture or covering is enough to boost your surroundings. Choose your colour carefully – different colours bring different energies:

6

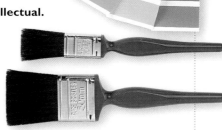

▶ **Green represents healing and balance.**

▶ **Red is physically stimulating.**

▶ **Yellow boosts optimism.**

▶ **Orange increases security.**

▶ **Purple increases spiritual awareness.**

▶ **Blue is calming and intellectual.**

▶ **Pink is caring and nurturing.**

COUNTRY CUISINE

When was the last time your home was filled with the smell of freshly baked bread? Has it been years since you prepared home-made soup? Dig out your old family recipes, pick up a few cook books and try some adventurous home cooking. Keep it healthy (see Chapter 2) and invite some friends round to join you.

7

Get back to Nature

Incorporate natural things into your surroundings. Natural-fibre soft furnishings can add a sense of calm to your home. Flowers and plants make a room look inspiring. Cook with fresh ingredients and wear clothes made from natural materials.

8

CHANGE YOUR ENVIRONMENT REGULARLY

According to research, people are happier and healthier if they can express themselves through their environment. Keep your home fresh and stimulating by changing it every week or so. Arrange fresh flowers in your kitchen, put a new photo on your desk, hang a picture, move the furniture around, try some do-it-yourself, play some different music or alter the lighting – try candlelight or a fragrancer.

9

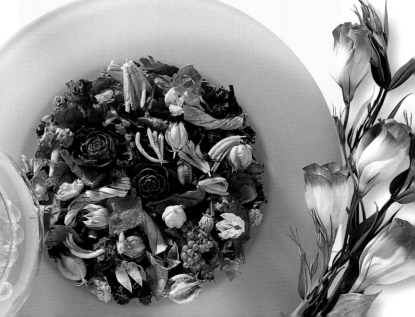

Family life

The average family is no longer Mum, Dad and two or three children. Whatever form your family takes, making it a cohesive unit takes a lot of time and effort; honest communication is essential.

In the past, couples traditionally started families in their 20s, and so by the time they reached their 40s and 50s the children were young adults, asserting their independence and leaving home. Parents then had to adapt to new family roles, no longer making all the decisions for their children, but being on hand to offer support when needed. Today, family relationships are more complicated.

An increasing number of people start a family later in life, and many have separated and divorced at least once by the time they reach middle age.

At its best, a family, no matter how large or small, is a supportive, loving network.

Children may be raised by a single parent or by a parent and step-parent. It is now quite common for families to be made up of children from two marriages (sometimes even more). All these situations demand a new approach to family life.

Family dynamics and individual roles within the family have undergone a transition; they are no longer based on traditional roles and gender stereotypes. In the West, there has been a gradual move towards equality of the sexes, which is reflected within the microcosm of the family unit. Women now find it easier to have careers and achieve financial independence, so they are less willing to take a passive, purely supportive role in family life or remain in an empty marriage or relationship. It's also the case that the man's career no longer automatically takes priority over the woman's. Most couples increasingly expect to share domestic tasks, such as parenting, cleaning and cooking.

As a result, men and women can no longer look to their parents' generation to find answers to the problems raised by today's complicated family dynamics. If couples take a flexible approach to gender issues, however, and are willing to compromise over their aims and priorities, changing family roles can provide opportunities for growth and development instead of conflict.

Remember that, as well as bringing up your children, you and your partner are looking for a loving relationship; a marriage needs work, time and commitment to succeed. Always talk about issues before they spiral out of control so that you can overcome areas of conflict. The joy and pride you experience in bringing up a family will form a strong bond in your relationship. Keep in regular touch with your children and your parents and encourage them to develop a close

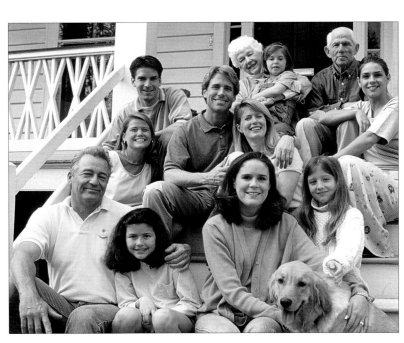

relationship. Grandchildren can learn a sense of responsibility and family history from their grandparents, and can, perhaps, perform modest tasks for them.

CHANGING RELATIONSHIPS

The relationship between parent and child changes radically over the years. Initially, children have to rely on their parents completely, but as they grow older and develop their own lives this dependence wanes and their independence flourishes. Encourage independent thinking in your children and stimulate them as much as possible so that they develop into well-rounded adults.

A child's journey towards independence can be immensely rewarding for the parents, but it can also be exceptionally trying.

Adolescence is a typically rebellious time of life, and some parents find the relationship with a son or daughter at this time particularly tough. Their children have increasingly adult bodies but without an adult's mental and emotional resources. Negotiating this transition can be a challenge, and positive and honest communication is essential. Set reasonable, consistent rules from an early age, so teenagers know them and that they should obey them; but listen to your child and be prepared to be flexible occasionally. Defiance tends to be more extreme if you set too few or too many inflexible rules. Consistency in discipline is vital, especially between partners.

A vital aspect of parenting is ultimately helping children to make their own decisions and take responsibility for their lives. If a late-adolescent or an adult son or daughter is about to make a bad decision, it can be hard not to intervene. But growing up is about making decisions, even bad ones, so the best option is to let your children learn from their mistakes. Try to be supportive, while behaving with dignity if your advice is not taken. Don't expect disaster – your child's decision may have been the right one after all.

From late adolescence on, the golden rule about voicing opinions and giving advice is: if in doubt, don't – unless asked. Unsolicited advice, however well meaning, tends to be rejected automatically. Constantly disapproving of a choice of partner, for example, only fuels rebellion and your son's or daughter's commitment to the relationship. It's only natural that you may equally want to give advice to your parents, too. Again, unless they are no longer legally capable of managing their own affairs, the same guidelines apply.

STARTING A FAMILY LATER IN LIFE

Thanks to medical technology (see pages 242–243) and the lifestyle changes that followed the women's movement, having a baby in your 40s is not unusual. By the

Family ties

Encourage communication between the generations of your family to create a supportive group.

Attend get-togethers Family events offer an opportunity for socialising in an informal atmosphere. It's particularly beneficial for children to get to know their cousins, aunts and uncles, who they are less likely to see regularly.

Support each other You expect your family to be there for you, so make sure you are there for them. Your love and support should be unconditional; it doesn't matter what's happened or who's done what, you don't even have to ask – just let them know you care and that you're there if they need you. For family members living away from home, a postcard

or quick phone call may be all that is necessary.

Keep in touch Encourage members of your family to keep in contact with one other. Remembering birthdays and sending a card is just one of many ways to let family members know that you are thinking of them. Younger children may ask Mum or Dad to send a drawing or painting they have done for Grandma or Grandpa. As parents, you may want to think about sending photos to keep far-away relations up to date with your children's ever-changing lives.

year 2000, statistics suggest that 1 baby in 12 will be born to a mother aged 35 or over.

The emotional maturity and increased life experience that often come with age are useful assets when coping with the challenges of parenthood. Many couples find they have more patience in later life, and more time to devote to their children.

Some women wait until they have established their professional careers before having children. With a secure financial base, they have an increased choice in childcare, schools, housing and whether or not to return to work. Women near or at the top of their professions may be able to name their own terms for maternity leave and return to work. Not all women in their 40s have rocketing careers, however, and pregnancy may interrupt job prospects for some women. It

DYNAMIC FAMILIES

The UK has the highest proportion of lone parents in Europe. In 1996 21 per cent of all families with dependent children were headed by a single parent.

Children
About 3 million children in the UK are being brought up in a one-parent family – that is about 1 in 5 of all dependent children.

Mum
About 91 per cent of single parents are women, 35 per cent of whom have never been married.

Dad
Single fathers tend to be older than single mothers and 25 per cent of them are alone because their partner has died.

might prompt thoughts on a change of direction, perhaps combining parenthood with studying at home. Many women are marrying later in life, so starting a family after 40 is the natural outcome. Likewise, the increased incidence of divorce and remarriage means that a couple may already have children but wish to start a 'new' family together.

THE CHANGING FAMILY UNIT

New partners may bring children from previous relationships. The stepfamily is an increasingly common phenomenon in Western society. According to the National Stepfamily Association in the UK, about one in three marriages every year is a remarriage. Around two and a half million children were living in stepfamilies in 1991, 800,000 of whom were under 16 years old, and this number is rising.

The success of a 'merged' or 'blended' family often depends on how the new partner and children are introduced and their developing reactions to each other. If you fall in love again, you still need to respect your children, so introduce any new partner gradually. If problems do arise, and undoubtedly there will be some feelings of ambivalence in the children or partner, talk them through. Tell your children that you cherish them but be firm about your own needs and those of your partner. Explain, too, that a new partner is not trying to replace their 'lost' parent and that their happiness is paramount, but at the same time they must be a little flexible.

Stepchildren may prove a joy or, alternatively, complicate your relationship with their parent.

Working dispassionately to make friends with a stepchild, allowing time for the relationship to develop, not assuming the mantle of parent and developing the ability to see through a stepchild's bitter behaviour are invaluable skills. Many step-parents are amazed at how jealous they feel of the time and attention their newly beloved pours into a relationship with children.

Demanding instant love, loyalty, respect or even friendship from a stepchild is doomed to failure. If a step-parent follows too quickly on the heels of the lost parent, he or she can impinge on the child's grief. Similarly, 'buying' love, through money, presents or treats, or tolerating unacceptable behaviour, is not in the child's best interests and may be counterproductive. Allow plenty of time for

ADJUSTING TO A NEW FAMILY

How children enter into a new family is incredibly important. It has a major effect on how successful the new family will be. For the wellbeing of the children, ensure that they have a continuing relationship with both parents, without feelings of divided loyalties. Prevent frustration and potential problems, by getting all parents and step-parents to agree on certain factors – you can then present a united front on issues such as bed-time, allowance and homework. Also agree on what name your children are going to give to a new partner. Will it be Mum or Dad or a first name? Children can be confused if they are not told how they should address someone new. Because children are sensitive to emotions, try to mask negative feelings, such as anger or resentment, and avoid criticising an ex-spouse within the children's earshot. If possible, keep on civil terms with your 'ex', and don't ask children to 'spy' on them and their new relationships, or ask children to carry messages or requests. Don't compete for your children's affection and loyalty at the expense of an ex-partner.

adjustment and be ready to provide support and encouragement when needed, without trying to force your help on the stepchildren. As children approach adolescence, traditional areas of conflict are liable to be intensified. There may be rivalry for power and control between a child and a step-parent.

HANDLING A SEPARATION INVOLVING CHILDREN

Separation is always a traumatic experience for children. When one parent leaves the family home for good, it can create a sense of loss akin to bereavement. Children can feel angry, anxious, insecure, depressed and even guilty – convinced that if they had behaved better their parents would never have parted.

Parents must take steps to protect children from the arguments, recriminations and turmoil of divorce.

No matter how bitter the separation, you should put their interests first and find a strategy that causes the least pain.

Older children may become angry and judgmental, and they could be rude, aggressive, sullen, resentful, withdrawn and lose interest in school, sports or hobbies. Younger children may be fearful and bewildered by the change and regress to more infantile behaviour – becoming clingy, uncooperative, moody, prone to nightmares and bedwetting.

Be upfront. Agree beforehand what you are going to say and who is going to explain what to the children, so they are not confused by conflicting versions.

Tell your children about the separation before there is any risk of them finding out from a third party. Do this when you can talk to them in a relaxed and unhurried manner.

You will probably be asked some difficult questions, so prepare well beforehand to anticipate these. Be honest in what you say and keep it simple to avoid burdening them with the rights and wrongs of the situation. A very important point to emphasise is that they are not the cause of the separation and are still loved and cherished.

Children love both parents and, for their emotional wellbeing, should not be forced to take sides. If custody arrangements have been agreed upon, then explain who they will live with and assure them that they will see both parents regularly. Never use access as a weapon against the other parent – it is the children who suffer most in a custody battle. If the situation becomes intense, know when to seek help. Turn to someone the children know and trust, but who is not directly involved in the separation, such as a family friend, close relative or teacher. It may help children adjust if they can spend some time in an emotionally neutral setting, such as a grandparent's home. Consult the family doctor, who may be able to help or recommend a psychologist or counselling organisation.

THE EMPTY NEST SYNDROME

Most young adults leave home at some point for university or work or to set up home themselves, sometimes well away from their family. For the children, leaving home is a welcome stage in the process of becoming independent. For parents, too, this can be a longed-for moment of liberation, yielding more freedom, available money, increased privacy and space. But for some parents, children leaving home may be an unsettling and even frightening experience – the 'empty nest syndrome'. Women who saw being a wife, homemaker and mother as their full-time careers may well feel a loss of purpose, identity and personal worth. If this coincides with menopause, such feelings may be intensified. The empty nest syndrome can be especially challenging for single parents, and for their children, who may feel guilty at seeming to abandon their parent.

Ironically, adult children who don't leave home, perhaps because they can't get a job or find affordable housing, can cause resentment and conflict at home.

Don't push your children out of the door, but be honest about your desire for privacy and need for time to yourself.

You may be thinking 'Wonderful, we're a couple again!' Back are the days of doing what you want when you want, taking more exotic holidays and having more of your own free time. A lot of couples view the time they're child-free and alone again as exciting and full of possibilities. Others, however, can find being just a couple for the first time in

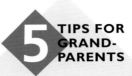

5 TIPS FOR GRAND-PARENTS

1. Always treat boys and girls – and grandchildren and stepgrandchildren – fairly and even-handedly.

2. Treat what grandchildren tell you in confidence, but if the information is serious, encourage them to tell their parents.

3. Don't try to compete with or take over the parental role.

4. Live your own life, not through your children or grandchildren. Treat invitations to spend time with them as a bonus, not a right.

5. Never attach 'strings' to offers of financial support.

years traumatic. It can be especially painful if the relationship is troubled. Children can provide a joint focus for parents who have little else in common. Once the children leave, conflicts that may have lain dormant for years often surface, leading to frustration, disappointment and anger. Parents who stayed together 'for the sake of the children' may decide this is the time to separate.

It helps if both partners take a thoughtful look at the health of the relationship before the last child leaves. This period also offers a chance to improve a relationship (or establish a new one), since couples inevitably change over the years. Take this opportunity to rediscover the level of sexual intimacy that you might have lost during the demanding years of child rearing. Look for household projects you can undertake together or joint leisure pursuits (see pages 234–235).

If you are having difficulty adjusting to your new-found coupledom, you and your partner may want to consider counselling. Your doctor may be able to refer you to an agency or private counsellor; some churches and synagogues also offer such counselling.

For many women, the option of returning to the career they left to start a family or of increasing the number of hours they work is an attractive one. Some fields have refresher courses, particularly for teaching and nursing careers, where age and experience are especially valued. Consider, too, courses for new careers, adult education classes and voluntary charity work (see pages 228–229).

BECOMING A GRANDPARENT

Grandparents play a very special role in family life – they provide a link with another generation. How you feel at the news that there's a grandchild 'on the way' is entirely dependent on you and your circumstances. Most people are overjoyed, brimming with excitement and anticipation. Some, however, may feel that they're not ready to be a grandparent: they're too young and not up to the task. If you feel this way, try instead to view it as an opportunity to provide love and support and as a new link in your family.

For many people, grandparenting offers a second chance at parenting. As a grandparent you probably have time, energy and money to lavish on grandchildren.

Young parents commonly have heavy demands on their energy – careers, financial commitments and home maintenance, as well as full-time parenting. Grandparenting, on the other hand, can offer the best of both worlds: the opportunity to spend time with children without the distractions of work and the moral responsibility for their upbringing.

As a grandparent, you are likely to be more philosophical, tolerant and sympathetic. Bringing up your own children means you've learned the knack of handling children with ease, and so you often enjoy grandchildren and their development in a more relaxed way. Moderate spoiling of grandchildren is considered 'part of the deal', but too many treats, and too few expectations of good behaviour, are counterproductive.

Watching your child, or daughter- or son-in-law make what you consider major parenting errors without intervening can be hard. From pregnancy onwards, differing attitudes towards marriage, child rearing and education can be potentially explosive. Remaining silent, even if it means leaving the room, is often best. Emotional, physical or sexual abuse, however, requires direct intervention, followed, if necessary, by contacting the child's doctor, a childcare agency or the police.

LOOKING AFTER ELDERLY PARENTS

Many older people can expect to maintain a high degree of independence until very late in life. By planning the logistics in advance, elderly parents can more easily maintain their dignity and independence – to the benefit of you and your children.

You can help your parents adapt their home to their changing needs by, for example, installing safety grab-rails on stair walls or handrails in the bathroom. You could hire a cleaner or odd-job person to help out with household tasks. It may eventually be in your parents' best interest to sell their home. Acknowledge sympathetically that 'moving down' into more compact accommodation may bring a sense of loss, but also emphasise the many benefits.

A longed-for 'second honeymoon' might not materialise if elderly parents need care just as grown-up children are leaving home and running their own lives.

People who find themselves having to care for parents while they're still bringing up their own family – the 'sandwich generation' – often suffer extreme stress.

Making sure elderly parents are looking after themselves or being cared for puts a lot of pressure on you and your family. Don't expect too much of yourself; you can't do everything. Share responsibility for your parents' care with brothers and sisters, if possible.

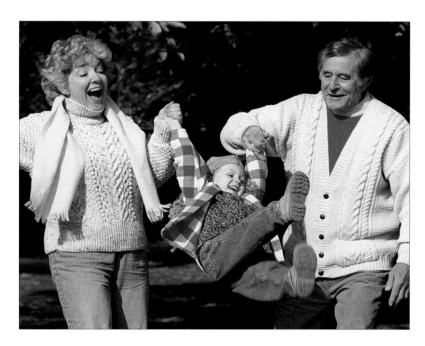

If full-time care is necessary, you'll have to consider the options of hiring a live-in nurse or moving your parent(s) to a nursing home. Whatever the solution, try to involve your parents in the decision.

Grandchildren can help forge a closer relationship between different generations.

ASSISTING FERTILITY
and conception

Technological advances in the medical treatment of fertility problems mean that couples having difficulties conceiving and couples deciding to have a family later in life can have the children they so dearly want.

The ability to have children is often seen as a birthright. Most people assume that they'll conceive without a problem, although this isn't always the case. Now, thanks to progress in medical technology, people in their 30s, 40s and even 50s can become parents.

While most men remain fertile well into their 50s or 60s, women over the age of 35 normally begin to ovulate less regularly, gradually reducing their chances of having a baby by natural means. If one or the other partner has reduced fertility or is infertile, for whatever reason, treatment may be necessary to help them start a family.

If you have been trying for a baby for about six months without success or suspect you may have trouble conceiving, consult your

Assisted reproductive technologies

The first baby to be conceived outside the mother's body — using a technique called *in-vitro* fertilisation — was born in 1978. Since then, over 300,000 babies have been conceived worldwide using this method. Other assisted reproductive technologies have also proved successful. Here is a rundown of the best-known techniques.

TECHNIQUE	THE PROCEDURE
ARTIFICIAL INSEMINATION	
This is the oldest, and simplest, method of assisted conception. The woman's partner, but in some cases an anonymous donor, supplies the sperm. The technique is most often used if normal sexual intercourse cannot be performed, or the man has too few healthy sperm for normal conception to be achieved.	The sperm are introduced using a syringe or catheter into the woman's cervical canal or, sometimes, uterus, from where they swim into the Fallopian tube and fertilise an egg. The exact nature of the timing of insemination is coordinated with the woman's ovulation cycle.
***IN-VITRO* FERTILISATION (IVF)**	
This involves removing one or more eggs from a woman's ovaries and mixing them with specially treated sperm in a culture dish. IVF is used for problems arising from blocked or damaged Fallopian tubes, poor-quality sperm, hostile cervical mucus and unexplained causes of infertility.	In most cases, the woman is given hormones to increase the number of eggs produced. An egg is fertilised and, usually after two days, the resulting embryo is placed in the uterus, where it continues to develop as normal. Up to three embryos may be placed in the uterus at one time to enhance the chance of successful implantation.

A form of IVF known as ZIFT – zygote intrafallopian transfer – uses the same procedure but implants the egg as soon as it has been fertilised, rather than waiting the few days it takes for the zygote to become an embryo. |

doctor, who can advise you on ways to improve your chances or refer you to a fertility clinic. Specialists there will be able to investigate the cause of any problems and, if appropriate, offer treatment. Before you embark on a course of fertility treatment, carefully consider the implications of such treatment. Many expensive, high-tech treatments have relatively low success rates.

Using hormones and other drugs, it is now possible to boost the fertility of older women so that they ovulate and are able to conceive. At present, however, most fertility clinics worldwide set an age limit – typically 50–55 years. However, in 1998, a 60-year-old widow in London gave birth after undergoing fertility treatment. She had told the doctors she was 49.

Aware of the decline in natural fertility with age, an increasing number of couples are making use of freezing techniques so that they can delay starting a family until later. In 1998, a 52-year-old mother gave birth to a boy after being implanted with a fertilised egg which had been frozen and stored for eight years. The boy's 'twin' had been born seven years earlier.

TYPE	THE PROCEDURE
GAMETE INTRAFALLOPIAN TRANSFER (GIFT)	
GIFT is a simpler alternative to IVF and is generally more successful because it better recreates the natural conditions necessary for successful implantation. GIFT can be used if there is a blockage in the Fallopian tubes or if the causes of infertility are unexplained.	Like IVF, GIFT involves mixing the sperm and eggs outside the woman's body. Unlike IVF, however, the mixture is immediately inserted into the Fallopian tube, which is where fertilisation normally occurs before the egg travels to the uterus.
MICROMANIPULATION	
In cases where the man produces few viable sperm, or sperm appear unable to penetrate the egg, micromanipulation can improve the chances of conception. These techniques are designed to bypass the shell that surrounds the egg (the zona pellucida), thereby allowing better access for the sperm. Men who have blocked or absent sperm ducts may be able to have their sperm extracted directly from their testicles.	One method known as SUZI – subzonal insemination – involves injecting a few specially selected sperm into the space between the zona pellucida and the egg using a very fine tube. Once a sperm enters the egg and fertilises it, the resulting embryo is implanted into the uterus. A more modern technique called ICSI – intracytoplasmic sperm injection – involves inserting a single sperm directly into the egg.
EGG OR EMBRYO TRANSFER	
Women who no longer ovulate can carry and deliver a baby using techniques that transfer an egg or embryo. An older couple who have previously donated eggs, sperm or embryos and had them frozen and stored for the future can use them to start that much wanted family using transfer techniques.	Usually, this involves a younger donor's egg being mixed with sperm (the older woman's partner's or a donor's) and transplanting the embryo into the uterus.

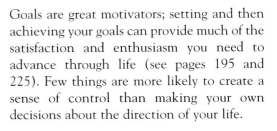

Looking ahead

Keep living life to the full. Take control of the direction and pace of your life by looking ahead, making plans and setting goals. Think positively and you could reach that exclusive group – the over-100 club.

You've heard the saying 'Life begins at 40'. Well, with people's ever-increasing life expectancy, you may not have even reached the half-way mark in your life. Aim to make the upcoming decades as fulfilling and happy as you possibly can, by maximising your time and cultivating a variety of interests – mentally and physically stimulating ones.

If you are among the 'empty nesters' with grown children, you have more time to focus on yourself. Look back at long-lost hobbies or activities and take a refresher course. Try to strike a balance between home-based activities and those that get you out, so that you meet and mix with others.

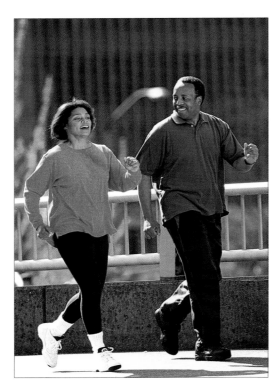

A positive attitude is key to staying healthy and looking forward to a long and happy life.

TAKING CONTROL OF YOUR LIFE

Some people feel more in command of their lives than others. Does this mean they're smarter than you? Probably not, but the odds are they're more focused. People in charge of their destiny formulate plans, pursue goals and make their own decisions.

By planning for the future, financially and otherwise, you will have less anxiety and stress.

Goals are great motivators; setting and then achieving your goals can provide much of the satisfaction and enthusiasm you need to advance through life (see pages 195 and 225). Few things are more likely to create a sense of control than making your own decisions about the direction of your life.

Research has linked a higher income and a higher socioeconomic status with a longer lifespan.

The reasons for this are multifaceted but a major factor is probably the level of long-term stress (see pages 192–197) suffered by poorer families or people, compared with those who are better off. Like a good income, a well-trained mind can help you stay relaxed and confident. Your most powerful anti-aging weapon is your mind, so actively expand your knowledge base to empower yourself.

PLANNING FOR YOUR FUTURE

Time is of the essence. You want to make the best use of all your time, so look forward. Try to foresee and solve potential problems, rather than sticking your head in the sand and pretending pitfalls don't exist – be proactive, not reactive. It's often the case that people who don't plan or anticipate future events are overwhelmed and suffer acute depression. So, get into action now.

Important areas to plan for include: health care; finances; work; and living arrangements. If you have private health insurance, check that your level of cover is appropriate for your changing needs and look into altering your policy if necessary. You may belong to your employer's health insurance plan. If this is the case, you will need to look into whether and how payments will change when you retire. Discuss the situation with your employer and discuss your options so that you can sort things out beforehand and have peace of mind.

Retirement is one of the most obvious necessities to plan for as we grow older. Many people look forward to that magic age when they can have the freedom, money and time to do whatever they desire. However, lack of foresight can take the gilt off the 'golden years'. When you retire is usually, but not always, up to you – but by planning ahead you can see how everything will fit into place, and if it doesn't, you've got time to sort out alternative arrangements.

TAKING STOCK OF YOUR FINANCES

You probably look forward with great relish to the day when you no longer have a mortgage – what you can do with all that money! – but you may also have worries about how you are going to support yourself when you stop working.

If you started a pension fund early, you may retire with a reassuringly sized nest egg.

Most pension companies now have built-in systems, whereby someone monitors your fund and sends a request for top-up contributions, if necessary, as you move towards your retirement date. Make an appointment with your bank manager or financial adviser to discuss how much income you can expect from your pension and how frequently the payments will be made.

Practically, you should consider how much money you will need to fund travel opportunities and to maintain the same lifestyle.

Now is probably a good time to review your savings accounts, life insurance, and stocks and shares as well.

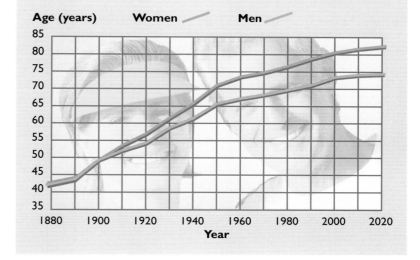

LIFE EXPECTANCY

Thanks to improved standards of living and health care, life expectancy has risen steadily during the last century. For example, a woman born in the 1990s will live almost twice as long as her counterpart born in the mid-nineteenth century. The data also show that women consistently live longer than men.

Age (years)　　Women ⟋　　Men ⟋

MAKING OR UPDATING A WILL

Another practical consideration is a will. Do you have one? When was the last time you looked at it? Don't put off making a will. Even if you aren't well off, making your wishes official is important. Who do you want to provide for in the event of your death? Don't feel morbid thinking about death – it's a practicality of life. It may take some time to think through all the options and decide exactly how you would like your estate divided. Ask your solicitor for advice.

RETHINKING HOW YOU WORK

Research has shown that long-lived people work hard every day of their lives but, more important, they like what they do. It's also been shown that women with demanding jobs have a lower risk of heart attack than women who don't work.

When planning ahead, work is often a critical consideration. Do you enjoy your work? When do you want to retire? How you feel about your job or career has great bearing on how you approach retirement. If you've been in a job you dislike just to get the children through university, now could be the time for an exciting change of direction (see pages 228–229).

You may be in the prime of your career and earning potential, and intellectually you have never been more capable. Practical problem-solving skills peak during your 40s, so you have a lot to offer in the world of work.

Nevertheless, it's worth spending some time thinking about the future and how you might ultimately want to reduce the amount of time you spend at work. For some women, now may be the first time they've had to return to the workplace after raising a family or to rethink how they want to spend their time. Consider what it is you want to get from working – money, job satisfaction, personal advancement, camaraderie?

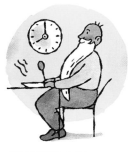

ORDER OF THE DAY
The secret of longevity, as revealed in a survey of 1200 centenarians, seems to be having order and routine in day-to-day life.

If you are considering retirement but you are unsure of how you'll manage it, try a 'retirement rehearsal' by taking a leave of absence from work. Many employers recognise that flexibility is the key to keeping valued employees as long as possible, so ask whether your company has flexible policies, such as job-sharing, flexitime or part-time positions.

Taking early retirement can be a very attractive option. After quitting work, you may decide that you want to try your hand at something new, perhaps reflexology or teaching one or two days a week. Be assertive, though, and decide exactly how much time you want to spend in which activities – don't get drawn into committing more time than you want. As a couple retiring together, try to make sure that you develop and cultivate interests and activities separately as well as jointly. It is vital to a healthy relationship that you enjoy doing things independently of your partner, so that you don't spend 100 per cent of your time together.

Fancy a change of scene?

Before deciding to move to a new area, there are several factors to consider:

▶ **Finances** Obviously, your available income will restrict your choice to some degree. Be realistic about what your needs are and look within your price range.

▶ **Preferred lifestyle** Are you a solitary person or a gregarious one? Are you fiercely independent or are you happy to rely on others? Also, think about what environment you prefer – city or country?

▶ **Neighbourhood** If you don't drive, what public transport is available? You need to be within easy distance of all the services you need, such as shops, a doctor and a dentist and some kind of entertainment facilities. You need to feel safe and secure in your new home, so, if necessary, check out local crime rates. You may also want to find out what type of people

(young couples, families, older people) make up the majority of those living in that area.

▶ **Family ties and responsibilities** Will you be near enough to your family and friends? You may feel pressure about being able to offer child care (perhaps for your grandchildren) or about moving to be nearer a particular relative. Remember it's what's you want that's important – keep things in perspective.

▶ **Type of accommodation** Do you want an apartment or a house? If it's a house, you may want to look at one on a single level. Make sure your new home has enough space for all your things and for visitors, if you want them. Find out how it's heated and maintained, and what sort of access it has if it's in an apartment building – how many lifts are there?

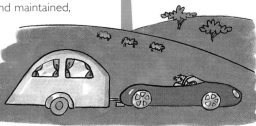

Retirement often gives time for foreign travel – it may be the first chance you have had to travel outside your own country. Because you have more time and freedom during retirement, you can often pick up great deals by travelling off peak or off season.

MOVING HOME

When you stop working, you may decide you want a complete change of scene. How about warm, sunny weather all year round? You may want to consider moving to a warmer climate, or to the beach or the country. There is nothing holding you in the city now – you could make a whole new start for yourself or realise a dream. Think carefully, however, and consider all the options before you pack up and move somewhere new.

If you are still living in the family home, you may feel you rattle around inside it once your children have left home. Selling your home and moving to a smaller house or apartment makes sound financial sense: the profits made on the sale can be invested so that they provide you with a very useful retirement income. Also, having a smaller home means that your heating and electricity bills will be lower and you will have fewer rooms to clean and redecorate – giving you more time, energy and money to get out and enjoy your life.

Leaving a long-time home can be traumatic, but instead of dwelling on the past, look to the future and concentrate on all of the advantages that moving to a smaller place brings.

Of course, not everyone wishes to move house – but it's an option you may want to keep open. To help decide if you want to move or not, make a list of all the things you currently enjoy that you couldn't transport to a new house, such as happy memories that are kept alive in familiar surroundings or good neighbours on whom you can rely. If you find any element that is essential to your happiness, then stay put.

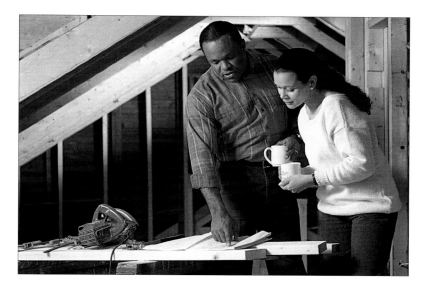

YOUR ATTITUDE TOWARDS AGING

Age isn't a number – it's an attitude. Having the right attitude can help you live longer and keep you younger. How old do you feel? If you're positive about life, it's probably younger than your actual age. Nevertheless, your physical, mental and social age is far more important than your chronological age.

Research into aging has shown that people who age best share similar characteristics: they have a good sense of humour, are active and tend to be forward looking (see page 225).

Rather than looking back at what you did or didn't do, focus on what's ahead, whether it's seeing your grandchildren or the next Test series. If you are feeling anxious about growing old, you need to take steps to help you think positively (see pages 178–179). Humans as a species would be badly adapted if we hadn't worked out how to make each stage of our lives successful and happy.

Your 40s and 50s are the most stable time of life emotionally. Successes at work and social relations combine to promote mature love, true friendship, freedom to make independent choices, self-respect and a fulfilling lifestyle. Be confident and assertive; life is still about getting what you want from it.

Strengthen your relationship by planning projects together.

AGING THEORIES
anti-aging therapies

Since ancient times, humans have endeavoured to find the secret of immortality and a cure for old age. Dozens of aging theories and anti-aging treatments have been proposed, but science has yet to find a universal answer.

One of the biggest questions is: Why do we age? The obvious next one is: How can we stop or, at least, delay it? Scientists believe that aging is a mechanism to ensure that, as a species, human beings continue to survive.

There are two major theories of aging – programmed aging and accidental aging. Programmed aging proposes that human development is governed by a biological 'clock', which sets the time for bodily changes to take place, such as the accelerated loss of calcium in bones (osteoporosis) and hearing loss. This clock could be controlled by your hormones or predetermined by your genes. According to the theory of accidental aging, as organisms grow older they are damaged by random events, such as attack from free radicals and general wear and tear. The basics of the principal theories of aging are outlined opposite.

A look at future possibilities

Scientific technology is constantly advancing. Some potential techniques, real and theoretical, include:

Cryonics You are probably familiar with the concept of suspended animation from sci-fi movies. It may be science fiction now, but techniques such as cryonics – using liquid nitrogen to freeze and store dead organisms, mainly for research at this stage – may become commonplace in the future. Fertility treatments, such as *in-vitro* fertilisation (IVF, see page 242) can use sperm, eggs or an embryo that have previously been frozen and then 'brought back to life'. Whether and how this technique, now used only on single cells, can be applied to whole people is uncertain, but people have already had their bodies frozen in the hope that one day the technology will exist to thaw and cure them and give them new life.

Genetic engineering Current research using genetic engineering techniques has shown that portions of DNA can be manipulated to restore a gene's function or to replace a disease-causing gene. It is unclear how soon these techniques could be used to help prevent the effects of aging, but it is probably not a treatment that will be available in your lifetime.

Nanotechnology A nanometer is 1/1,000,000 of a metre – which is very small indeed. Scientists have hypothesised that in the future, various biological structures or organs could be built or repaired at the molecular level – this is nanotechnology. For the present, however, the idea of building such incredibly refined machines remains a theory, but who knows what is waiting for us just around the corner?

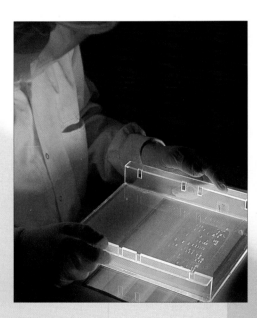

In the future, genetic techniques may enable doctors to determine if a baby carries aging-related disease genes before it's born.

Theories on aging and current therapies

Over the last five years, astonishing progress has been made in the field of biogerontology – the study of the biology of aging. If further research can identify and understand the processes that cause aging, the human lifespan could be extended enormously. Here, we explain the principal theories and the current therapies available.

THEORY	TREATMENTS AVAILABLE
HORMONE THEORY	
Hormones are chemical messengers secreted in specialised endocrine glands around the body. They regulate bodily functions, ranging from metabolism and reproduction to damage repair. Certain hormone levels appear to decline with age, and result in weakening of bones, muscles and some organ functions. Research has shown that boosting these levels using synthetic hormones can reduce or even reverse signs of aging or age-related diseases.	Treatments include taking hormone supplements (see pages 140–141). Melatonin, for example, has been shown to stimulate the immune system. In a study of men over 60, growth hormone turned the clock back 20 years: middle-age spreads disappeared, body composition changed (less fat, more muscle) and bones became stronger. Hormone supplements should only be taken under medical supervision – taking too high a dose or supplementing for too long can have disastrous effects on your body.
GENETIC CONTROL THEORY	
Your genes control everything that happens in your body. Each person is born with a unique set of genes encoded in DNA. Every time body cells divide, tiny pieces at the tips of your chromosomes (the structures in your cells that contain your genes) are lost. Initially, these regions are not essential to your body's function, but with each division the area of loss moves closer to your functional genes. Once these are affected, your body function starts to suffer and decline.	Using biotechnology and genetic engineering, research is underway to isolate an 'immortalising' enzyme – telomerase – that will repair and replace the lost pieces of DNA. Unfortunately, you may not see the fruits of this research in your lifetime.
FREE RADICAL THEORY	
Without free radicals, your body would not be able to produce energy, maintain immunity, transmit nerve impulses or synthesise hormones. Nevertheless, free radicals attack the structure of cell membranes and create waste products as they do so. As you grow older, the accumulation of free-radical damage take its toll on your body.	Many researchers and nutritionists recommend taking antioxidant supplements because they counteract free radicals. Antioxidants come in various guises: as vitamins A, C and E, as beta-carotene and as enzymes (coenzyme Q-10 and catalase). By including them in your diet or by taking supplements, researchers believe that you may prevent age-related diseases, such as cancer, atherosclerosis and heart disease – three of the biggest premature killers in the Western world.
WEAR AND TEAR THEORY	
First proposed in 1882, this theory is based on the belief that your body and cells are damaged by overuse and abuse. Vital body organs, such as the skin, liver, stomach and kidneys, are worn down by toxins in your diet and environment. Excess consumption of fat, sugar, caffeine, alcohol and nicotine, and damage caused by the sun's ultraviolet radiation and other physical and emotional stresses, also contribute. When you're young, your body can compensate, but with age you can succumb to factors that were easily fought off in youth.	Having a prevention strategy is the key here, rather than treating the problems as they arise. Taking nutritional supplements and living a healthy lifestyle can help keep you young and reverse some of the aging process by stimulating the body's ability to repair and maintain itself once more.

Index

Acknowledgements

Carroll & Brown would also like to thank the following for their assistance in the production of this book:

Editorial
Dawn Henderson, Richard Emerson
Design
Julie Bennett, Dorian Cassidy
Studio photography
Jules Selmes, David Murray
Picture research
Richard Soar
Make-up artist
Kym Menzies
Illustrators
Kim Dalziel, Sally Kindberg, Tony Graham
Proofreader
Clare Hacking
Indexer
Anne McCarthy
Equipment
John Bell & Croyden, London, for the loan of medical equipment

Photo credits
Title page (bottom left) **& 137** Telegraph Colour Library; **title page** (top middle) **& 212** Telegraph Colour Library; **6–7 & 230** The Stock Market; **7** (right) **& 99** (top) Tony Stone Images; **8 & 34** Images Colour Library; **8–9 & 42** Robert Harding Picture Library; **9** (right) **& 50** Scimat/Science Photo Library; **12** (top) **& 244** Telegraph Colour Library; **19** (bottom) Tony Stone Images; **24** Tony Stone Images; **28** The Image Bank; **38** (bottom) Tony Stone Images; **39** Hulton Getty; **40** (background) Tony Stone Images; **52** Pictor International; **57** (middle) Tony Stone Images; **67** (top) The Stock Market; **68** (background) Rex Interstock Ltd; **68** (top) The Stock Market (bottom) Robert Harding Picture Library; **70** (insert) Prof. P. Motta/Dept. of Anatomy/University "La Sapienza", Rome/Science Photo Library; **72** (left) Tony Stone Images; **78** Prof. Arthur Lesk/Science Photo Library; **84** (top & bottom) The Sun/Rex Features; **91** (left) The Stock Market (middle) Images Colour Library (right) Tony Stone Images; **100** (right) Dr Jeremy Burgess/Science Photo Library;

105 BSIP Laurent/Science Photo Library; **107** (left) Manfred Kage/Science Photo Library; **110** (background) The Stock Market (top & bottom) Howard Stean/Aesthetic Dentistry and Professional Testing; **112** Tony Stone Images; **124** Tony Stone Images; **129** (top) Carroll & Brown Ltd; **130** Telegraph Colour Library; **131** Petit Format/Science Photo Library; **134–5** Tony Stone Images; **140** Images Colour Library; **142** Tony Stone Images; **144** Tony Stone Images; **148** Tony Stone Images; **150** Telegraph Colour Library; **153** (right) Tony Stone Images; **154** (background) The Image Bank (top & bottom) Tony Stone Images; **156** Rex Interstock Ltd; **157** Tony Stone Images; **161** Tony Stone Images; **168** (left) Tony Stone Images; **170** (left) Tony Stone Images; **173** (left) Waterlily Pond, 1899/ MONET Claude/National Gallery, London/The Bridgeman Art Library, London (right) The Japanese Bridge, 1918–24/ MONET Claude/Galerie Daniel Malingue: Paris/The Bridgeman Art Library, London; **174** Dr. G. Oran Bredberg/Science Photo Library; **176** (background) Carroll & Brown Ltd; **176** (bottom) BSIP Laurent/Science Photo Library; **183** The Stock Market; **189** (top) Tony Stone Images; **192** The Stock Market; **198** (all) Carroll & Brown Ltd; **200** Images Colour Library; **201** (top & bottom) Carroll & Brown Ltd; **202** (top) Telegraph Colour Library; **204** Tony Stone Images; **205** (top) The Stock Market; **209** Tony Stone Images; **211** Telegraph Colour Library; **214** (all) Carroll & Brown Ltd; **215** (left) Carroll & Brown Ltd; **219** John Greim/Science Photo Library; **221** (top left) A prince and a lady in a combination of two canonical erotic positions listed in the "Kama Sutra", Bundi, Rajput School, 1790/Private Collection/The Bridgeman Art Library, London; **222** (bottom) Tony Stone Images; **224** Tony Stone Images; **228** (bottom) Tony Stone Images; **229** (top) Tony Stone Images; **234** (right) Jules Selmes; **235** (top left) Telegraph Colour Library (top right & bottom) Carroll & Brown Ltd; **236** The Stock Market; **242–243** Tony Stone Images; **247** Telegraph Colour Library; **248** (bottom) Simon Fraser/Science Photo Library; **248–9** (background) Tony Stone Images.

Recommended daily vitamin and mineral intakes

Vitamins and minerals are an essential part of your diet, as your body cannot manufacture most of them itself. Each nutrient has a specific function, as outlined in Chapter 2 (together with the best sources). Deficiencies can lead to ill health, so be sure to include adequate amounts of each nutrient in your diet. Refer to the chart below for the daily intakes recommended in your country.

VITAMIN	UNITED KINGDOM		AUSTRALIA AND NEW ZEALAND		SOUTH AFRICA	
	MEN	WOMEN	MEN	WOMEN	MEN	WOMEN
A	700 µg	600 µg (950 µg in lactation)	750 µg	750 µg (1200 µg in lactation)	1000 µg	800 µg (1300 µg in lactation)
B₁ (thiamin)	1.0 mg	0.8 mg	1.1 mg	0.8 mg	1.5 mg	1.1 mg
B₂ (riboflavin)	1.3 mg	1.1 mg	1.7 mg	1.2 mg	1.7 mg	1.3 mg
B₃ (niacin)	17 mg	13 mg	19 mg	13 mg	19 mg	15 mg
B₅ (pantothenic acid)	3.0–7.0 mg	3.0–7.0 mg	—	—	4.0–7.0 mg	4.0–7.0 mg
B₆ (pyridoxine)	1.4 mg	1.2 mg	1.3–1.9 mg	0.9–1.4 mg	2.0 mg	1.6 mg
B₁₂ (cyanocobalamin)	1.5 µg	1.5 µg	2.0 µg	2.0 µg	2.0 µg	2.0 µg
C (ascorbic acid)	40 mg (smokers at least 80 mg)	40 mg	40 mg (smokers at least 80 mg)	30 mg	60 mg (smokers at least 80–120 mg)	60 mg
D (calciferols)	Enough is made when skin is exposed to sunlight. People confined indoors require 10 µg from food.					
E (alphatocopherol)	At least 4.0 mg	At least 3.0 mg	10 mg	7.0 mg	10 mg	8.0 mg
Folic acid (folate)	200 µg	200 µg (400 µg in pregnancy)	200 µg	200 µg (400 µg in pregnancy; 350 µg in lactation)	200 µg	180 µg (400 µg in pregnancy
H (biotin)	10–200 µg	10–200 µg	—	—	30–100 µg	30–100 µg
K (phylloquinone, menadione)	70 µg	65 µg	—	—	70–80 µg	60–65 µg

MINERAL	UNITED KINGDOM		AUSTRALIA AND NEW ZEALAND		SOUTH AFRICA	
	MEN	WOMEN	MEN	WOMEN	MEN	WOMEN
Calcium	700 mg	700 mg	800 mg	800 mg (1000 mg after menopause)	800 mg	800 mg
Chloride	2500 mg	2500 mg	—	—	750 mg	750 mg
Chromium	25 µg	25 µg	—	—	50–200 µg	50–200 µg
Copper	1.2 mg	1.2 mg	—	—	1.5–3.0 mg	1.5–3.0 mg
Iodine	140 µg	140 µg	150 µg	120 µg	150 µg	150 µg
Iron	8.7 mg	14.5 mg	7.0 mg	12–16 mg (5.0–7.0 mg after menopause)	10 mg	15 mg
Magnesium	300 mg	270 mg	320 mg	270 mg	350 mg	280 mg
Manganese	1.4 mg	1.4 mg	—	—	2.0–5.0 mg	2.0–5.0 mg
Molybdenum	50–400 µg	50–400 µg	—	—	75–250 µg	75–250 µg
Phosphorus	550 mg	550 mg	1000 mg	1000 mg	800 mg	800 mg
Potassium	3500 mg	3500 mg	50–140 mmol	50–140 mmol	2000 mg	2000 mg
Selenium	75 µg	60 µg	85 µg	70 µg	70 µg	55 µg
Sodium	1600 mg	1600 mg	40–140 mmol	40–140 mmol	500 mg	500 mg
Zinc	9.5 mg	7.0 mg	12 mg	12 mg	15 mg	12 mg

Pregnant, lactating and postmenopausal women require a slightly higher intake of certain vitamins and minerals, and should be guided by their doctor. 1 µg (microgram) is 0.001 mg (milligram). — No daily requirement is yet established.